Working with Families in Speech-Language Pathology

Working with Families in Speech-Language Pathology

EDITED BY

Nicole Watts Pappas and Sharynne McLeod

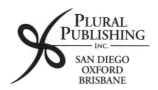

PLURAL
PUBLISHING
INC.
SAN DIEGO
OXFORD
BRISBANE

MW

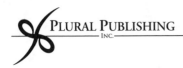
PLURAL PUBLISHING
INC.

5521 Ruffin Road
San Diego, CA 92123

e-mail: info@pluralpublishing.com
Web site: http://www.pluralpublishing.com

49 Bath Street
Abingdon, Oxfordshire OX14 1EA
United Kingdom

Copyright © by Plural Publishing, Inc. 2009

Typeset in 11/13 Garamond by Flanagan's Publishing Services, Inc.
Printed in the United States of America by McNaughton and Gunn, Inc.

For permission to use material from this text, contact us by
Telephone: (866) 758-7251
Fax: (888) 758-7255
e-mail: permissions@pluralpublishing.com

*Every attempt has been made to contact the copyright holders for material originally
printed in another source. If any have been inadvertently overlooked, the publishers
will gladly make the necessary arrangements at the first opportunity.*

Library of Congress Cataloging-in-Publication Data

Working with families in speech-language pathology / [edited by] Nicole Watts Pappas and Sharynne McLeod.
    p. ; cm.
Includes bibliographical references and index.
ISBN-13: 978-1-59756-241-6 (alk. paper)
ISBN-10: 1-59756-241-6 (alk. paper)
    1. Speech therapy. 2. Speech therapy for children. 3. Speech disorders in chil-
dren—Patients & family relationships. I. Pappas, Nicole Watts. II. McLeod, Sharynne.
    [DNLM: 1. Rehabilitation of Speech and Language Disorders—methods. 2. Child.
3. Professional-Family Relations. WL 340.2 W926 2008]
    RC423.W67 2008
    616.85'5—dc22
                                                          2008027856

4/22/10

Contents

Foreword

When I was a graduate student (long ago!) we received a few lectures on the importance of family participation in assessment and treatment, the emphasis being on how much more quickly treatment proceeded when a child's family was involved. If I had better understood the crucial importance of working with families, my notes for those lectures would have been more detailed, and the heading "Families" would have been in red ink with large arrows and huge stars circling around it.

As I discovered when I began working, family is the pivot of a child's life, essential as air. Essential because human infants are born too helpless to survive without caregivers and require long apprentices under protective guardians to learn all they must know to survive. I soon learned that families differed enormously in disposition, composition, and child-rearing ability. Some were a "comfort zone" from which a child explored the world, and others a place from which a child needed to escape. Some families included a single parent, other two parents, two women, two men, a grandparent, or parents unrelated biologically to the child. Child-rearing skills of families ranged from awe inspiring to awful. To illustrate, I remember working with two couples. One couple, both of who were mildly retarded, were particularly conscientious parents, and the other couple, both professionals, were so consumed by career goals as to border on inflicting child abuse.

If I were a student today, I would want *Working with Families in Speech-Language Pathology* as a textbook. For a clinician, educator, or researcher *Working with Families* is an invaluable reference. The editors and authors are experienced clinicians and fine writers, and they have assembled an outstanding international cadre of chapter authors. The first part of *Working with Families* provides an excellent description of the editors' theoretical framework. The second and main part consists of eight strong chapters, each focusing on a particular child population, including family issues arising in the care of children with language impairment, speech impairment, stuttering, AAC devices, dysphagia, hearing loss, and emergent literacy.

Working with Families in Speech-Language Pathology has something for everyone. Whether as a textbook or a reference, it is an excellent resource that likely will be read and reread for a long time to come.

Ken M. Bleile

Preface

Parent and family involvement in intervention for young children has increased in recent years. Legislation in the United States and United Kingdom now mandates that the family is involved in services for children requiring early intervention. This increase in parent and family involvement means that speech-language pathologists are now working with parents and families more than ever before. Therefore, knowing how to most effectively interact with and involve families in intervention is of increasing importance to clinicians. *Working with Families in Speech-Language Pathology* provides a comprehensive guide for speech-language pathologists, audiologists, teachers, and other professionals about working with parents and families in intervention for young children.

Working with Families in Speech-Language Pathology is organized into two sections. Part I outlines the history of speech-language pathologists' work with families and reviews the literature on allied health professionals' and parents' perceptions of family involvement in intervention. Four models of working with parents and families are explained: therapist-centered, parent-as-therapist aide, family-centered, and family-friendly practice. Extensive tables summarize the evidence for working with families.

Part II of *Working with Families in Speech-Language Pathology* contains eight chapters covering parent and family involvement in different areas of speech-language pathology clinical practice. Each chapter has been written by internationally renowned experts in their specific discipline. Elizabeth Crais has written about identification and assessment issues when working with families of young children with communication and language impairments. Complementing Dr. Crais' chapter, Luigi Girolametto and Elaine Weitzman have written about intervention issues for the same population of children (young children with communication and language impairments). In Chapter 6 Ann Packman and Marilyn Langevin have clearly outlined evidence-based practices for working with families of children who stutter, and we (the book's editors) have written about working with families of children with speech impairments in Chapter 7. Julie Marshall and Juliet Goldbart have considered the complex issues of working with families of children who use Augmentative and Alternative Communication (AAC), and have included perspectives based on their extensive cross-cultural experiences. In Chapter 9 Bernice A. Mathisen provides an interdisciplinary perspective to working with families of children with dysphagia. Alice Eriks-Brophy outlines the many issues of diagnosis, assessment, and intervention when working with families of children with hearing loss. In the final chapter A. Lynn Williams and Martha J. Coutinho outline methods for working with families of young children with language impairment to facilitate emergent literacy skills.

Each chapter in Part II is organized in the following way:

- Research: Historical overview of parent/family involvement
- Clinical practice: Speech-language pathologists' involvement of families
- Families' views of involvement in speech-language pathology
- Nexus between research, clinical practice, and families' views
- Case study of family involvement

Thus, each chapter informs readers of what methods of parental involvement have been proven to increase child and family outcomes. Each chapter also links research to clinical practice with studies of parents' perceptions of their involvement in their child's intervention and their relationship with the speech-language pathologist being used to inform clinicians of the most effective ways of interacting with and involving parents in speech-language pathology intervention. Each chapter in Part II concludes with a case study to facilitate the readers' knowledge of how to work with families in professional practice.

It is our wish that readers of this book will feel more confident in their work with families in speech-language pathology intervention. Armed with a knowledge of: the evidence of the effectiveness of family involvement in different clinical populations, practical strategies for involving families, and an understanding of how parents and families view their involvement in intervention, we hope that readers will be able to enhance their work with families.

Nicole Watts Pappas and Sharynne McLeod

Acknowledgments

It has been my great fortune to continue working with Sharynne McLeod after the submission of my Ph.D. I would like to acknowledge her as the driving force behind the publication of this book. Her incredible energy, organizational ability, and passion for speech-language pathology are always an inspiration for me.

I would also like to acknowledge my wonderful husband, John Pappas, my parents Ron and Marilyn Watts, and all my friends and family who are so supportive of my research and academic endeavours. I would particularly like to acknowledge my very good friends Rebecca Peng and Belinda Wade for their support throughout the writing of this book. Thank you!

Nicole Watts Pappas

It has been a pleasure to write and edit this book with Nicole Watts Pappas. I would like to acknowledge her brilliant insights into working with families, continuous zeal, and thorough exploration of this important topic.

The writing and editing of this book was supported by a key researcher fellowship from the Research Institute for Professional Practice, Learning and Education (RIPPLE) at Charles Sturt University, Australia.

As always, I sincerely thank my family, David, Brendon, and Jessica, who are my constant source of inspiration and support.

Sharynne McLeod

Contributors

Martha J. Coutinho, East Tennessee State University, USA
Martha Coutinho, Ph.D. is a Professor in Special Education at East Tennessee State University. Her research interests include emergent literacy, students with high functioning autism and Asperger's syndrome, the transition of young adults with special needs to successful life outcomes, and the human-animal bond.
Chapter 11

Elizabeth R. Crais, University of North Carolina at Chapel Hill, USA
Elizabeth Crais, Ph.D. is a Professor in the Division of Speech and Hearing Sciences of the Department of Allied Health Sciences at the University of North Carolina at Chapel Hill School of Medicine. She has published a number of articles and book chapters and is co-author with P. J. McWilliam and Pam Winton of *Practical Strategies for Family-Centered Early Intervention*.
Chapter 4

Alice Eriks-Brophy, University of Toronto, Canada
Alice Eriks-Brophy, Ph.D. is Assistant Professor at the Department of Speech-Language Pathology at the University of Toronto, where she teaches courses in aural rehabilitation and articulation development and disorders. Her research interests include the role of parental involvement in communication outcomes for children with hearing loss as well as the provision of culturally appropriate speech-language pathology services to minority culture children. Prior to embarking on an academic career, Alice worked as an itinerant teacher for the Montreal Oral School for the Deaf and as an elementary classroom teacher on several First Nations reserves in northern and southern Québec.
Chapter 10

Luigi Girolametto, University of Toronto, Canada

Luigi Girolametto, Ph.D. is an Associate Professor in the Department of Speech-Language Pathology at the University of Toronto. He has practiced as a speech-language pathologist and worked with parents of children with language disorders at The Hanen Centre and the Hospital for Sick Children in Toronto. His university teaching and research focuses on language intervention for young children. His research interests include the efficacy of parent-focused language intervention, the prevention of language disorders, and the promotion of language and literacy skills in educational settings. His research is funded by the Social Sciences and Humanities Research Council, the Canadian Language and Literacy Network, and the Australian Medical Research Council. *Chapter 5*

Juliet Goldbart, Manchester Metropolitan University, United Kingdom

Juliet Goldbart, Ph.D. is a Reader in Psychology at Manchester Metropolitan University (MMU), UK. She has taught on the speech and language therapy course at MMU for over 25 years. Her research and teaching interests include explanatory models of communication development/disorders, communication in people with severe and profound intellectual impairment, exploring and developing the evidence base in communication impairment, Augmentative and Alternative Communication (AAC), and service delivery models in countries of the south. She has been involved in developing and running workshops for parents of children with severe and profound disability on communication, both in the United Kingdom and in India, where she has collaborated on a number of projects with the Indian Institute for Cerebral Palsy. *Chapter 8*

Marilyn Langevin, University of Alberta, Canada

Marilyn Langevin, Ph.D. is Assistant Professor, Fluency Disorders (Research) at the Institute for Stuttering Treatment and Research (ISTAR), Faculty of Rehabilitation Medicine, University of Alberta. She recently completed her Ph.D. at The University of Sydney after having extensive experience in treating stuttering. She has made major contributions to the development of the *Comprehensive Stuttering Programs* for teens, adults, and school-age children and the associated clinical training programs. She also authored *Teasing and Bullying: Unacceptable Behaviour*, a school program designed to educate school-age students about stuttering and change attitudes toward teasing and bullying. Her research interests include evidence-based practice and the impact of stuttering on children and families. *Chapter 6*

Julie Marshall, Manchester Metropolitan University, United Kingdom

Julie Marshall, Ph.D. is a speech and language therapist and a Senior Research Fellow/Senior Lecturer in Speech and Language Therapy, at Manchester Metropolitan University, UK. She has research and teaching interests in explanatory models of communication development/disorders, cross-cultural competence, parents' perspectives of the impact of the communication environment, and Augmentative and Alternative Communication. She has lectured on two speech and language therapy courses in Manchester, UK for 17 years and has also worked as a speech and language therapist and trainer in Tanzania, Kenya and in Manchester, with a range of professional and client groups. *Chapter 8*

Bernice Mathisen, University of Newcastle, Australia

Bernice Mathisen, Ph.D. is the Speech Pathology Program Convenor at The University of Newcastle and former Director of its Interdisciplinary Dysphagia Clinic (IDC) from 2001 to 2006. She has 35 years' experience in the profession, in Australia and in the United Kingdom (University College, London) with a broad spectrum of research, teaching, clinical service, and senior administrative roles. She obtained her initial undergraduate degree and Ph.D. at The University of Queensland, Australia and her Masters degree in Human Communication at the City University, London. She has published widely in speech pathology with a particular interest in dysphagia (especially in infants and children), complex communication needs and disability across the life span, and, more recently, spirituality and health, meditation, and creative writing, in particular, poetry. She received The University of Newcastle Excellence in Teaching Award in 2001 and is regarded as an innovator in interdisciplinary professional education in Australia. *Chapter 9*

Lindy McAllister, Charles Sturt University, Australia

Lindy McAllister, Ph.D. is Associate Professor in Speech Pathology at Charles Sturt University (CSU), a Key Researcher in the Research

Institute for Professional Practice, Learning, and Education (RIPPLE), and Deputy Director of CSU's Education for Practice Institute. Dr. McAllister was National President of Speech Pathology Association of Australia in 2003 and 2004, and currently serves as a senior council member of the association's ethics board. In 2002, she was the recipient of the association's highest honor—The Eleanor Wray Award for Outstanding Contribution to the Profession, and in 2006 was made a Life Member. She is the co-author of three books on clinical education: *Facilitating Learning in Clinical Settings* (Nelson Thornes), *Clinical Education in Speech Pathology* (Whurr), and *Communication in the Health and Social Sciences* (Oxford University Press).
Chapter 1

Sharynne McLeod, Charles Sturt University, Australia

Sharynne McLeod, Ph.D. is Associate Professor of speech and language acquisition at Charles Sturt University, Australia. She is vice president of the International Clinical Linguistics and Phonetics Association, Fellow the American Speech-Language-Hearing Association and of Speech Pathology Australia, and editor of the *International Journal of Speech-Language Pathology*. She recently provided advice to the World Health Organization about the *International Classification of Functioning, Disability and Health—Children and Youth Version*. Her research promotes the rights of children and their families to participate fully in society. Recent books include *The International Guide to Speech Acquisition* (Thomson, 2007) and *Speech Sounds: A Pictorial Guide to Typical and Atypical Speech* (Plural, 2008).
Chapters 1, 2, 3, 7

Ann Packman, The University of Sydney, Australia

Ann Packman, Ph.D. is Associate Professor at The University of Sydney, Australia. She has worked with people who stutter and their families for over 35 years, as a clinician and a researcher, and as advisor to Speak Easy, the Australian self-help and advocacy association for people who stutter. She is currently Senior Research Officer at the Australian Stuttering Research Centre at The University of Sydney. She regularly presents her work at national and international conferences and has published three books and over 80 papers in the field of stuttering.
Chapter 6

Nicole Watts Pappas, Charles Sturt University and Queensland Health, Australia
Nicole Watts Pappas, Ph.D. is an adjunct lecturer at Charles Sturt University as well as a senior speech pathologist at the Upper Mt. Gravatt Children's Development Centre in Brisbane. She recently completed her Ph.D. in working with families in intervention for speech impairment. She is the recipient of the Mitchell Search Grant, the Nadia Verrall Memorial Grant, and a Charles Sturt University scholarship. She is co-editor for *ACQuiring Knowledge in Speech, Language and Hearing* (2004). Her continuing area of research and clinical practice is in working with families of young children with communication impairments.
Chapter 1, 2, 3, 7

Elaine Weitzman, The Hanen Centre, Canada
Elaine Weitzman, M.Ed., Executive Director of The Hanen Centre in Toronto, Canada is a speech-language pathologist and co-author of two guidebooks on facilitating young children's language and emergent literacy development: *It Takes Two to Talk*, for parents of children with language delays and *Learning Language and Loving It*, for early childhood professionals. Ms. Weitzman is an Assistant Professor in the Department of Speech-Language Pathology, University of Toronto, where she collaborates on research studies on how early childhood educators facilitate the language and literacy development of young children in child care settings, as well as on the efficacy of caregiver training programs.
Chapter 5

A. Lynn Williams, East Tennessee State University, USA
Lynn Williams, Ph.D. is a professor at East Tennessee State University. She has conducted federally funded research that has been the basis of several published articles, book chapters, and a book, and developed an National Institutes of Health funded intervention software program. Dr. Williams served as associate editor of *Language, Speech, and Hearing Services in Schools*. She is a Fellow of the American Speech-Language-Hearing Association.
Chapter 11

This book is dedicated to our families

Chapter 1

Models of Practice Used in Speech-Language Pathologists' Work with Families

Nicole Watts Pappas, Sharynne McLeod, and Lindy McAllister

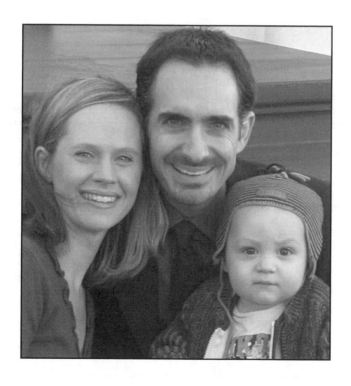

Introduction

Speech-language pathologists' (SLPs') work with families in pediatric intervention has changed significantly over the past 50 years. Recommended practice for SLPs and other allied health professionals has shifted from very limited involvement with parents to a collaborative relationship with the child's whole family (Andrews & Andrews, 1986; Crais, 1991; Hanna & Rodger, 2002). Three sequential phases of parent and family involvement have been advocated by policy makers and discussed in the literature. These include the therapist-centered model, the parent-as-therapist aide model, and the family-centered model. The models vary, primarily in relation to the extent of parent and family involvement, the focus of the intervention on the child or family, and the amount of family participation and power in the decision-making process. This book introduces a new model of practice in working with families in pediatric intervention, the family-friendly model (Watts Pappas, 2007). Table 1-1 summarizes the four different models and their major similarities and differences.

Table 1–1. The Four Models of Practice

Model	Family Involvement in Intervention Provision	Family Involvement in Intervention Planning	Primary Decision-Maker	Primary Client
Therapist-centered	No	No	Professional	Child
Parent-as-therapist aide	Yes	No	Professional	Child
Family-centered	Varies according to families' wishes	Varies according to families' wishes	Family	Usually the family (varies according to families' wishes)
Family-friendly	Families supported to be involved in the intervention	Varies according to families' wishes	Professional	Usually the child (varies according to families' wishes)

In this chapter each of the four models of practice is described, outlining the foundation for each model, their *theorized* advantages and disadvantages, and the existing evidence base for each model's effectiveness. Although the models are discussed historically in order of emergence in professional practice, any of the four may currently be in use in intervention services for young children. Actual practice may not always be aligned with recommended practice. The information presented here therefore is a reflection of the discussion of family-professional relationships in the literature rather than actual practices of professionals, which may vary between services (Mahoney & O'Sullivan, 1990; McWilliam, Synder, Harbin, Porter, & Munn, 2000). For a discussion of the literature on the reported practices and beliefs of SLPs and other allied health professionals regarding working with parents and families see Chapter 2. Chapter 3 includes a discussion of the literature on parents' views of working with SLPs and other allied health professionals. The remaining chapters in this book discuss working with families of children presenting with language impairment, stuttering, speech impairment, hearing impairment, complex communication needs, dysphagia, and early literacy concerns.

Therapist-Centered Model

Description

Traditionally, intervention services for young children were provided using a therapist-centered model of service delivery (Bailey, McWilliam, & Winton, 1992a; Bazyk, 1989). In the therapist-centered model or, as it is also known, the expert model of practice, professionals assume hierarchical control over the planning and provision of intervention services for young children (Rosenbaum, King, Law, King, & Evans, 1998) (Table 1–2). The professional assesses, diagnoses and treats the child and the family has little or no involvement in either the planning or provision of the intervention (Lawlor & Mattingly, 1998). Using this model, professionals considered the child in isolation rather than in the context of the family and parents were seen as part of the problem rather than the solution (Leviton, Mueller, & Kaufmann, 1992; Wehman, 1998). For example, in his article on parental influences on speech production, Wood (1946, p. 272) stated, "Functional articulatory defects of children are definitely and significantly associated with

Table 1–2. Contextualizing the Therapist-Centered Model

Model	Family Involvement in Intervention Provision	Family Involvement in Intervention Planning	Primary Decision-Maker	Primary Client
Therapist-centered	No	No	Professional	Child
Parent-as-therapist aide	Yes	No	Professional	Child
Family-centered	Varies according to families' wishes	Varies according to families' wishes	Family	Usually the family (varies according to families' wishes)
Family-friendly	Families supported to be involved in the intervention	Varies according to families' wishes	Professional	Usually the child (varies according to families' wishes)

maladjustment and undesirable traits on the part of the parents, and such factors are usually maternally centered". This view, although no longer prevalent, supported a therapist-centered approach.

Advantages

No advantages for the therapist-centered model of practice have been discussed in the literature, perhaps because the practice was taken for granted at the time, and because practice itself was not seen as a topic of investigation. However, some studies of parents' and professionals' perceptions of family involvement in intervention for young children have indicated a preference for selected features of the therapist-centered model of practice. For example, a number of researchers have found that parents prefer the professional to take the lead in intervention planning for their child (MacKean, Thurston, & Scott, 2005; McBride, Brotherson, Joanning, Whiddon, & Demmitt, 1993; Piggot,

Hocking, & Patterson, 2003; Watts Pappas, McAllister, & McLeod, 2009b) and that professionals believe that parents need and/or want this guidance (Bailey et al., 1992a; Litchfield & MacDougall, 2002; McBride et al., 1993; Minke & Scott, 1995; Watts Pappas, McAllister, & McLeod, 2009a). Both of these beliefs are compatible with the therapist-centered model of practice.

Disadvantages

Some disadvantages to the therapist-centered model of practice have been theorized in the literature. For example, in the therapist-centered model, parents' knowledge about their child is not utilized. This loss of parental perspective means that intervention goals and plans may be irrelevant to the child and family (Appleton & Minchom, 1991) and intervention effectiveness may be diminished by a lack of knowledge about the child's skills in contexts outside the clinic. The therapist-centered model also gives parents limited opportunity to participate in the intervention and thereby acquire new skills to help their child (Dunst & Trivette, 1996). This encourages families to be dependent on the professional, placing parents in a position of powerlessness and perhaps engendering a lack of confidence in their caregiving skills (Dunst, 1985).

Evidence Base

The many intervention efficacy studies that have been conducted without mention of parent involvement in service planning or delivery testify to the fact that intervention for young children without family involvement can be effective. For example, intervention approaches for children with speech impairment (Gierut, 1989; Williams, 2000), phonological awareness difficulties (Gillon, 2000), and language impairment (Goldstein, 1984; Wilcox, Kouri, & Caswell, 1991) have all been demonstrated to be effective without parental involvement.

However, other studies have demonstrated parent dissatisfaction with the therapist-centered model of service delivery. Parents in a number of studies have reported discontent with professionals' disregard for their opinions and knowledge about their child (Baxter, 1989; Case-Smith & Nastro, 1993; Glogowska & Campbell, 2000; Minke &

Scott, 1995), which can be associated with the limited parental involvement of the therapist-centered model. For an in-depth review of parents' perceptions of intervention see Chapter 3.

Parent-as-Therapist Aide Model

As parents became dissatisfied with the expert model of service delivery, they campaigned for more involvement in their child's intervention (Turnbull & Turnbull, 1982). Partly due to the pressure applied by these parent groups as well as legislative changes in the United States, professionals began giving parents greater involvement in their child's intervention (Bailey et al., 1992a; Bazyk, 1989; Hanna & Rodger, 2002; Rosenbaum et al., 1998). The parent-as-therapist aide model of working with parents in intervention for young children has been described by previous authors as the "transplant model" (Appleton & Minchom, 1991, p. 28), "parents as teachers and therapists" (Bazyk, 1989, p. 724), and the "family-allied model" (McBride et al., 1993, p. 415). In this book the model is identified as the parent-as-therapist aide model. This redefinition was made on the basis of the limited parental involvement in decision-making in the model, thereby placing the parent in the position of therapist's aide.

Description

Although the legislation in the United States mandated that parents should have a decision-making role in intervention services for their child, this appeared to be actualized as a role in the delivery of intervention, mostly by requesting that parents conduct home activities (Bazyk, 1989). As Andrews and Andrews (1986, p. 359) commented in their description of speech-language pathology practice at this time, "Input from the client is of course appreciated but it is the expert professional who evaluates the problem, sets the goals, and determines the course of treatment."

In the parent-as-therapist aide model, parents mostly participate in intervention by conducting activities at home which are planned and designed by the professional (Appleton & Minchom, 1991) (Table 1–3). These activities could be given in conjunction with intervention sessions or as a complete replacement, with the professional acting as a consultant and the parent as the primary agent of intervention. The

Table 1–3. Contextualizing the Parent-as-Therapist Aide Model

Model	Family Involvement in Intervention Provision	Family Involvement in Intervention Planning	Primary Decision-Maker	Primary Client
Therapist-centered	No	No	Professional	Child
Parent-as-therapist aide	Yes	No	Professional	Child
Family-centered	Varies according to families' wishes	Varies according to families' wishes	Family	Usually the family (varies according to families' wishes)
Family-friendly	Families supported to be involved in the intervention	Varies according to families' wishes	Professional	Usually the child (varies according to families' wishes)

intervention is still child-centered in that it focuses on the child in isolation rather than in the context of their family (Andrews & Andrews, 1986) and although parents were now given the opportunity to be involved in their child's intervention provision, they still had limited participation in decision-making about their child's care (Case-Smith & Nastro, 1993; McBride et al., 1993).

Advantages

Many benefits of involving parents in intervention provision have been theorized in the literature. As parents had the ability to work with their child in natural settings such as the home environment, it was considered that family involvement could facilitate generalization of skills to settings outside of the clinic (Bazyk, 1989; Costello & Bosler; 1976; Jansen, Ketelaar, & Vermeer, 2003; Shelton, Johnson, Willis, & Arndt, 1975; Wing & Heimgartner, 1973). Parental involvement was also suggested as a strategy to increase the cost-effectiveness of intervention, as the professional was not required to give all the intervention to the child (Dodd & Barker, 1990; Fey, 1986; McPherson, Morris, & Ferguson, 1987). Advantages for the parent and family were also suggested. Authors surmised that if parents learned how to help their child it would decrease parental stress (Turnbull, Turnbull, & Wheat, 1982) and provide them with greater knowledge and confidence in their caregiving role (Jansen et al., 2003). Professionals working in a clinical setting also supported parental involvement in intervention, with many studies indicating that professionals believed parental involvement in intervention for young children was important and could improve intervention outcomes (Hinojosa, Anderson, & Ranum, 1988; Hinojosa, Sproat, Mankhetwit, & Anderson, 2002; Iversen, Poulin Shimmel, Ciacera, & Meenakshi 2003; Leiter, 2004; MacKean et al., 2005).

Disadvantages

Some disadvantages of the parent-as-therapist aide model of service delivery have been discussed. For example, a study of parents' perceptions of home programs revealed that some parents found participation in these programs difficult and time consuming (Hinojosa & Anderson, 1991). Many authors cautioned professionals about having unrealistic expectations of parental involvement in their child's intervention (Allen & Stefanowski Hudd, 1987; Bazyk, 1989; Rodger, 1986; Turnbull & Turnbull, 1982). It was suggested that when parents adopt the role of the professional it may affect child-parent relationships by making the parent-child interaction take on the role of work (Allen & Stefanowski Hudd, 1987). Additionally, the authors cautioned that attempting to implement a home program could increase the stress of a family that already had the additional time requirements of caring for a child with a disability (Rodger, 1986).

Additionally, the parent-as-therapist aide model assumed that all parents would wish to take an active role in intervention for their child. However, a number of studies have demonstrated that this was not true for all parents (Andrews, Andrews, & Shearer, 1989; McKenzie, 1994; Piggot et al., 2003). Although the model gave parents an opportunity to be involved in the intervention, it did not give them a choice about whether to be involved or not, or in what way to be involved (Turnbull & Turnbull, 1982). The parent-as-therapist aide model also did not consider the individual needs and preferences of families, labeling parents as noncompliant if they did not do the activities requested of them (Giller Gajdosik & Campbell, 1991; Mayo, 1981; Short, Schkade, & Herring, 1989). For example, Short and colleagues (1989, p. 446) wrote: "Some mothers seemed to respond negatively to the increased performance demands with apparent avoidance behaviors."

Evidence Base

Numerous studies have been conducted to investigate the effect of parental involvement in intervention provision for young children. A number of reviews of this body of research have also been conducted (Table 1–4). Most of the studies have focused on the effect of parental involvement on specific intervention outcomes for the child.

Table 1–4. Reviews of the Effect of Parental Involvement on Intervention Outcomes

Review	Number of Studies Reviewed	Children's Difficulty (as Specified in Review)	Age of Children	Service Provided (as Specified in Review)
Ketelaar, Vermeer, Helders, & Hart, 1998	7	Cerebral palsy	Younger than 5 years	Early intervention services
Law, Garret, & Nye 2003a	33 (15 of which involved parents' opinions/ involvement)	Speech/language delay/disorder	0–15 years	Speech-language pathology
Shonkoff & Hauser-Cram, 1987	31	"Disabled"	Younger than 3 years	Early intervention services
White, 1985	27 involving parents compared to 80 with no parental involvement	Disabled, disadvantaged, or at risk	Not specified	Early intervention services
White, Taylor, & Moss, 1992	172	"Disabled, disadvantaged, or at risk"	Not specified	Early intervention services

Few have included investigation of the effect of parental involvement on outcomes for the parents and family. Three different types of question primarily have been addressed in these studies:

1. Are intervention programs that incorporate parental involvement effective?
2. Are parent-administered interventions as effective as professional-administered interventions?
3. Can parental involvement increase the effectiveness of intervention provided by a professional?

Research addressing the above three questions is briefly reviewed here. Due to the large number of studies investigating these questions, the discussion is limited to consideration of previous systematic reviews of the research, rather than critique of individual studies. Where possible, the review focuses on studies incorporating speech-language pathology intervention. However, intervention generally was provided by a combination of allied health and other professionals such as nurses and teachers, rather than a specific professional discipline.

Are Intervention Programs Incorporating Parental Involvement Effective?

A substantial evidence base exists to support the proposition that intervention incorporating parental involvement can be effective (Law, Garrett, & Nye, 2003a; White, 1985). For example, in a review of parental involvement in intervention for young children, White (1985) listed 27 studies demonstrating the effectiveness of intervention programs involving parent participation. However, when compared to studies which did not involve parents, the effect sizes were similar. In the field of speech-language pathology, a Cochrane review of the effectiveness of speech-language pathology intervention (Law et al., 2003a) included a total of 27 studies, four of which compared parent-administered intervention to no intervention (Gibbard, Coglan, & MacDonald, 1994; Girolametto, Steig Pearce, & Weitzmen, 1996a; Girolametto, Steig Pearce, & Weitzmen 1996b; Shelton, Johnson, Ruscello, & Arndt, 1978). The review found that in three of these studies, the intervention involving parents was more effective than no intervention (Gibbard et al., 1994; Girolametto et al., 1996a; Girolametto et al., 1996b). For example, in a study of parent-administered intervention for young children with expressive vocabulary delays (Girolametto et al., 1996a), the 12 children in the experimental group exhibited a larger increase in expressive vocabulary than the 13 children in the control group who received no intervention over the 4-month time period of the study. However, in the study conducted by Shelton and colleagues (1978), a parent-administered program did not improve the children's receptive phonological knowledge in comparison to no intervention. Although the majority of these studies demonstrated that intervention involving parents could be effective, they did not investigate the effectiveness of the intervention in comparison to intervention provided by professionals.

Is Parent-Administered Intervention as Effective as Professional-Administered Intervention?

The Cochrane review study (Law et al., 2003a) also incorporated studies that compared primarily parent-administered intervention to primarily professional-administered intervention. This review found that intervention conducted by parents was just as effective as intervention conducted by a SLP (Law et al., 2003a). Of the 27 studies that met the criteria for the review, five compared parent-administered to SLP-administered intervention (Fey, Cleave, & Long, 1993; Gibbard, 1994; Lancaster, 1991 [unpublished], cited in Law et al., 2003a; Law, 1999 [unpublished], in Law et al., 2003a; Tufts & Holliday, 1959). Three of the studies focused on intervention for early language delay (Fey et al., 1993; Gibbard, 1994; Law, 1999 [unpublished], cited in Law et al., 2003a) and two of the studies on intervention for speech impairment (Lancaster, 1991 [unpublished], cited in Law et al., 2003a; Tufts & Holliday, 1959). These studies all demonstrated similar improvements in the outcomes of intervention provided by trained parents as compared to that provided by SLPs. For example, Gibbard (1994) compared the outcomes of a parental training group to individual direct speech-language pathology treatment for a group of children with early language delay. At the end of the 6-month period of the study the two groups showed similar gains in their expressive language skills. The Cochrane review suggested therefore that intervention programs primarily conducted by trained parents can be just as effective as professional-conducted intervention.

Can Parental Involvement Increase the Effectiveness of Intervention Provided by a Professional?

Research investigating whether the involvement of parents can make intervention provided by a professional more effective has produced differing findings. For example, Ketelaar, Vermeer, Helders, and Hart (1998) reviewed seven studies of parental involvement in intervention for children with cerebral palsy. They concluded that parental participation mostly had a positive effect on child-related outcomes. Additionally, in a meta-analysis of intervention for young children with disabilities conducted by Shonkoff and Hauser-Cram (1987), pediatric intervention programs that included work with parents and children together were found to be more successful than programs that did not encourage parental involvement.

However, conflicting results have also been reported. For example, a second review conducted by White and colleagues (1992) of 172 intervention studies, reported no evidence of larger effect sizes for intervention programs that included parental involvement. The only exception was intervention for speech impairment in which one reviewed study (Eiserman, McCoun, & Escobar, 1990) demonstrated that parental involvement had a positive effect on speech intervention outcomes. (A comprehensive review of the effectiveness of parental involvement in intervention for speech impairment [including further details of the study conducted by Eiserman and colleagues] is provided in Chapter 7.) Additionally, whereas the White (1985) review found that intervention programs involving parents were effective, it showed that the programs that included parents were no more effective than those that did not involve parents.

The reasons for the differences in the findings of these reviews are unclear. The much larger number of studies included in the reviews conducted by White (1985) and White and colleagues (1992) may have provided a broader picture of the effect of parental involvement in pediatric intervention. Alternatively, both the reviews by Shonkoff and Hauser-Cram (1987) and Ketelaar and colleagues (1998) exclusively included studies of young children (under 5 or 3 years of age). It is possible that the effects of parental involvement are greater in intervention for younger children, thus explaining the larger effects of parental participation reported by these reviews.

It should be noted that the studies reviewed by the authors in Table 1–4 evidenced a number of limitations, including nonrandomization of groups, nonblinded examiners, and limited longitudinal measures. The studies also differed vastly in terms of the intervention provided, the type and amount of parental involvement, the age, difficulties, and severity of the children serviced, and the characteristics of the parents. The diversity of the studies makes it difficult to draw conclusions about their group findings. However, it appears that although there is evidence to suggest that parent-administered intervention can be just as effective as that administered by a professional, it has not been proven that parental involvement in allied health intervention provided by a professional makes that intervention any more effective.

Family-Centered Model

In the 1990s, the family-centered model emerged as a new model of practice and basis for relationships between families and professionals (Rosenbaum et al., 1998). Although this model was initially developed for use in the disability field, the family-centered movement has influenced all areas of SLP and other pediatric allied health intervention, including services for children in hospital (Franck & Callery, 2004). Two major factors influenced the development of this model of practice:

1. Theories of child development, such as human ecological theory (Bronfenbrenner, 1979), that highlight the role of the family and the community in a child's development and health and well-being. Human ecological theory suggests that a child's development is not only determined by properties innate to the child but is also influenced by the child's interaction with the immediate environment and the larger contexts in which that environment is embedded. For example, children's development may be influenced by their interactions with their immediate family, their participation in other environments (such as preschool), the impact of environments in which they do not participate but are linked to their immediate environment (for example, their parent's place of work), and, finally, the culture of the society in which they live. Therefore, for children with developmental difficulties, focusing intervention on the family as well as the child was postulated to facilitate the child's development.

2. A series of legislative acts which were passed in the United States beginning with the Education for All Handicapped Children Act of 1975 (Turnbull & Turnbull, 1982) and later the Individuals with Disabilities Education Act (IDEA) of 1990 (Wehman, 1998) that extended the role of families in decision-making in intervention for young children and introduced the concept of the family as client rather than solely the child. A similar trend occurred in the United Kingdom, with government policy mandating the use of family-centered practices in intervention for children from 1991 (Franck & Callery, 2004).

Description

Family-centered practice is a model of practice in intervention for young children that focuses on supporting and strengthening the child's whole family. In Table 1-5 the features of family-centered practice

Table 1–5. Contextualizing the Family-Centered Model

Model	Family Involvement in Intervention Provision	Family Involvement in Intervention Planning	Primary Decision-Maker	Primary Client
Therapist-centered	No	No	Professional	Child
Parent-as-therapist aide	Yes	No	Professional	Child
Family-centered	Varies according to families' wishes	Varies according to families' wishes	Family	Usually the family (varies according to families' wishes)
Family-friendly	Families supported to be involved in the intervention	Varies according to families' wishes	Professional	Usually the child (varies according to families' wishes)

with regard to the extent of parent involvement in intervention provision and intervention planning and the focus of services (i.e., who
is considered the primary client) are outlined in comparison with the
therapist-centered and parent-as-therapist aide model. The practices
in this table refer to the usual way in which family-centered practice is
conducted. However, considering that another major feature of family-
centered service is family choice-making, it should be considered that
the family's involvement in intervention planning and the identity of
the primary client may vary according to the family's wishes.

Several terms have been used to refer to pediatric intervention
practices that are synonymous with the family-centered model. The
most notable of these include family empowerment (Dunst, Trivette
& Deal, 1988), family-focused intervention (Bailey et al., 1986), and
family-centered service, practice, or care (Bailey et al., 1992a). The
term *family-centered* has become the most widely used and accepted
of these labels (Dunst, 2002). In this book, application of the family-
centered model is referred to as family-centered service or practice.
Descriptions of the family-centered model vary and no universal definition has been agreed on in the literature. However, some major
assumptions are similar in all approaches. These features are now
discussed.

Family as Client

One of the key concepts of family-centered practice is the acceptance
of the family as the client rather than just the child. Based on the view
that change to one family member affects all other family members,
intervention then focuses not only on making direct changes to the
child but also on helping the child's whole family (Andrews & Andrews,
1986; Goetz, Gavin, & Lane, 2000).

Positive Parent-Professional Relationships

Some authors have suggested that the cornerstone of family-centered
practice is the formation of positive relationships between parents and
professionals (Hanna & Rodger, 2002; McWilliam, Tocci, & Harbin,
1998). This is achieved by professionals' interpersonal skills (such as
being caring and empathetic) and their attitudes toward parents—
treating them as capable and deserving of respect (Dunst, 2002).

Parental Decision-Making

Family-centered service acknowledges the parents' and family's right to make the final decisions about their child's intervention and these choices are supported and accepted by professionals even if they do not agree with them (Bailey et al., 1992a; Bazyk, 1989; King, Rosenbaum, & King, 1997; Leviton et al., 1992). Professionals act as consultants and are responsible for providing parents with information and support for their decision-making role (Dinnebail & Rule, 1994). Underlying this process is the professionals' belief that parents are capable of making decisions about their child and have the right to do so (Dunst & Trivette, 1996; Viscardis, 1998).

Parent Choice of the Level of Involvement

Although family-centered practice encourages parents and families to be involved in all aspects of intervention, this involvement is not considered mandatory. The extent of the family's involvement in any aspect of intervention planning or provision is always their choice (Brown, Humphry, & Taylor, 1997; Rosenbaum et al., 1998). For example, if a family decides they do not wish to be involved in intervention provision this would be accepted by professionals.

Individualization of Services

Family-centered practice recognizes the individuality and diversity of parents and families and adapts services to take into account each family's beliefs, culture, and the environment in which they live (Crais, 1991; Law et al., 1998). Family-centered services are designed to fit the needs of families and are flexible and accessible (Dunst, 2002).

Empowering and Enabling Families

Family-centered services reflect an enabling model of helping, thereby fostering the skills of families to care for their child with special needs (Dunst & Trivette, 1996). The aim of family-centered practice is to identify and enhance child and family strengths rather than focusing on weaknesses, and to promote competence rather than dependence on service providers (Andrews & Andrews, 1986).

Advantages

Many advantages of family-centered practice have been suggested in the literature. It has been theorized that providing services to the child's whole family indirectly facilitates the child's development (Mahoney & Bella, 1998). For example, organizing housing support for a family would also benefit the child, relieving stress on the family and allowing more time to be spent on the child's intervention. It has also been suggested that allowing parents choice and control over their child's intervention may increase their satisfaction with the service (Viscardis, 1998). The model's focus on providing participatory experiences for parents has been hypothesized to encourage parental competency-building and feelings of empowerment (Dunst & Trivette, 1996). In addition, the utilization of parents' knowledge about their child and parental involvement in service planning may result in intervention activities and outcomes that are more relevant to the child and family (Crais, 1991; Hanna & Rodger, 2002). Finally, the focus of the family-centered practice model on forming positive relationships between professionals and parents has been proposed to increase the outcomes of intervention. For example, Kalmanson and Seligman (1992, p. 48) stated, "The success of all interventions will rest on the quality of provider-family relationships."

Disadvantages

Many of the disadvantages of family-centered practice that have been discussed in the literature center around the concept of parental decision-making. Whether parents are capable of making appropriate decisions regarding their child's health is a concern that has been voiced by a number of researchers and clinicians (Allen & Stefanowski Hudd, 1987; Appleton & Minchom, 1990; Bailey et al., 1992a; Brotherson & Goldstein, 1992; Litchfield & MacDougall, 2002). These studies have suggested that parents need and want the guidance of an expert professional in determining intervention plans for their child and that allowing parents to make the final, possibly inappropriate decisions about intervention could be unethical. It has also been suggested that not all families may want the best for their children. As Allen and Stefanowski Hudd (1987, p. 135) stated, "The occurrence of child abuse is a harsh reminder that the needs of parents and their children are not always isomorphic."

Parent and family advocates have highlighted another potential disadvantage of family-centered practice relating to parental decision-making. Considering that families are a heterogeneous rather than a homogeneous group and have different time, abilities, priorities, and beliefs, Viscardis (1998) argued that not all families may wish to participate in the planning or delivery of their child's intervention. Although true family-centered practice advocates family choice of level of involvement, if misconstrued, involvement in intervention may be considered a parental responsibility rather than a right. Professionals may then require parents to take a lead role in their child's intervention, even if this is not the parents' wish (Espezel & Canam, 2003; MacKean et al., 2005).

From an administrative perspective, using a family-centered approach to service delivery has been suggested to be more time-intensive than traditional approaches because of the need to negotiate the content of intervention goals and activities with parents (Lawlor & Mattingly, 1998). The use of this form of service therefore may be

Table 1–6. Details of Studies Investigating Outcomes of Family-Centered Intervention

Study	Outcomes Evaluated	Type of Investigation	Control Group	No. of Participants
Law et al., 1998	Child intervention outcomes	Experimental study	No	12 children
Mahoney & Bella, 1998	Child intervention outcomes Parent stress and well-being	Experimental study	No	47 families

at odds with the current focus on effectiveness and accountability in allied health practice (Litchfield & MacDougall, 2002).

Evidence Base

Although the advantages of family-centered practice have been theorized in the literature and gained widespread acceptance, limited empirical evidence exists as to the effect of this service model on intervention outcomes (Franck & Callery, 2004; Hanna & Rodger, 2002; Jansen et al., 2004; Mahoney & Bella, 1998). Table 1–6 provides a summary of studies that reported allied health intervention outcomes (or allied health intervention in combination with other intervention) of family-centered practice for children with developmental delays or disabilities. The first studies investigating family-centered intervention were conducted in the late 1990s. In the studies identified, the outcome measures investigated included child intervention outcomes, parental satisfaction, and parental well-being. Results relating to each of these outcomes is discussed in the following sections.

(in Chronologic Order)

Discipline of Professionals	Child's Difficulty	Age of Children	Family-Centered Aspects of Service	Major Findings
Physio-therapists and occupational therapists	Cerebral palsy	1–4 years	Family involvement in all aspects of planning and provision	Eleven of the 12 children demonstrated changes that were considered by the researchers to be clinically important
Early intervention staff	A variety of conditions, the most prevalent being Down syndrome	0–3 years	Varied	Family-centered service not associated with better intervention outcomes for child, decreased parent stress or improved parent-child attachment

continues

Table 1–6. *continued*

Study	Outcomes Evaluated	Type of Investigation	Control Group	No. of Participants
King, King, Rosenbaum & Goffin, 1999	Parent stress and well-being Parent satisfaction with service	Survey	No	164 parents
Van Riper, 1999	Parent stress and well-being Parent satisfaction with service	Survey	No	94 parents
Ketelaar, Vermeer, Hart, Beek, & Helders, 2001	Child intervention outcomes	Experimental study	Yes Randomized	55 children
Law et al., 2003b	Parent satisfaction with service	Survey	No	494 parents, 411 service providers, 15 managers
McGibbon Lammi & Law, 2003	Child intervention outcomes	Experimental study	No	3 children

Discipline of Professionals	Child's Difficulty	Age of Children	Family-Centered Aspects of Service	Major Findings
Early intervention staff	Non-progressive neuro-developmental disorders (primarily spina bifida, cerebral palsy or hydrocephalus)	3–5 years	Not specified	Family-centered service found to be positively related to parental satisfaction, stress and well-being
Health professionals	Down syndrome	0–22 years	Not specified	Parents' perception of relationship with health professionals linked to satisfaction with care and emotional well-being
Physio-therapists	Cerebral palsy	2–7 years	Family involvement in all aspects of planning and provision	Children in functional therapy group (family-centered) improved more on functional outcomes than control group receiving traditional intervention
Early intervention professionals, most frequent being occupational therapists, SLPs, and physio-therapists	A variety of conditions, the most prevalent being cerebral palsy	Majority between 3–8 years	Not specified	Satisfaction linked to parents' perception of the family-centeredness of the service
Occupational therapists	Cerebral palsy	3–3.5 years	Family involvement in all aspects of planning and provision	Improvement on at least one of the two targeted tasks for all three of the children in the study

Effect of Family-Centered Practice on Intervention Outcomes

Although a number of researchers have investigated the effect of the parent-as-therapist aide model on child intervention outcomes (see Table 1-5), fewer have investigated child intervention outcomes when family-centered practice has been used (see Table 1-6), particularly in the area of allied health. A few studies have examined child intervention outcomes of family-centered allied health intervention (Ketelaar, Vermeer, Hart, Beek, & Helders, 2001; Law et al., 1998; Mahoney & Bella, 1998; McGibbon Lammi & Law, 2003). To date, only one of these studies (Mahoney & Bella, 1998) has included SLP intervention. Three of the four studies in Table 1-6 involved experimental designs that did not include control groups (Law et al., 1998; Mahoney & Bella, 1998; McGibbon Lammi & Law, 2003). The four studies are reviewed below.

Law and colleagues (1998) used a family-centered approach to occupational and physiotherapy intervention labeled "family-centered functional therapy" for a group of 12 children with cerebral palsy. This intervention was determined to be family-centered in that families were integrally involved in the planning and provision of the intervention. Measurements of the targeted skills were taken at baseline and after a 3-month period of intervention. Eleven of the 12 children demonstrated changes that were considered by the researchers to be clinically important. However, statistical significance of these changes was not evaluated.

McGibbon Lammi and Law (2003) conducted a study of the effectiveness of family-centered practice in occupational therapy intervention for three young children with cerebral palsy. Family-centered functional therapy was again used. The outcomes were measured by the children's performance on functional tasks identified as priorities by their family. Improvement was reported on at least one of the two targeted tasks for all three of the children. Both these studies demonstrated improvements in children's targeted skills over the duration of family-centered intervention. However, as no control groups were included it is not known whether the improvements were attributable to maturation or whether similar results would have been achieved with a more traditional model of service delivery.

The third study (Mahoney & Bella, 1998) investigated children and their families who received differing levels of family-centered service. However, as defined groups were not identified, the study could not be considered to have a control group. The study investigated 47 families of children with "significant disabilities" to determine whether the degree of family-centeredness of the intervention they received affected intervention outcomes. The children were aged between 1 and 3 years and presented with disabilities such as Down syndrome and cerebral palsy. Tests of child functioning and parent stress were conducted at the beginning and end of the 12-month intervention period. The children and their families all received intervention services from an early intervention center in their state, 36 different early intervention centers being represented in the study. After 6 months of intervention the parents were asked to fill in a survey that determined the level of family-centeredness of the service they were receiving. At the end of the study, the researchers compared the children's intervention outcomes to the family-centeredness of the service their parents reported receiving. No relationship was found between the perceived level of family-centeredness of the service and the intervention outcomes of the child (the results for the parent-stress outcomes measure are reported later in this chapter).

Finally, Ketelaar and colleagues (2001) conducted a physiotherapy intervention study of 55 children with mild-moderate cerebral palsy. The purpose of the study was to determine if functional therapy (similar to the intervention programs used in the studies conducted by Law et al. [1998] and McGibbon Lammi and Law [2003]) was more effective than a traditional model of intervention for cerebral palsy. The traditional model involved less parental consultation. The 55 children were randomized into the two intervention groups. Assessments were conducted 6, 12, and 18 months after the pretest. The results demonstrated no difference between groups in the children's movement on a standardized test. However, the children receiving the functional therapy made greater gains in their ability to do functional tasks in daily situations than children in the traditional group. It is unclear whether this improvement was due to the focus of the intervention on functional skills or the family-centered nature of the intervention. No other measures (such as parental stress or satisfaction) were taken.

The studies reviewed above have reported differing findings. Although intervention that is family-centered in nature was demonstrated to be effective for young children with disabilities, it was not entirely clear whether the family-centeredness of the intervention was the factor that affected intervention outcomes. Three of the studies investigated the same intervention program, functional therapy, and included children with severe disabilities only (Ketelaar et al., 2001; Law et al., 1998; McGibbon Lammi & Law, 2003). Only one study included a broader range of intervention programs and agents and children with (possibly) milder difficulties (Mahoney & Bella, 1998). That study reported different results from the other three, demonstrating that the family-centeredness of the service had no impact on the intervention outcomes of the children. The type of intervention provided and the nature of the child's difficulties therefore may be a factor in the relative effectiveness of family-centered intervention.

Effect of Family-Centered Practice on Parental Satisfaction

Three of the studies listed in Table 1–6 investigated the impact of family-centered practice on parental satisfaction with service (King, King, Rosenbaum, & Goffin 1999; Law, Hanna, Hurley, King, Kertoy, & Rosenbaum 2003b; Van Riper, 1999). These studies involved general intervention services that incorporated other services in addition to allied health intervention. None included a control group in their experimental design.

Van Riper (1999) conducted a survey of 89 mothers of children with Down syndrome. The study evaluated the mothers' perceptions of the family-centeredness of the care they had received from their child's health care providers (including allied health) (these perceptions are analyzed in detail in Chapter 4). The relationships of those perceptions to the mothers' satisfaction with the services they received and their general well-being were also investigated (the well-being component of the study is described in detail in the following section). Both the mothers' perceptions of the family-centeredness of the service and their satisfaction with service were measured using the Family-Provider Relationships Instrument, an assessment developed specifically for the study. The results demonstrated that mothers who believed the intervention services they were receiving were family-centered reported greater satisfaction with their child's care.

A second survey study was conducted by Law and colleagues (2003b) of 494 parents of children with a disability. The study was conducted to determine the factors that influenced parents' perceptions of the family-centeredness of care and the relationship of those factors to parental satisfaction with service (aspects of the parents' perceptions of family-centeredness of care are discussed in detail in Chapter 3). The children all attended early intervention services in Ontario, Canada. A questionnaire containing elements of the Measures of Processes of Care (MPOC) (King, King, & Rosenbaum, 1996) was used to measure parental perceptions of the family-centeredness of the service they received. The Client Satisfaction Questionnaire (Larsen et al., 1979, cited in Law et al., 2003b) measured the parents' satisfaction with the early intervention service. The results indicated that the parents' perceptions of receiving family-centered practice strongly influenced their satisfaction with service.

Finally, King and colleagues (1999) evaluated the effect of family-centered practice on parent satisfaction with service (among other measures including parents' stress and emotional well-being which are discussed in the following section). Parents of children with chronic difficulties (such as spina bifida and cerebral palsy) responded to a survey. The children of the 164 parents had received early intervention services from one of six publicly funded children's rehabilitation centers in a state in Canada. Satisfaction with care was assessed using the Client Satisfaction Questionnaire (Larsen et al., 1979, cited in Law et al., 2003b) and the parents' perceptions of the family-centeredness of the service were evaluated using the MPOC (King et al., 1996). Structural equation modeling demonstrated a relationship between family-centered practice (as reported by parents) and parent satisfaction with service. Although these three studies reported positive outcomes for family-centered practice, they relied on parents' perceptions of the family-centeredness of the service they received. It is therefore unknown how family-centered the intervention actually was.

Effect of family-Centered Practice on Parental Stress and Well-Being

Three of the previously described studies in Table 1–6 also included measures of parental stress and/or well-being in their experimental design (King et al., 1999; Mahoney & Bella, 1998; Van Riper, 1999). All involved general intervention services which incorporated other services in addition to allied health intervention.

The survey study conducted by King and colleagues (1999) of 164 parents of children with chronic disabilities (see previous section for details) also evaluated the parents' stress and well-being. Parental stress and well-being was measured using eight different indicators including, for example, The Centre for Epidemiological Studies Depression Scale (Radloff, 1977, cited in King et al., 1999). The results indicated that family-centered service delivery (as reported by the parents) was positively associated with parental well-being and negatively associated with parental stress.

Second, the survey study conducted by Van Riper (1999) of 89 mothers of children with Down syndrome also investigated the effect of family-centered service provision on parent well-being. As described previously, the mothers' perceptions of the family-centeredness of the service they received was evaluated using the Family-Provider Relationships Instrument (Van Riper, 1999). Maternal well-being was measured using the Ryff's Measure of Psychological Well-being (Ryff, 1989, cited in Van Riper, 1999) and The Centre for Epidemiological Studies Depression Scale (Radloff, 1977, cited in Van Riper, 1999). The results indicated that mothers who believed they had family-centered relationships with their health providers reported higher levels of well-being.

Finally, the previously described study conducted by Mahoney and Bella (1998) also investigated the effect of family-centered service provision on parent stress. This study reported results contrary to the first two studies. The 47 mothers who participated in this study were asked to complete an abridged version of the Questionnaire on Resources and Stress (Holroyd, 1974, cited in Mahoney & Bella, 1998) at the beginning and end of a 12-month period of intervention. At the end of the study no significant differences in maternal stress were found. There were also no significant differences in maternal stress between parents who received services they identified as family-centered (using the MPOC measurement instrument) and those who received services that were identified as not family-centered.

The studies reviewed appear to indicate that the provision of family-centered service increases parental satisfaction with service and in some cases increases parental well-being. However, it is unknown which aspects of the family-centered practice the parents felt they received were important in achieving these outcomes. There is to date only limited evidence to indicate that family-centered practice leads to improved child intervention outcomes. Again, it is unclear which elements of the model are responsible for this change.

Family-Friendly Model

Although the family-centered model has been recommended by policy makers and the literature as best practice in intervention for young children an increasing number of studies have found that both professionals and parents do not agree with some aspects of the model

(Bailey, Buysee, Edmondson, & Smith,1992b; Bruce, Letourneau, Ritchie, Larocque, Dennis, & Elliott, 2002; Litchfield & MacDougall, 2002; MacKean et al., 2005; McBride et al., 1993; Minke & Scott, 1995; Piggot et al., 2003; Thompson, 1998; Watts Pappas et al., 2008; Watts Pappas et al., 2009a, 2009b). Parents in some studies have shown a preference for a child-centered, predominantly therapist-led approach to intervention (MacKean et al., 2005; McBride et al., 1993; Piggot et al., 2003; Thompson, 1998; Watts Pappas et al., 2009b) and professionals also support this form of practice (Bailey et al., 1992b; Bruce et al., 2002; Litchfield & MacDougall, 2002; McBride et al., 1993; Minke & Scott, 1995; Watts Pappas et al., 2009a). Most particularly, professionals have highlighted ethical concerns regarding allowing parents to have the final say in decisions about their child's intervention. In family-centered practice professionals are required to follow the parents' lead even if they do not agree with their decisions. Bailey et al. (1992b, p. 299), for example, stated, "professionals should attend to family priorities for goals and services even when those priorities differ substantially from professional priorities" and Brown et al. (1997, p. 600) argued that "by shifting the power to the family, the clinician implies that what constitutes best practice is determined by the family, which may not be what the clinician would select." In situations in which parents request intervention which is contraindicated for the child it has been questioned whether professionals can fulfill their ethical responsibilities to provide care that is effective and evidence-based using the family-centered model (Watts Pappas et al., 2009a).

Much of the literature on family-centered practice is located in the disability field, with little research focusing on children with milder difficulties. Studies investigating parents and professionals' views of intervention for children with milder difficulties have indicated that these families may have different needs to those of children with pervasive disabilities (King et al., 1996; Watts Pappas et al., 2009b). Considering these issues an adapted model of practice to guide SLPs' work with families with both subtle and pervasive difficulties, the family-friendly model is introduced in this book.

Description

Family-friendly practice (Watts Pappas, 2007) is a model in which parents are supported to be involved in intervention provision and are given the opportunity to be involved in intervention planning. However, in family-friendly practice SLPs retain the responsibility as primary decision-makers and use their expertise to guide the intervention process (Table 1–7).

The family-friendly practice model includes many of the features of family-centered practice that have been accepted by professionals and demonstrated to be desired by parents. These include the following components:

- Establishing positive relationships with parents and families
- Respecting families' ideas and opinions
- Communicating effectively with families
- Acknowledging parents' and families' individuality
- Considering the child in the context of the family
- Supporting and encouraging family members to be involved in the intervention if they wish.

As in the family-centered model, family-friendly practice acknowledges the important role of the family in the child's life and places great importance on establishing positive professional/parent rela-

Table 1–7. Contextualizing the Family-Friendly Model

Model	Family Involvement in Intervention Provision	Family Involvement in Intervention Planning	Primary Decision-Maker	Primary Client
Therapist-centered	No	No	Professional	Child
Parent-as-therapist aide	Yes	No	Professional	Child
Family-centered	Varies according to families' wishes	Varies according to families' wishes	Family	Usually the family (varies according to families' wishes)
Family-friendly	Families supported to be involved in the intervention	Varies according to families' wishes	Professional	Usually the child (varies according to families' wishes)

tionships. Parents' opinions are listened to and respected by professionals and family members are invited and supported to be a part of the intervention if they wish. In family-friendly practice professionals share information with parents openly and communicate clearly and consistently. Intervention is flexible to take into account the needs of individual parents and families, and children are considered in the context of their individual family (Watts Pappas et al., 2009a).

The family-friendly model also involves some differing elements to family-centered practice. These include:

- An increased focus on child rather than family-centered goals
- The professional as the primary decision-maker
- Supported family involvement in intervention provision if this is optimal for the effectiveness of the intervention
- A focus on ensuring intervention is a positive experience for the child.

In contrast to family-centered practice, in which the whole family is usually considered the client, family-friendly practice acknowledges that not all families may want intervention to center on them, particularly families of children with subtle delays as opposed to pervasive disabilities. Rather, they may place greater importance on the intervention being focused on the child. Therefore, in family-friendly practice there may be an increased focus on child rather than family-centered goals. Additionally, in family-friendly practice, although the families wishes are accommodated as much as possible and the family is invited to be involved in the goal-setting process, the professional retains the responsibility of making the final decisions regarding intervention. This allows professionals to fulfill their ethical obligation to provide care that they judge to be evidence-based and effective.

Unlike family-centered practice in which families may choose to not be involved in their child's intervention, family-friendly practice recognises that some intervention approaches are dependent on family involvement to be effective. Consequently, in family-friendly practice, parents and other family members are supported to be involved in the intervention if required, using family/professional problem-solving to identify ways in which individual families can most easily be involved. Finally, in response to research indicating the importance that parents place on the intervention being a positive experience for their child (Carrigan, Rodger, & Copely, 2001; MacKean et al., 2005; McKenzie, 1994; Watts Pappas et al., 2009b), family-friendly practice particularly focuses not only on positive parent/professional relationships but also on establishing positive relationships between the professional and the child.

Advantages

The family-friendly practice model is supportive of parental involvement in intervention planning and provision. Similar to the family-centered model, inclusion of families in these activities may lead to intervention which more closely meets the child's and families' needs (Hanna & Rodger, 2002). Placing the professional in the role of primary decision-maker and providing support for families to be involved in the intervention provision if required ensures children are provided with care which is evidence-based and effective and safeguards the rights of the child as separate to their family (Allen & Stefanowski Hudd, 1997). By not dictating that professionals respond to all requests made by families the professional integrity of SLPs is also protected. In intervention for children with milder difficulties, centering intervention on the family may be unnecessary and even intrusive to families (Watts Pappas et al., 2009b). The family-friendly intervention model, in which the focus may be on the child rather than the family, may be more acceptable for families in this clinical population (Packman & Langevin, 2008 [Chapter 6 of this volume]).

Disadvantages

Although family-friendly practice involves the family in intervention planning, the professional makes the final decisions regarding the intervention. This decreases the control the family has over the intervention process and may lead to families feeling disempowered (Dunst, 1985). Additionally, family-friendly practice could be misinterpreted by professionals who may interpret "taking the lead" as "taking over" the intervention and excluding families from the decision-making process.

Evidence Base

As the family-friendly model has only recently been developed no evidence exists regarding its impact on outcomes in allied health intervention for young children. Preliminary investigation of SLPs and parents of children with speech impairment indicate that professionals and parents of children with more subtle difficulties may prefer a family-friendly approach to intervention (Watts Pappas et al., 2009a, 2009b). Additionally, as outlined in other chapters of this book, some established intervention programs for young children could be considered to be family-friendly in their approach to working with parents and families. For example, the Lidcombe program for children who stutter (Onslow, Packman & Harrison, 2003) could be classified as family-friendly in that, although families are involved in the intervention provision and planning, intervention goals center on the child and the intervention is still predominantly therapist directed. As outlined in Chapter 6, the Lidcombe program is the only intervention for early stuttering that has been demonstrated to be more effective than no intervention in a randomized control trial. Another intervention program that could be considered to be family-friendly is the Parents and Children Together (PACT) (Bowen & Cupples, 1999) approach to speech intervention. As discussed in Chapter 7, this approach also has been demonstrated to be more effective than no intervention. Although these possibly family-friendly intervention programs have been demonstrated to be effective, more specific investigation is required to determine the impact of the family-friendly model on intervention outcomes for young children.

Summary

Models of practice in intervention for young children have undergone major changes over the past 50 years. These changes have required a significant redefinition of practice for SLPs and other allied health professionals in their work with parents and families. The models have varied according to the level of parental involvement in the intervention, the focus of the intervention on the child or family, and the level of parental involvement and power in the decision-making process. Further research is required to establish the relative effectiveness of the four models of care and their acceptability to clinicians and families. The following two chapters review the research on the practices and perceptions of SLPs and other allied health professionals and families regarding family involvement in pediatric intervention.

Chapters 4 through 11 consider working with families of children with differing diagnoses. In each of these chapters, the four models of intervention are considered in relation to work with these different clinical populations.

References

Allen, D. A., & Stefanowski Hudd, S. (1987). Are we professionalizing parents? Weighing the benefits and pitfalls. *Mental Retardation, 25*(3), 133–139.

Andrews, J. R., & Andrews, M. A. (1986). A family-based systemic model for speech-language services. *Seminars in Speech and Language, 7*(4), 359–365.

Andrews, J. R., Andrews, M. A., & Shearer, W. M. (1989). Parents' attitudes toward family involvement in speech-language services. *Language, Speech, and Hearing Services in Schools, 20*, 391–399.

Appleton, P., & Minchom, P. (1991). Models of parent partnership and child development centres. *Child: Care, Health and Development, 17*, 27–38.

Bailey, D. B., Buysee, B., Edmondson, R., & Smith, T. M. (1992b). Creating family-centered services in early intervention: Perceptions of professionals in four states. *Exceptional Children, 58*, 298–309.

Bailey, D. B., McWilliam, P., & Winton, P. J. (1992a). Building family-centered practices in early intervention: A team-based model for change. *Infants and Young Children, 5*(1), 73–82.

Bailey, D. B., Simeonsson, R. J., Winton, P. J., Huntington, G. S., Comfort, M., Isbell, P., O'Donnell, K., & Helm, J. M. (1986). Family-focused intervention: A functional model for planning, implementing and evaluating individualized family services in early intervention. *Journal of the Division for Early Childhood, 10*, 156–171.

Baxter, C. (1989). Parent-perceived attitudes of professionals: Implications for service providers. *Disability, Handicap and Society, 4*(3), 259–269.

Bazyk, S. (1989). Changes in attitudes and beliefs regarding parent participation and home programs: An update. *American Journal of Occupational Therapy, 43*(11), 723–728.

Bowen, C., & Cupples, L. (1999). Parents and children together (PACT): A collaborative approach to phonological therapy. *International Journal of Language and Communication Disorders, 34*, 35–83.

Bronfenbrenner, U. (1979). *The ecology of human development.* Cambridge, MA: Harvard University Press.

Brotherson, M., & Goldstein, B. (1992). Time as a resource and constraint for parents of young children with disabilities: Implications for early intervention services. *Topics in Early Childhood Special Education, 12*(4), 508–527.

Brown, S., Humphry, R., & Taylor, E. (1997). A model of the nature of family-therapist relationships: Implications for education. *American Journal of Occupational Therapy, 51*(7), 597–603.

Bruce, B., Letourneau, N., Ritchie, J., Larocque, S., Dennis, C., & Elliott, M. R. (2002). A multisite study of health professionals' perceptions and practices of family-centered care. *Journal of Family Nursing, 8,* 408–429.

Carrigan, N., Rodger, S., & Copley, J. (2001). Parent satisfaction with a paediatric occupational therapy service: A pilot investigation. *Physical and Occupational Therapy in Pediatrics, 21*(1), 51–76.

Case-Smith, J., & Nastro, M. (1993). The effect of occupational therapy intervention on mothers of children with cerebral palsy. *American Journal of Occupational Therapy, 47*(9), 811–817.

Costello, J., & Bosler, S, (1976). Generalization and articulation instruction. *Journal of Speech and Hearing Disorders, 41,* 359–373.

Crais, E. (1991, September). Moving from "parent involvement" to family-centered services. *American Journal of Speech-Language Pathology,* pp. 5–8.

Dinnebeil, L. A., & Rule, S. (1994). Variables that influence collaboration between parents and service coordinators. *Journal of Early Intervention, 18,* 349–361.

Dodd, B., & Barker, R. (1990). The efficacy of utilizing parents and teachers as agents of therapy for children with phonological disorders. *Australian Journal of Human Communication Disorders, 18*(1), 29–45.

Dunst, C. J. (1985). Rethinking early intervention. *Analysis and Intervention in Developmental Disabilities, 5,* 165–201.

Dunst, C. J. (2002). Family-centered practices: Birth through high school. *Journal of Special Education, 36*(3), 139–147.

Dunst, C. J., & Trivette, C. M. (1996). Empowerment, effective helpgiving practices and family-centered care. *Pediatric Nursing, 22*(4), 334–337.

Dunst, C. J., Trivette, C. M., & Deal, A. G. (1988). *Enabling and empowering families.* Cambridge, MA: Brookline Books.

Eiserman, W., McCoun, M., & Escobar, C. (1990). A cost-effectiveness analysis of two alternative program models for serving speech-disordered preschoolers. *Journal of Early Intervention 14*(4), 297–317.

Espezel, H., & Canam, C. (2003). Parent-nurse interactions: Care of hospitalized children. *Journal of Advanced Nursing, 44*(1), 34–41.

Fey, M. E. (1986). *Language intervention with young children.* Needham Heights, MA: Allyn and Bacon.

Fey, M. E., Cleave, P. L., & Long, S. H. (1993). Two models of grammar facilitation in children with language impairments: Phase 2. *Journal of Speech and Hearing Research, 40,* 5–19.

Franck, L. S., & Callery, P. (2004). Re-thinking family-centered care across the continuum of children's healthcare. *Child: Care, Health and Development, 30*(3), 265–277.

Gibbard, D. (1994). Parental-based intervention with pre-school langauge-delayed children. *European Journal of Disorders of Communication, 29*, 131-150.

Gibbard, D., Coglan, L., & MacDonald, J. (1994). Cost-effectiveness analysis of current practice and parent intervention for children under three years presenting with expressive language delay. *International Journal of Language and Communication Disorders, 39*(2), 229-244.

Gierut, J. A. (1989). Maximal opposition approach to phonological treatment. *Journal of Speech and Hearing Disorders, 54*, 9-19.

Giller Gajdosik, C. G., & Campbell, S. K. (1991). Effects of weekly review, socioeconomic status, and maternal belief on mother's compliance with their disabled children's home exercise program. *Physical and Occupational Therapy in Pediatrics, 11*(2), 47-65.

Gillon, G. (2000) Facilitating phoneme awareness development in 3- and 4-year-old children with speech impairment. *Language, Speech, and Hearing Services in Schools, 36*, 308-324.

Girolametto, L., Steig Pearce, P., & Weitzman, E. (1996a). Interactive focused stimulation for toddlers with expressive vocabulary delays. *Journal of Speech and Hearing Research, 39*, 1274-1283.

Girolametto, L., Steig Pearce, P., & Weitzman, E. (1996b). The effects of focused stimulation for promoting vocabulary in young children with delays: A pilot study. *Journal of Children's Communication Development, 17*(2), 39-49.

Glogowska, M., & Campbell, R. (2000). Investigating parental views of involvement in pre-school speech and language therapy. *International Journal of Language and Communication Disorders, 35*(3), 391-405.

Goetz, A. L., Gavin, W., & Lane, S. (2000). Measuring parent/professional interaction in early intervention: Validity and reliability. *Occupational Therapy Journal of Research, 20*, 221-241.

Goldstein, H. (1984). Effects of modeling and corrected practice on generative language learning of preschool children. *Journal of Speech and Hearing Disorders, 49*, 389-398.

Hanna, K., & Rodger, S. (2002). Towards family-centered practice in pediatric occupational therapy: A review of the literature on parent-therapist collaboration. *Australian Occupational Therapy Journal, 49*, 14-24.

Hinojosa, J., & Anderson, J. (1991). Mother's perceptions of home treatment programs for their preschool children with cerebral palsy. *American Journal of Occupational Therapy, 45*, 273-279.

Hinojosa, J., Anderson, J., & Ranum, G. (1988). Relationships between therapists and mothers of preschool children with cerebral palsy: A survey. *Occupational Therapy Journal of Research, 8*, 285-297.

Hinojosa, J., Sproat, C. T., Mankhetwit, S., & Anderson, J. (2002). Shifts in parent-therapist partnerships: Twelve years of change. *American Journal of Occupational Therapy, 56*(5), 556-563.

Iversen, M., Poulin Shimmel, J., Ciacera, S., & Meenakshi, P. (2003). Creating a family-centered approach to early intervention services: Perceptions of parents and professionals. *Pediatric Physical Therapy, 15*, 23-31.

Jansen, L., Ketelaar, M., & Vermeer, A. (2003). Parental experience of participation in physical therapy for children with physical disabilities. *Developmental Medicine and Child Neurology, 45*, 58-69.

Kalmanson, B., & Seligman, S. (1992). Family-provider relationships: The basis of all interventions. *Infants and Young Children, 4*(4), 46-52.

Ketelaar, M., Vermeer, A., Hart, H., Beek, E., & Helders, P. (2001). Effects of a functional therapy program on motor abilities of children with cerebral palsy. *Physical Therapy, 81*(9), 1534-1545.

Ketelaar, M., Vermeer, A., Helders, P., & Hart, H. (1998). Parental participation in intervention programs for children with cerebral palsy: A review of the research. *Topics in Early Childhood Special Education, 18*(2), 108-117.

King, G. A., King, S. M.., & Rosenbaum, P. (1996). How mothers and fathers view professional caregiving for children with disabilities. *Developmental Medicine and Child Neurology, 38*, 397-407.

King, G., Rosenbaum, P., & King, S. (1997). Evaluating family-centered service using a measure of parents' perceptions. *Child: Care, Health and Development, 23*(1), 47-62.

King, G., King, S., Rosenbaum, P., & Goffin, R. (1999). Family-centered caregiving and well-being of parents of children with disabilities: Linking process with outcome. *Journal of Pediatric Psychology, 24*, 41-53.

Law, J., Garrett, Z., & Nye, C. (2003a). Speech and language therapy interventions for children with primary speech and language delay or disorder. *Cochrane Database of Systematic Reviews, 3*, Art. No.: CD004110. DOI: 10.1002/14651858.CD004110.

Law, M., Darrah, J., Pollock, N., King, G., Rosenbaum, P., Russell, D. Palisano, R., Harris, S., & Watt, J. (1998). Family-centered functional therapy for children with cerebral palsy: An emerging practice model. *Physical and Occupational Therapy in Pediatrics, 18*(1), 83-102.

LLaw, M., Hanna, S., Hurley, P., King, S., Kertoy, M., & Rosenbaum, P. (2003b). Factors affecting family-centered service delivery for children with disabilities. *Child: Care, Health and Development, 29*, 357-366.

Lawlor, M., & Mattingly, C. (1998). The complexities embedded in family-centered care. *American Journal of Occupational Therapy, 52*, 259-267.

Leiter, V. (2004). Dilemmas in sharing care: Maternal provision of professionally driven therapy for children with disabilities. *Social Science and Medicine, 58*, 837-849.

Leviton, A., Mueller, M., & Kauffman, C. (1992). The family-centered consultation model: Practical applications for professionals. *Infants and Young Children, 4*(3), 1-8.

Litchfield, R., & MacDougall, C. (2002). Professional issues for physiotherapists in family-centered and community-based settings. *Australian Journal of Physiotherapy, 48*, 105–112.

MacKean, G., Thurston, W., & Scott, C. (2005). Bridging the divide between families and health professionals' perspectives on family-centered care. *Health Expectations, 8,* 74–85.

Mahoney, G., & Bella, J. M. (1998). An examination of the effects of family-centered early intervention on child and family outcomes. *Topics in Early Childhood Special Education, 18*(2), 83–101.

Mahoney, G., & O'Sullivan, P. (1990). Early intervention practices with families of children with handicaps. *Mental Retardation, 3,* 169–176.

Mayo, N. (1981). The effect of a home visit on parental compliance with a home program. *Physical Therapy, 61*(1), 27–32.

McBride, S., Brotherson, M., Joanning, H., Whiddon, D., & Demmitt, A. (1993). Implementation of family-centered services: Perceptions of families and professionals. *Journal of Early Intervention, 17*(4), 414–430.

McGibbon Lammi, B., & Law, M. (2003). The effects of family-centered functional therapy on the occupational performance of children with cerebral palsy. *Canadian Journal of Occupational Therapy, 70*(5), 285–297.

McKenzie, S. (1994). Parents of young children with disabilities: Their perceptions of generic children's services and service professionals. *Australian Journal of Early Childhood, 19*(4), 12–17.

McPherson, E., Morris, M., & Ferguson, A. (1987, March). What do parents think of home programs? *Australian Communication Quarterly,* pp. 16–20.

McWilliam, R. A., Synder, P., Harbin, G., Porter, P., & Munn, D. (2000). Professionals' and families' perceptions of family-centered practices in infant-toddler services. *Early Education and Development, 11*(4), 519–538.

McWilliam, R. A., Tocci, L., & Harbin, G. L. (1998). Family-centered services: Service providers' discourse and behaviour. *Topics in Early Childhood Special Education, 18,* 206–221.

Minke, K., & Scott, M. (1995). Parent-professional relationships in early intervention: A qualitative investigation. *Topics in Early Childhood Special Education, 15*(3), 335–352.

Onslow, M., Packman, A., & Harrison, E. (2003). *The Lidcombe Program of early stuttering intervention: A clinician's guide.* Austin, TX: Pro-Ed.

Packman, A. & Langevin, M. (2008). Working with families of children who stutter. In N. Watts Pappas & S. McLeod (Eds.), *Working with families in speech-language pathology* (pp. 171–188). San Diego, CA: Plural.

Piggot, J., Hocking, C., & Paterson, J. (2003). Parental adjustment to having a child with cerebral palsy and participation in home programs. *Physical and Occupational Therapy in Pediatrics, 23*(4), 5–29.

Rodger, S. (1986). Parents as therapists: A responsible alternative or abrogation of responsibility? *Exceptional Child, 33,* 17–27.

Rosenbaum, P., King, S., Law, M., King, G., & Evans, J. (1998). Family-centered service: A conceptual framework and research review. *Physical and Occupational Therapy in Pediatrics, 18,* 1–20.

Shelton R. L., Johnson A. F., Ruscello D. M., & Arndt W. B. (1978). Assessment of parent-administered listening training for preschool children with articulation deficits. *Journal of Speech and Hearing Disorders, 18,* 242–254.

Shelton, R., Johnson, A., Willis, V., & Arndt, W. (1975). Monitoring and reinforcement by parents as a means of automating articulatory responses: II. Study of preschool children. *Perceptual and Motor Skills, 40,* 599–610.

Shonkoff, J. P., & Hauser-Cram, P. (1987). Early intervention for disabled infants and their families: A quantitative analysis. *Pediatrics, 80*(5), 650–658.

Short, D., Schkade, J., & Herring, J. (1989). Parent involvement in physical therapy: A controversial issue. *Journal of Pediatric Orthopaedics, 9,* 444–446.

Thompson, K. (1998). Early intervention services in daily family life: Mothers' perceptions of 'ideal' versus 'actual' service provision. *Occupational Therapy International, 5*(3), 206–221.

Tufts, L. C., & Holliday, A. R. (1959). Effectiveness of trained parents as speech therapists. *Journal of Speech and Hearing Disorders, 24,* 395–401.

Turnbull, A. P., & Turnbull, H. (1982). Parent involvement in the education of handicapped children: A critique. *Mental Retardation, 20,* 115–122.

Turnbull, H. R., Turnbull, A. P., & Wheat, M. J. (1982, August). Assumptions about parental participation: A legislative history. *Exceptional Education Quarterly,* pp. 1–8.

Van Riper, M. (1999). Maternal perceptions of family-provider relationships and well-being in families of children with Down syndrome. *Research in Nursing and Health, 22,* 357–368.

Viscardis, L. (1998). The family-centered approach to providing services: A parent perspective. *Physical and Occupational Therapy in Pediatrics, 18,* 41–53.

Watts Pappas, N. (2007). *Parental involvement in intervention for speech impairment.* Unpublished doctoral dissertation, Charles Sturt University, Bathurst, Australia.

Watts Pappas, N., McAllister, L., & McLeod, S. (2009a). *Working with families in paediatric speech intervention: Speech-language pathologists' beliefs and practices* (manuscript in preparation).

Watts Pappas, N., McAllister, L., & McLeod, S. (2009b). *Family involvement in paediatric speech intervention: What do parents think?* (manuscript in preparation).

Watts Pappas N., McLeod, S., McAllister, L., & McKinnon, D. H. (2008). Parental involvement in speech intervention: A national survey. *Clinical Linguistics and Phonetics, 22*(4), 335–344.

Wehman, T. (1998). Family-centered early intervention services: Factors contributing to increased parent involvement and participation. *Focus on Autism and Other Developmental Disabilities, 13*(2), 80–86.

White, K. R. (1985). Efficacy of early intervention. *Journal of Special Education, 19*(4), 401–416.

White, K. R., Taylor, M. J., & Moss, V. D. (1992). Does research support claims about the benefits of involving parents in early intervention programs? *Review of Educational Research, 62*(1), 91–125.

Wilcox, M. J., Kouri, T. A., & Caswell, S. B. (1991). Early language intervention: A comparison of classroom and individual treatment. *American Journal of Speech-Language Pathology, 1,* 49–62.

Williams, A. L. (2000). Multiple oppositions: Case studies of variables in phonological intervention. *American Journal of Speech-Language Pathology, 9,* 289–299.

Wing, D. M., & Heimgartner, L. M. (1973). Articulation carryover procedure implemented by parents. *Language, Speech, and Hearing Services in Schools, 4,* 182–195.

Wood, K. S. (1946). Parental maladjustment and functional articulatory defects in children. *Journal of Speech Disorders, 11,* 255–275.

Chapter 2

Speech-Language Pathologists' and Other Allied Health Professionals' Perceptions of Working with Parents and Families

Nicole Watts Pappas and Sharynne McLeod

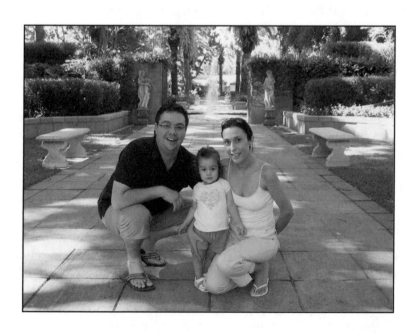

Introduction

Chapter 1 outlined the changing models of professional/parent inter-action that have been proposed in the literature. However, changes in theory do not automatically lead to changes in the beliefs and prac-tices of professionals. Professional beliefs about what constitutes ideal practice and their actual practice may also differ, especially if barriers to using ideal practice exist. How SLPs and other allied health profes-sionals have responded to changing recommendations for working with families has been investigated over the last 25 years, with the first stud-ies appearing in the late 1980s. A systematic literature search located 30 studies that included discussion of allied health professionals' percep-tions of working with families in pediatric intervention (Table 2–1). Nineteen of the studies also investigated the perceptions of other pro-fessionals (i.e., nonallied health) working with children in early inter-vention, such as educators (e.g., teachers) and medical professionals (e.g., doctors, nurses). Of interest to the readers of this book, few studies have involved only SLPs (Keilmann, Braun, & Napiontek, 2004; Watts Pappas, McAllister, & McLeod, 2009; Watts Pappas, McLeod, McAllister, & McKinnon, 2008). Table 2–1 provides an outline of the studies. This chapter reviews the findings of these studies and identi-fies common themes in the professionals' experiences and beliefs.

Parental Involvement in Intervention Provision

Professionals place great importance on working with parents and families in intervention for young children. Parental involvement in intervention *provision* is considered particularly important by some professionals, who believe that parental participation increases the effectiveness of the intervention (Hinojosa, Anderson, & Ranum, 1988; Hinojosa, Sproat, Mankhetwit, & Anderson 2002; Iversen, Poulin Shim-mel, Ciacera, & Meenakshi, 2003; Leiter, 2004; Watts Pappas, 2007; Watts Pappas et al., 2009; Watts Pappas et al., 2008). For example, 98% of SLPs who participated in a survey about working with parents in speech intervention identified parental involvement as essential to the intervention's effectiveness (Watts Pappas et al., 2008).

Professionals working within a variety of allied health professions report they involve parents in intervention provision in a variety of ways including: asking parents to conduct home activities, participate in the intervention and assessment sessions, and occasionally, act as a coordinator and conveyer of information between services. Many professionals expect that parents will be part of the intervention process and in some cases strategize to obtain this involvement (Iverson et al., 2003; Leiter, 2004; MacKean, Thurston, & Scott, 2005; Mahoney & O'Sullivan, 1990; Piggot, Hocking, & Patterson, 2003; Watts Pappas et al., 2009; Watts Pappas et al., 2008). For example, the professionals in a study by Iverson and colleagues (2003) described various techniques they used to "promote active family involvement in care" (p. 28). These included being flexible, including parental goals in the intervention, and providing positive support and encouragement toward family involvement. Some professionals view parents negatively if they do not wish to be involved in their child's intervention (Leiter, 2004; Litchfield & MacDougall, 2002; MacKean et al., 2005; Watts Pappas et al., 2009; Watts Pappas et al., 2008). For instance, early intervention professionals in a study conducted by Leiter (2004, p. 841) perceived parents who were not involved in their child's intervention as "less committed to their child's development." Other professionals involve parents to a lesser extent. For example, 44% of the professionals who responded to a survey conducted by Simeonsson, Edmonson, Smith, Carahan, and Bucy (1995, p. 206) endorsed asking parents to "wait in the lobby" while their child was assessed. In the same study, parent participation in the assessment was perceived as helpful by only 19% of professionals.

Parental Involvement in Intervention Planning

Professionals' views about parental involvement in intervention planning vary. Some professionals embrace family-centered decision-making (MacKean et al., 2005; McBride, Brotherson, Joanning, Whiddon, & Demmitt, 1993; Minke & Scott, 1995; Summers, Dell'Oliver, Turnbull, Benson, Santelli, & Campbell, 1990; Washington & Schwartz, 1996). For example, some of the early intervention professionals who participated in a study conducted by Minke and Scott (1995, p. 344) indicated that parents should be allowed to "control" the content of their child's intervention. In another example, the professionals who participated in the focus group interviews conducted by Summers et al. (1990, p. 82) acknowledged parents as the "ultimate decision-makers" in their child's care.

Table 2–1. Studies of Allied Health Professionals' Perceptions of Working with

Study	Focus of Study	Type of Investigation	Country of Focus	No. of Participants
Hinojosa, Anderson, & Ranum, 1988	Occupational therapists' views of their relationship with parents	Survey	USA	257 occupational therapists
Mahoney & O'Sullivan, 1990	How early intervention activities focus on the family	Survey	USA	989 professionals
Summers et al., 1990	Family and professional preferences regarding the individualized family service plan process	Focus groups	USA	51 family members (majority mothers), 51 early intervention professionals
Bailey, Palsha, & Simeonsson, 1991	Professionals' skills, concerns and perceived importance of work with families in early intervention	Survey	USA	142 early intervention professionals

Families (in Chronologic Order)

Discipline of Professionals	Children's Difficulty (as stated in article)	Age of Children	Intervention Setting (as stated in article)	Major Themes
Occupational therapists	Cerebral palsy	3–5 years	Majority preschool environment	Professionals' beliefs: Parental involvement was important to progress University training was inadequate for work with families
Majority teachers, SLPs, occupational therapists, physiotherapists	Young children with handicaps	0–6 years	Home-based and center-based services	Professionals spent limited time with families; most goals were child-centered; professionals found time a limitation for working with families
Early intervention professionals	Ranged from prematurity (at risk) to severe/profound multiple disabilities	6 months–33 years (majority under 5 years)	Early intervention program	Need for emotional sensitivity, information, and social support from early intervention professionals
Early intervention professionals (including allied health staff)	Children with disabilities	Infants and toddlers	Early intervention programs	Professionals: • valued working with families • felt more competent with children than families • were concerned about impact of family-centered practice on themselves and families

continues

Table 2–1. *continued*

Study	Focus of Study	Type of Investigation	Country of Focus	No. of Participants
Brotherson & Goldstein, 1992	Time as a resource and constraint for parents of young children with disabilities: implications for early intervention services	Focus groups	USA	21 parents: 18 mothers, 2 fathers, and 1 grandmother; 19 professionals
Bailey, Buysee, Edmondson, & Smith, 1992	Perceptions of professionals regarding family-centered practice in early intervention	Survey	USA	180 professionals
McBride, Brotherson, Joanning, Whiddon, & Demmitt, 1993	Family and professional perceptions of the family-centeredness of services	Semi-structured interviews	USA	15 families: mostly mothers, some fathers and grandparents; 14 professionals
Minke & Scott, 1995	Parent-professional relationships in early intervention	Semi-structured interviews Observation of individual family service plan meetings	USA	9 families represented by 10 parents; 4 administrators; 10 direct service providers

Discipline of Professionals	Children's Difficulty (as stated in article)	Age of Children	Intervention Setting (as stated in article)	Major Themes
Six disciplines represented including SLPs	Nine types of handicapping conditions ranging from mild to severe	16 months –15 years	Both center-based and home-based early intervention services	Professionals cited decreased time and knowledge of how to work with families as barriers
Mostly teachers, therapists, psychologists or social workers	Worked with young children with disabilities	Not specified	Various	Gap between ideal versus actual practice Identified family and agency barriers to provision of family-centered service
Special educators, social worker, and an occupational therapist	Various disabilities including Down syndrome, cerebral palsy, hearing loss, and brain damage Two children with language delay	Mean age 16.2 months	Primarily home-based program for children aged 0–3 years with disabilities	Incongruence between family-centered attitudes and actual practice
Teaching and therapy staff	Various disabilities ranging from mild to severe	0–3 years	Center- and home-based services for children aged 0–3 years with disabilities or at risk for developing disabilities	Professionals had close relationships with parents but struggled allowing them a decision-making role in intervention

continues

Table 2–1. *continued*

Study	Focus of Study	Type of Investigation	Country of Focus	No. of Participants
Simeonsson, Edmonson, Smith, Carnahan, & Bucy, 1995	Professional and parent perspectives of family involvement in assessment	Survey	USA	39 parents; 81 professionals
Crais & Wilson, 1996	Professionals' views and practices of parental involvement in assessment	Survey	USA	336 professionals
Washington & Schwartz, 1996	Perceptions on the affect of physiotherapy and occupational therapy services on care giving competency	Semi-structured interviews	USA	2 adoptive mothers; 1 physiotherapist; 1 occupational therapist
King, Law, King ,& Rosenbaum, 1998	Family and service providers' perceptions of family-centeredness of service	Survey	Canada	436 parents; 309 service providers
McWilliam, Tocci, & Harbin, 1998	Family-centered service providers discourse and behavior	Interviews	USA	6 service providers identified as family-centered from a previous study

Discipline of Professionals	Children's Difficulty (as stated in article)	Age of Children	Intervention Setting (as stated in article)	Major Themes
Variety of service providers including SLPs	Known or suspected disabilities	10 months –16 years	Not specified	Substantial variability in individual parents and professionals perceptions of their roles in child assessment.
Half SLPs Other—special educators, physiotherapists, occupational therapists, and psychologists	Not specified	Birth– 3 years	Variety including home-based settings, health departments, community clinics, regional centers, and research facilities	Respondents mostly family-centered in their assessment practices Respondents identified time and parent barriers to working with families
Physiotherapist and occupational therapist	Cerebral palsy Meningo-myelocele	18 months –3 years	Center and home-based services	Professionals allowed parents to take the lead in decision-making Professionals felt relationship with parent is important
Service providers in early intervention center	Chronic, mostly neuro-developmental disorders	7 months– 20 years	Rehabilitation centers	Both parents and therapists identified information provision as weak area
Three teachers, one occupational therapist, one SLP, one social worker	Worked with young children with disabilities	Not specified	Early intervention agency or educational setting	Themes: Family orientation Thinking the best of families Sensitivity Responsiveness Friendliness Child and community skills

continues

Table 2–1. *continued*

Study	Focus of Study	Type of Investigation	Country of Focus	No. of Participants
Crais & Belardi, 1999	Family participation in child assessment: Perceptions of families and professionals	Survey	USA	23 families; 58 professionals
McWilliam, Synder, Harbin, Porter, & Munn, 2000	Professionals' and families' perceptions of family-centered practices	Survey	USA	198 professionals; 118 families
O'Neil & Palisano, 2000	Attitudes towards family-centered care among physiotherapists	Survey	USA	25 physiotherapists
Wilkins, Pollock, Rochon, & Law, 2001	Professionals' perceptions of implementing client and family-centered practice	Survey	Canada	13 service providers

Discipline of Professionals	Children's Difficulty (as stated in article)	Age of Children	Intervention Setting (as stated in article)	Major Themes
Service providers in early intervention services	Not specified	0–3 years	Early intervention services Center and home-based programs	Gap between ideal and typical practices Families and professionals both feel many family-centered assessment practices are ideal
Teachers, administrators, and therapists	Developmental delays to severe disabilities	Average age 24.9 months	Home and center-based early intervention services	Both families and professionals felt that services were family-centered Professionals felt ideally that family-centered practice could occur more
Physiotherapists	Not provided	Under 3 years	Early intervention agency	Therapists supported family-centered practice but did not always make clinical decisions which supported this Described agency barriers to family-centered practice
Variety of service providers including occupational therapists	Pediatric clients attending one of seven children's rehabilitation centers	Not specified	Children's rehabilitation centers	Professionals identified barriers at a system, parent and client level to family-centered practice

continues

49

Table 2–1. *continued*

Study	Focus of Study	Type of Investigation	Country of Focus	No. of Participants
Bruce, Letourneau, Ritchie, Larocque, Dennis, & Elliott, 2002	Health professionals' perceptions and practices of family-centered care	Survey	Canada	483 health professionals
Litchfield & MacDougall, 2002	Professional issues for physiotherapists in family-centered and community based settings	Semi-structured interviews	Australia	10 physiotherapists
Hinojosa, Sproat, Mankhetwit, & Anderson, 2002	Occupational therapists views of working with parents	Survey	USA	202 occupational therapists
Iversen, Poulin Shimmel, Ciacera, & Pabhakar, 2003	Perceptions of parents and professionals about the effectiveness of early intervention	Survey	USA	18 parents; 11 service providers

Discipline of Professionals	Children's Difficulty (as stated in article)	Age of Children	Intervention Setting (as stated in article)	Major Themes
Variety of health professionals including SLPs	The health professionals worked with pediatric clients	Not specified	Tertiary care children's hospitals	Professionals had understanding of concepts of family-centered practice but did not consistently apply these to their practice, particularly with regard to parent decision-making
Physiotherapists	Worked with children with disabilities	Not specified	Community-based setting	Professionals felt a loss of professional identity and control with parental decision-making Felt that parents wanted professionals to take the lead
Occupational therapists	Worked with children with "developmental disabilities"	Not specified	Not specified	Professionals considered working with parents to be important to outcomes of intervention
Early intervention staff including SLPs	Developmental disabilities	Not specified	Early intervention programs	Professionals valued parent involvement and strategized to increase collaboration with families Many professionals felt uncomfortable interacting with families

continues

Table 2–1. *continued*

Study	Focus of Study	Type of Investigation	Country of Focus	No. of Participants
Iversen et al. *continued*				
Edwards, Millard, Praskac, & Wisniewski, 2003	Factors that encourage or inhibit family-centered practice	Interviews	USA	6 mothers; 4 occupational therapists
Piggot, Hocking, & Paterson, 2003	Parental perception of having a child with cerebral palsy and their involvement in their child's intervention	In-depth interviews and participant observations	New Zealand	8 parents, 1 father and 7 mothers of seven children; 3 physiotherapists; 1 occupational therapist
Leiter, 2004	Professionals' and mothers' perceptions of parental involvement in their child's intervention	In-depth interviews and observation of home visits	USA	31 families: majority mothers interviewed; 19 early intervention staff

Discipline of Professionals	Children's Difficulty (as stated in article)	Age of Children	Intervention Setting (as stated in article)	Major Themes
				Professionals outlined many barriers to collaboration
Occupational therapists	Special needs: cerebral palsy, micro-encephalitis, developmental delay	0–3 years	Early intervention service	Importance of considering individuality of families Time barriers to family-centered practice Professionals adapted activities to daily routine to increase family ability to be involved in care
Physiotherapy and occupational therapy	Cerebral palsy	2–10 years	Child development centers	Professionals see "being on board" as parents complying with their directions Professionals may not realize parents are not doing home activities
Early intervention staff including SLPs	May have had established diagnosis or be biologically vulnerable	0–3 years	Home-based early intervention program	Professionals create a therapeutic imperative for parents to be involved in intervention. When parents do not wish to be involved they are seen as noncompliant

continues

Table 2–1. *continued*

Study	Focus of Study	Type of Investigation	Country of Focus	No. of Participants
Keilmann, Braun, & Napiontek, 2004	Satisfaction of parents and SLPs with outcomes of intervention	Survey	Germany	169 parents; 140 SLPs
MacKean, Thurston, & Scott, 2005	Parents' and professionals' perceptions of their role in early intervention	Focus groups + semi-structured interviews	Canada	37 parents; 16 health care providers
Crais, Poston Roy, & Free, 2006	Professionals' and parents' perceptions of family-centered practices in child assessments	Survey	USA	134 professionals; 58 family members
Dyke, Buttigieg, Blackmore, & Ghose, 2006	Professionals and families' perceptions of the family-centeredness of an intervention service	Survey	Australia	43 professionals; 158 families

Discipline of Professionals	Children's Difficulty (as stated in article)	Age of Children	Intervention Setting (as stated in article)	Major Themes
SLPs	Speech and language delays	2–9 years	Not specified	More experienced SLPs involved parents less in the intervention
Health and allied health professionals including SLPs	19 autism; 12 Down syndrome; 6 developmental delay	Not specified	Developmental services at a children's hospital	Professionals want parents to take lead role, parents not always comfortable in this role
A range of disciplines with most prevalent being SLPs, special educators, and psychologists	Working in agency for 'children with disabilities'	Mean age 26.8 months	Center- and home-based services providing evaluation or evaluation and intervention	Agreement between parents and professionals as to ideal and actual practices Implementation gap between ideal and actual family-centered practices
A range of disciplines including SLPs, occupational therapists, physiotherapists, and social workers	Cerebral palsy	Not specified	Not specified	Professionals rated showing interpersonal sensitivity as occurring most often and providing general information occurring least often

continues

Table 2–1. *continued*

Study	Focus of Study	Type of Investigation	Country of Focus	No. of Participants
Watts Pappas, McLeod, McAllister, & McKinnon, 2008	SLPs' practices and perceptions of parental involvement in intervention for speech impairment	Survey	Australia	277 SLPs
Watts Pappas, McAllister, & McLeod, 2008	SLPs' perceptions of parental involvement in intervention for speech impairment	Focus Group	Australia	6 SLPs

SLP = speech-language pathologist.

Discipline of Professionals	Children's Difficulty (as stated in article)	Age of Children	Intervention Setting (as stated in article)	Major Themes
SLPs	Speech Impairment	Not specified	SLPs worked in a variety of settings including education, health and private practice settings	SLPs involved parents more frequently in intervention provision than planning SLPs believed parental involvement in intervention was important. Gaps existed between ideal and actual practice
SLPs	Speech impairment	3;0 to 6;0 years	Community health clinics	SLPs considered parental involvement in speech intervention important and strategized to obtain parental involvement Although they supported parental involvement in intervention planning they believed that the SLP should take the lead in the intervention planning and provision

Other professionals involve parents in intervention planning but may not give parents the opportunity to make the final decisions about the intervention; in line with family-friendly practices. For example, although 67% of SLPs surveyed by Watts Pappas and colleagues (2008) indicated they involved families in intervention planning only 38% reported they gave the family the opportunity to make the final decisions about their child's care.

In contrast, some professionals do not actively involve parents in intervention planning and decision-making, supporting therapist-centered or parent-as-therapist aide practices (Bruce, Letourneau, Ritchie, Larocque, Dennis, & Elliott 2002; Crais, Poston Roy, & Free, 2006; McBride et al., 1993; Minke & Scott, 1995). For example, parent/professional collaboration was one of the elements of family-centered service least believed in and practiced in a study conducted by Bruce and colleagues (2002). In another study, only 53% of professional pairs agreed that they asked family members to identify goals for their child (Crais et al., 2006). In some cases, although professionals allow parents to make decisions, they experience concern about parents' ability to act in this role (Bailey, Buysee, Edmondson, & Smith, 1992; Litchfield & MacDougall, 2002; Minke & Scott, 1995). These professionals report feeling anxious about the possibility of parents making inappropriate intervention decisions for their children. Other professionals believe that not all parents wish to be involved in decision making about their child's intervention and instead want and expect the professional to take the lead role (Bailey et al., 1992; Litchfield & MacDougall, 2002; Watts Pappas et al., 2009).

Focus of Services: Child or Family

In theoretical discussions of family-centered practice, the whole family is considered the client rather than just the child (Rosenbaum, King, Law, King, & Evans, 1998). However, the issue of who should be considered the client is rarely discussed in the research literature. Some professionals report they consider the whole family the client (McBride et al., 1993; McWilliam, Tocci, & Harbin, 1998). For example, all the professionals (purposively sampled by the authors to be family-centered) interviewed by McWilliam and colleagues (1998) perceived that their role was to orient services not only to the child but also to the child's family. Other professionals believe that their first priority for intervention is the child (Hinojosa et al., 2002; Mahoney & O'Sullivan, 1990). For example, the professionals in a study conducted by Mahoney and O'Sullivan (1990) reported that they mostly worked on child-focused goals in their intervention and spent very little time with parents. In addition, Hinojosa and colleagues (2002) reported that although their occupational therapist participants were aware that family issues could affect the child they tended to "avoid involvement with family issues in treatment" (p. 561).

Parent/Professional Relationships

From the studies in Table 2–1 it is apparent that establishing positive, trusting relationships with parents is valued by professionals (Brotherson & Goldstein, 1992; Bruce et al., 2002; King, Law, King, & Rosenbaum, 1998; MacKean et al., 2005; Minke & Scott, 1995; Piggot et al., 2003; Summers et al., 1990; Washington & Schwartz, 1996; Watts Pappas et al., 2009), and it is acknowledged that these relationships require time to develop. Professionals often believe that strong professional/parent relationships facilitate joint problem-solving, increase parent willingness to try new ideas (Minke & Scott, 1995), and make parents feel comfortable in honestly sharing information (Piggot et al., 2003). Although professionals' views of the skill-base necessary to develop good relationships with parents have not been directly addressed in much of the literature, professionals have identified a number of skills which may affect the parent/professional relationship. These include the relationship outlined below.

Sensitivity to Families' Individuality

Many professionals believe that individualizing services for each family is important (Brotherson & Goldstein, 1992; Bruce et al., 2002; Edwards, Millard, Praskac & Wisniewski, 2003; Leiter, 2004) and often accomplish this by incorporating home activities within each family's daily routine (Brotherson & Goldstein, 1992; Edwards et al., 2003; Leiter,

2004). For example, the occupational therapists in a study conducted by Edwards and colleagues (2003) incorporated the children's siblings into the intervention activities, thereby facilitating the use of the activities in the home environment.

Communicating Effectively with Families

Many professionals feel that communication skills are important to their work with families (Iversen et al., 2003; MacKean et al., 2005; Piggot et al., 2003; Watts Pappas et al., 2009). The ability to listen to families' perspectives and provide families with information are seen as important components of establishing positive parent/professional relationships. For example, professionals in a study conducted by MacKean and colleagues (2005, p. 78) believed that one of their major roles and "relational competencies" in working with parents was as a provider of information.

Respecting Parents' Knowledge and Choices

Professionals often state the importance of recognizing the expertise that parents provide to early intervention and responding to parents' needs and wishes (Brotherson & Goldstein, 1992; Dyke, Buttigieg, Blackmore, & Ghose, 2006; King et al., 1998; McWilliam et al., 1998; O'Neil & Palisano, 2000; Watts Pappas et al., 2009). For example, the majority of physiotherapist participants in the survey study by O'Neil and Palisano (2000, p. 179) rated the respectful and supportive care items as "very important."

Friendliness—Treating Parents as Friends

Some professionals acknowledge the importance of not only being approachable to parents but treating them as friends rather than clients (McWilliam et al., 1998; Summers et al., 1990). For example, one of the major themes from the McWilliam et al. (1998, p. 217) study was "Friendliness: Treating parents as friends." These professionals reported they shared a close relationship with the parents and families they served, more like a friendship than a professional relationship.

Factors Affecting Professionals' Work with Parents and Families

When professionals are asked what affects their work with parents and families, three major factors emerge from the studies in Table 2–1: parent factors, workplace factors, and professional factors.

Parent Factors

There are three parent factors that professionals' report affect their work with parents and families: parents' skills and priorities, parents' time, and parents' wish to be involved.

Parents' Skills and Priorities

Sometimes professionals question whether parents possess the knowledge and skills to be involved in the provision and especially the planning of their child's early intervention; they see parent education level as a barrier to working with families (Bailey et al., 1992; Brotherson & Goldstein, 1992; Crais & Wilson, 1996; McBride et al., 1993; Minke & Scott, 1995; Watts Pappas et al., 2008). Some professionals also doubt whether all parents can be relied on to act in their child's best interests. For example, two professionals in a study conducted by McBride and colleagues (1993) indicated that parents could not be trusted to know what was best for their child. Minke and Scott (1995) described a "feeling among most staff members that at least some parents cannot be relied upon to act in the best interests of their children" (p. 345). As parents are seeking advice from a professional they may not possess the skills and knowledge to make final intervention decisions for their children.

Parents' Time

Another factor that professionals believe affects their work with families is the family's available time (Bailey et al., 1992; Edwards et al., 2003; Iversen et al., 2003; Watts Pappas et al., 2008). Busy family schedules and the presence of other siblings can make conducting intervention and organizing appointments difficult and can decrease the amount of involvement parents are able to have in their child's intervention.

Parents' Wish to Be Involved in the Intervention

Parent inclination to be involved in their child's intervention is identified by professionals as a possible barrier to working with families (Crais & Wilson, 1996; Hinojosa et al., 1988, 2002). For example, 47% of respondents to a survey conducted by Crais and Wilson (1996, p. 132) indicated that "lack of interest by parents" was a barrier to working more closely with parents. Additionally, two survey studies conducted by Hinojosa and colleagues (1988, 2002) identified the occupational therapists' concern about parents' commitment to involvement in their child's intervention. The professionals reported that inconsistent parental attendance at their child's intervention sessions, lack of respect for the professional's knowledge, and an expectation that the professional would assume care of the child were difficult issues to deal with when working with families.

Workplace Factors

Workplace factors such as lack of support for working collaboratively with families are described by professionals as impacting on their work with families (Bailey et al., 1992; Litchfield & MacDougall, 2002; O'Neil & Palisano, 2000; Piggot et al., 2003; Watts Pappas et al., 2008). For example, the physiotherapists in O'Neil and Palisano's survey (2000) highlighted workplace issues as one of the major barriers to collaborating with families in their workplace. In open-ended question responses they described an increased workplace focus on productivity (i.e., face-to-face sessions with the child) as decreasing the time for family-centered activities such as meeting with parents and families. Resource and time limitations are also identified by professionals as a significant barrier to working with families (Bailey et al., 1992; Brotherson & Goldstein, 1992; Litchfield & MacDougall, 2002; Piggot et al., 2003). For example, the professionals interviewed by Brotherson and Goldstein (1990) reported that staffing limitations at their workplace meant they found it difficult to provide family-centered services such as home visiting due to the additional time requirements of traveling to the family's home.

Professional Factors

Characteristics of professionals as factors impacting on working with parents and families are rarely mentioned in the literature. However, one factor that is highlighted by professionals is their lack of confidence and training in working with parents and families. This issue is mentioned predominantly in studies conducted in the 1990s (Bailey et al., 1992; Brotherson & Goldstein, 1992; Hinojosa et al., 1988 Mahoney & O'Sullivan, 1990; McBride et al., 1993). However, similar concerns are voiced by professionals in more recent studies, including a group of physiotherapists in a study reported in 2002 (Litchfield & MacDougall), a focus group interview of SLPs reported in 2009 (Watts Pappas et al., 2009) and a survey of a group of early intervention professionals reported in 2003 (Iversen et al.). In the study conducted by Iversen and colleagues only 59% of the professionals surveyed stated that they were confident working with families.

Professional Variables

Professionals' beliefs and practices in working with families vary greatly, with some demonstrating very family-centered or family-friendly beliefs and practice and others using a more therapist-centered or parent-as-therapist aide model of service. Selected studies have investigated the effect of demographic characteristics of professionals on their beliefs and practice. These studies have demonstrated some differences relating to the professionals' discipline, years of experience and intervention setting. For example, in a survey study conducted by Bruce and colleagues (2002) the effect of professional discipline was found to be a significant factor in the professionals' beliefs and practice. In this study, education professionals were more likely than allied health professionals to agree with family-centered service philosophies. In other studies, intervention setting was found to be related to the beliefs and practice of professionals. For example, SLPs working in an education setting were found to involve parents less in the intervention than SLPs working in health or private practice settings (Watts Pappas et al., 2008). McWilliam, Synder, Harbin, Porter, and Munn (2000) found clinic-based professionals reported the lowest family-centered ideals and practices compared with professionals working in an educational setting or a home-visiting service. In the same study, agencies that served a younger client group were found to be more family-centered than agencies serving older children. Corroborating the findings of this study, Mahoney and O'Sullivan (1990) found that professionals who worked with children in the 0- to 3-year-old age group spent more time with parents than those working in the 3- to 6-year-old age group. Increased time with parents could be considered to be indicative of family-centered or family-friendly practice but it also could be indicative of a parent-as-therapist aide model.

Some differences in practice have been noted according to the years of experience of professionals. In three studies in Table 2–1, the more experience the professionals had in working with parents and families, the less they used family-centered practices (Keilmann et al., 2004; McWilliam et al., 2000; Watts Pappas et al., 2008). For example, in a study of SLPs conducted by Keilmann and colleagues (2004), the more experienced professionals involved parents less in the intervention. A similar finding was reported in a survey study conducted by McWilliam and colleagues (2000): more experienced professionals working in a clinical setting were less family-centered in belief and practice than their less experienced counterparts. In a survey study conducted by Watts Pappas and colleagues (2008) more experienced SLPs were less likely to allow parents to have the final say regarding intervention decisions. Two studies, however, found no differences between the responses of less and more experienced professionals (Crais & Wilson, 1996; King et al., 1998) and in another study professionals who had more years of experience felt that working with parents had the greatest impact on the child's progress (Hinojosa et al., 2002). As each of these studies varied in terms of the client base served, the focus of the study (intervention or assessment practices), and the discipline of the professionals, the reasons for the differing results are unclear.

Comparison with Parents' Beliefs

A number of studies have investigated both professionals' and parents' views about family involvement in early intervention, giving researchers the opportunity to compare both groups' experiences and beliefs. In many cases professionals and parents are in agreement about actual and ideal practices in early intervention (Crais et al., 2006; Iversen et al., 2003; King et al., 1998). For example, in a study of parents' and professionals' perceptions of the use of family-centered practices in child assessment (Crais et al., 2006), a high agreement existed between the parents and professionals regarding both actual and ideal practices. However, in other studies, discrepancies exist between parents' and professionals' beliefs and perceptions (Brotherson & Goldstein, 1992; Leiter, 2004; MacKean et al., 2005; McWilliam et al., 2000; Piggot et al., 2003). For example, in a study conducted by McWilliam and colleagues (2000), professionals generally rated their practices as more family-centered than parents did.

Models of Practice

As outlined in Chapter 1, three major models of practice have been discussed in the literature, the therapist-centered model, the parent-as-therapist aide model, and the family-centered model. In addition, this book has introduced a new model of service, family-friendly practice. Many professionals indicate that they consider the family-centered model the ideal method of service provision. However, even though this belief is held, in practice professionals may be using a therapist-centered rather than family-centered approach. This is particularly prevalent in areas of practice such as parental involvement in decision-making, orienting services toward the whole family, and allowing parents choice regarding the extent of their involvement. In much of the research it is difficult to determine the actual model of practice the professionals are using. However, it appears that only rarely do professionals use models of service that are predominantly family-centered (McWilliam et al., 1998; Summers et al., 1990; Washington & Schwartz, 1996). This finding appears unrelated to the timing of the studies, with one of the earliest studies (Summers et al., 1990) reporting participants' adherence to the model of family-centered service whereas other, more recent studies reported participants' use of more traditional forms of service delivery such as the parent-as-therapist aide model (Bruce et al., 2002; Leiter, 2004). Some professionals use a family-friendly approach to intervention with parents involved in intervention planning and provision but the professional retaining the role as primary decision-maker (Watts Pappas et al., 2008; Watts Pappas et al.,

2009). It should be considered however that the majority of the research in this area has relied on professionals' reports of their practices or surveys in which the possible responses were limited. Thus, the practices identified as typical by the participants might not have been the actual practices they used in their work with families.

There is often a gap between idealized models of service and the way professionals actually work with parents and families (Bailey et al., 1992; Bruce et al., 2002; Crais et al., 2006; McBride et al., 1993; McWilliam et al., 2000; O'Neil & Palisano, 2000; Piggot et al., 2003; Watts Pappas et al., 2008). For example, a study of professionals' perceptions of ideal versus actual assessment practices found a significant difference in the professionals' perceptions of what ideal assessment practices would be and the services they actually provided to families (Crais et al., 2006).

Whereas discussion about family-centered practice has been evident in the literature for many years, actual practice may take longer to change (Hall, 1979). Some professionals may be attempting to adapt their practice to accommodate new models of service but continue to hold beliefs supporting a more traditional form of practice. These shifts in professional roles are sometimes associated with feelings of a loss of professional identity and control (Litchfield & MacDougall, 2002; Minke & Scott, 1995). For example, Litchfield and MacDougall (2002) discussed how the physiotherapists in their study adapted to allow parents to have more control over their child's intervention but simultaneously struggled with the fact that they had less control as a result. Studies of other health professionals such as nurses have revealed similar themes and feelings of allied health professionals in their attempt to implement family-centered practice in their work with families (Paliadelis, Cruickshank, Wainohu, Winskill, & Stevens, 2005).

Health professionals are under pressure to ensure that their practice with clients is not only family-centered but also evidence-based and productive (Reilly, 2004). With an increased focus on efficiency and accountability in health care, SLPs and other allied health professionals may be unsure which model of working with families will meet all the demands of current best practice as well as the policies and expectations of the agency in which they work. It has been suggested that professionals have a "moral" obligation to provide evidence-based intervention to their clients (Hancock & Eason, 2004, p. 189). When a parent requests interventions that the professional feels are ineffective or inappropriate for the particular child, it places the professional in an ethical dilemma. Should professionals adhere to family-centered philosophies and provide interventions the parents request, even if professionally they do not agree with this decision? This dilemma has been described by the ethics-in-health-care literature as a case of finding a "balance between autonomy and beneficence" (Berglund, 2004, p. 76). In this situation, the health provider must choose between upholding the parents' autonomy and providing the intervention they request, even if it is ineffective, or upholding the principles of professional autonomy and beneficence in which the health provider refuses to give intervention which he or she believes is not in the best interests of the child. Professionals may be reluctant to use family-centered practice when it contravenes other demands of their workplace such as providing service that is evidence-based and efficacious. Although academic literature and policy advocate a family-centered service delivery model in working with parents and families, allied health clinicians in this literature review were not uniformly using this model of service, with many appearing to use a parent-as-therapist's aide or family-friendly model instead.

Summary

SLPs and other allied health professionals who work with children in early intervention have been changing the way they interact with the parents and families. Many professionals have reported promoting and using family-centered practices such as establishing positive, respectful and supportive relationships with parents and orienting services toward the whole family. However, a number of other professionals continue to work in a parent-as-therapist aide or therapist-centered model of practice in intervention for young children (Bruce et al., 2002; Hinojosa et al., 2002; Keilmann et al., 2004; Leiter, 2004; Mahoney & O'Sullivan, 1990; McBride et al., 1993; Minke & Scott, 1995; Simeonsson et al., 1995).

A review of the literature revealed that most professionals generally believe that parental involvement in early intervention is important. Additionally, most professionals do involve parents and families in their child's intervention. However, a belief/practice implementation gap exists, with differences between perceived ideal and actual practice reported in a number of studies. This may be attributable to a number of factors that prevent professionals from working collaboratively with parents and families (such as family, workplace, and professional factors). However, some professionals continue to feel uncomfortable about putting into practice elements of family-centered service such as parental decision-making. This may be due to ethical concerns regarding parents making the final, possibly inappropriate, decisions about their child's care. Generally more experienced health professionals, those working in clinical rather than community-based settings, and those working with older children were the least family-centered in the service they provided to families. Conversely, the most family-centered professionals appear to be those who are less experienced, working in community-based settings and those working with younger children. The following chapter presents a review of the literature investigating the perceptions and practices of the family: the other participants in the phenomenon of family involvement in pediatric intervention.

References

Bailey, D. B., Buysee, B., Edmondson, R., & Smith, T. M. (1992). Creating family-centered services in early intervention: Perceptions of professionals in four states. *Exceptional Children, 58*, 298–309.

Bailey, D. B., Palsha, S. A., & Simeonsson, R. J. (1991). Professional skills, concerns, and perceived importance of work with families in early intervention. *Exceptional Children, 58*, 156–165.

Berglund, C. (2004). *Ethics for health care* (2nd ed.). New York: Oxford University Press.

Brotherson, M., & Goldstein, B. (1992). Time as a resource and constraint for parents of young children with disabilities: Implications for early intervention services. *Topics in Early Childhood Special Education, 12*(4), 508–527.

Bruce, B., Letourneau, N., Ritchie, J., Larocque, S., Dennis, C., & Elliott, M. R. (2002). A multisite study of health professionals' perceptions and practices of family-centered care. *Journal of Family Nursing, 8*, 408–429.

Crais, E., & Belardi, C. (1999). Family participation in child assessment: Perceptions of families and professionals. *Infant-Toddler Intervention: A Transdisciplinary Journal, 9*, 209–238.

Crais, E., Poston Roy, V., & Free, K. (2006). Parents' and professionals' perceptions of family-centered practices: What are actual practices vs. what are ideal practices? *American Journal of Speech-Language Pathology, 15*, 365–377.

Crais, E. R., & Wilson, L. B. (1996). The role of parents in child assessment: Self-evaluation by practicing professionals. *Infant-Toddler Intervention, 6*(2), 125–143.

Dyke, P. Buttigieg, P., Blackmore, A. M., & Ghose, A. (2006). Use of the Measure of Process of Care for families (MPOC-56) and service providers (MPOC-SP) to evaluate family-centered services in a paediatric disability setting. *Child: Care, Health and Development, 32*(2), 167–176.

Edwards, M., Millard, P., Praskac, L., & Wisniewski, P. (2003). Occupational therapy and early intervention: A family-centered approach. *Occupational Therapy International, 10*(4), 239–252.

Hall, G. E. (1979). The concerns-based approach to facilitating change. *Educational Horizons, 4*, 202–208.

Hancock, H. C., & Easen, P. R. (2004). Evidence-based practice: An incomplete model of the relationship between theory and professional work. *Journal of Evaluation in Clinical Practice, 10*(2), 187–196.

Hinojosa, J., Anderson, J., & Ranum, G. (1988). Relationships between therapists and mothers of preschool children with cerebral palsy: A survey. *Occupational Therapy Journal of Research, 8*, 285–297.

Hinojosa, J., Sproat, C. T., Mankhetwit, S., & Anderson, J. (2002). Shifts in parent-therapist partnerships: Twelve years of change. *American Journal of Occupational Therapy, 56*(5), 556–563.

Iversen, M., Poulin Shimmel, J., Ciacera, S., & Meenakshi, P. (2003). Creating a family-centered approach to early intervention services: Perceptions of parents and professionals. *Pediatric Physical Therapy, 15*, 23–31.

Keilmann, A., Braun, L., & Napiontek, U. (2004). Emotional satisfaction of parents and speech-language pathologists with outcome of training intervention in children with speech and language disorders. *Folia Phoniatrica et Logopaedica, 56*(1), 51–61.

King, G., Law, M., King, S., & Rosenbaum, P. (1998). Parents' and service providers' perceptions of the family centeredness of children's rehabilitation services. *Physical and Occupational Therapy in Pediatrics, 18*(1), 21–40.

Leiter, V. (2004). Dilemmas in sharing care: Maternal provision of professionally driven therapy for children with disabilities. *Social Science and Medicine, 58*, 837–849.

Litchfield, R., & MacDougall, C. (2002). Professional issues for physiotherapists in family-centered and community-based settings. *Australian Journal of Physiotherapy, 48*, 105–112.

MacKean, G., Thurston, W., & Scott, C. (2005). Bridging the divide between families and health professionals' perspectives on family-centered care. *Health Expectations, 8*, 74–85.

Mahoney, G., & O'Sullivan, P. (1990). Early intervention practices with families of children with handicaps. *Mental Retardation, 3*, 169–176.

McBride, S., Brotherson, M., Joanning, H., Whiddon, D., & Demmitt, A. (1993). Implementation of family-centered services: Perceptions of families and professionals. *Journal of Early Intervention, 17*(4), 414–430.

McWilliam, R. A., Synder, P., Harbin, G., Porter, P., & Munn, D. (2000). Professionals' and families' perceptions of family-centered practices in infant-toddler services. *Early Education and Development, 11*(4), 519–538.

McWilliam, R. A., Tocci, L., & Harbin, G. L. (1998). Family-centered services: Service providers' discourse and behaviour. *Topics in Early Childhood Special Education, 18*, 206–221.

Minke, K., & Scott, M. (1995). Parent-professional relationships in early intervention: A qualitative investigation. *Topics in Early Childhood Special Education, 15*(3), 335–352.

O'Neil, M., & Palisano, R. J. (2000). Attitudes toward family-centered care and clinical decision-making in early intervention among physical therapists. *Pediatric Physical Therapy, 12*, 173–182.

Paliadelis, P., Cruickshank, M., Wainohu, D., Winskill, R., & Stevens, H. (2005). Implementing family-centered care: An exploration of the beliefs and practices of paediatric nurses. *Australian Journal of Advanced Nursing, 23*(1), 31–36.

Piggot, J., Hocking, C., & Paterson, J. (2003). Parental adjustment to having a child with cerebral palsy and participation in home programs. *Physical and Occupational Therapy in Pediatrics, 23*(4), 5–29.

Reilly, S. (2004). The move to evidence-based practice within speech pathology. In S. Reilly, J. Douglas & J. Oates (Eds.), *Evidence-based practice in speech pathology* (pp. 3–17). London: Whurr.

Rosenbaum, P., King, S., Law, M., King, G., & Evans, J. (1998). Family-centered service: A conceptual framework and research review. *Physical and Occupational Therapy in Pediatrics, 18*, 1–20.

Simeonsson, R. J., Edmonson, R., Smith, T. M., Carahan, S., & Bucy, J. E. (1995). Family involvement in multidisciplinary team evaluation: Professional and parent perspectives. *Child: Care, Health and Development, 21*(3), 199–215.

Summers, J., Dell'Oliver, C., Turnbull, A., Benson, H., Santelli, E., Campbell, M., & Sigel-Causey, E. (1990). Examining the individualized family service plan process: What are family and practitioner preferences? *Topics in Early Childhood Special Education, 10*, 78–99.

Washington, K., & Schwartz, P. (1996). Maternal perceptions of the effects of physical and occupational therapy services on caregiving competency. *Physical and Occupational Therapy in Pediatrics, 16*(3), 33–54.

Watts Pappas, N. (2007). *Parental involvement in intervention for speech impairment.* Unpublished doctoral dissertation, Charles Sturt University, Bathurst, Australia.

Watts Pappas, N., McAllister, L., & McLeod, S. (2009). *Working with families in paediatric speech intervention: Speech language pathologists' beliefs and practices* (manuscript in preparation).

Watts Pappas N., McLeod, S., McAllister, L., & McKinnon, D. H. (2008). Parental involvement in speech intervention: A national survey. *Clinical Linguistics and Phonetics, 22*(4), 335-344.

Wilkins, S., Pollock, N., Rochon, S., & Law, M. (2001). Implementing client-centered practice: Why is it so difficult to do? *Canadian Journal of Occupational Therapy, 68*(2), 70-79.

Chapter 3

Parents' Perceptions of Their Involvement in Pediatric Allied Health Intervention

Nicole Watts Pappas and Sharynne McLeod

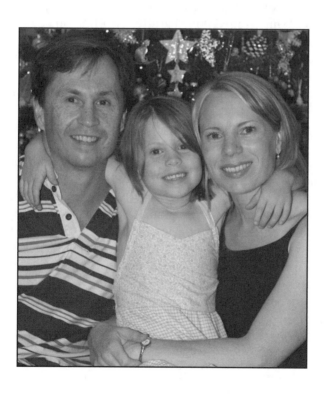

Introduction

As discussed in Chapters 1 and 2, changing models of working with parents and families in pediatric allied health intervention have led to an increase in parental involvement in their child's intervention. The advent of family-centered practice in particular has promoted parental involvement not only in intervention provision but also in the planning and coordination of services for children. However, despite this fact, research investigating parental views of involvement in their child's intervention is limited.

A systematic search of the literature located 39 studies investigating parental perceptions of pediatric intervention services involving some form of allied health intervention (Table 3-1). Of interest to the readers of this book, nine studies exclusively focused on parents' perceptions of their child's SLP intervention (Andrews, Andrews, & Shearer, 1989; Baxendale, Frankham, & Hesketh, 2001; Glogowska & Campbell, 2000, Glogowska & Roulstone, 2001; Goldbart & Marshall, 2004; Keilmann, Bruan, & Napiontek, 2004; Mirabito & Armstrong, 2005; Parette, Brotherson, & Huer, 2000; Watts Pappas, McAllister, & McLeod, 2009). The studies explored parents' satisfaction with pediatric intervention services, their feelings about their involvement in their child's intervention, and their views about their relationship with allied health professionals. It should be noted that the studies were primarily conducted in English-speaking countries and, as a result, the findings predominantly reflect western perspectives. This chapter reviews the findings from the studies and summarizes common themes in the parents' experiences.

The review of the literature reported in Chapter 2 highlighted that many allied health professionals believe that family involvement in intervention is important. As Marshall and Goldbart note in Chapter 8, however, believing that family involvement is important does not necessarily mean that professionals will work "appropriately and successfully" with families. The intention of the review of the literature in this chapter is to increase SLPs' understanding of parents' beliefs and feelings about their involvement in intervention and consequently the effectiveness of SLPs' work with families.

Parents' Overall Experience of Intervention

The studies reviewed indicated that generally, parents' experience of allied health intervention for their child is positive (Carrigan, Rodger, & Copely, 2001; Crais & Belardi, 1999; Glogowska & Campbell, 2000; Glogowska & Roulstone, 2001; Iversen, Poulin Shimmel, Ciacera, & Meenakshi, 2003; Keilmann et al., 2004; McBride, Brotherson, Joanning, Whiddon, & Demmitt 1993; McWilliam, Lang, Vandiviere, Angell, Collins, & Underdown, 1995; Mirabito & Armstrong, 2005; Watts Pappas et al., 2009). Outcomes that influence satisfaction include:

- parental skill acquisition (McBride et al., 1993; Mirabito et al., 2005; Piggot, Hocking, & Patterson, 2003; Washington & Schwartz, 1996; Watts Pappas et al., 2009),
- the child's enjoyment of the intervention (Carrigan et al., 2001; Watts Pappas et al., 2009), and
- the child's progress (Carrigan et al., 2001; Piggot et al., 2003).

Parents are also more satisfied with:

- services that are provided in a family-centered manner (Law, Hanna, Hurley, King, Kertoy, & Rosenbaum, 2003; Rosenbaum, King, & Cadman, 1992),
- accessible, coordinated services (Glogowska & Roulstone, 2001; Rosenbaum et al., 1992), and
- the provision of respectful and supportive care (Carrigan et al., 2001; King, Cathers, King, & Rosenbaum, 2001; Watts Pappas et al., 2009).

Dissatisfaction with services can be associated with:

- a lack of respectful and supportive care (Case-Smith & Nastro, 1993; King et al., 2001; Watts Pappas et al., 2009),
- poor information provision (Glogowska & Roulstone, 2001; Iversen et al., 2003; King, Law, King, & Rosenbaum, 1998; Rosenbaum et al., 1992), and
- service delivery issues such as difficulty accessing services (Goldbart & Marshall, 2004; Glogowska & Roulstone, 2001; King et al., 2001; Piggot et al., 2003; Watts Pappas et al., 2009).

Table 3–1. Studies of Parents' Perceptions of Working with Professionals (in

Study	Focus of Study	Type of Investigation	Country of Focus	No. of Participants
Winton & Turnbull, 1981	Parents' perspectives on their involvement in intervention	Interviews + survey	USA	31 mothers
Andrews, Andrews, & Shearer, 1989	Parents' attitudes to involvement in speech-language services	Survey	USA	1684 parents
Baxter, 1989	Parents' perspectives of the attitudes of service providers	Interviews	Australia	131 parents
Summers et al., 1990	Family and professional preferences regarding the individualized family service plan process	Focus groups	USA	51 family members (majority mothers), 51 early intervention professionals

Chronologic Order)

Discipline of Professionals	Child's Difficulty	Age of Children	No. of Interviews	Major Themes
Health and educational professionals working with the children	Intellectual, physical, visual or hearing impairment, autism or significant language delays	Preschool aged	Each parent interviewed once plus completed a survey	Mothers didn't always want to be involved in the intervention Valued good relationships with professionals
SLPs	Speech language delay, stuttering	4–12 years	—	Approximately half of respondents happy with the level of their involvement in intervention or would like to be involved more. Significant percentage would like to be involved less
Professionals working with children with intellectual impairment	Intellectual impairment	3–19 years	Each parent interviewed once	Themes: Helpfulness Professional interest Consideration and respect Professional commitment
Early intervention professionals	Ranged from prematurity (at risk) to severe/ profound multiple disabilities.	6 months–33 years (majority under 5 years)	Each parent attended one focus group	Need for emotional sensitivity, information and social support from early intervention professionals

continues

77

Table 3–1. *continued*

Study	Focus of Study	Type of Investigation	Country of Focus	No. of Participants
Hinojosa, 1990	Parents' perceptions of early intervention	Nonstructured Interviews	USA	8 mothers
Hinojosa & Anderson, 1991	Parents' perceptions of home programs	Nonstructured Interviews	USA	8 mothers
Able-Boone, Goodwin, Sandall, Gordon, & Martin, 1992	Parents' and professionals' perceptions of early intervention services	Survey	USA	290 parents (majority mothers) and 267 professionals
Brotherson & Goldstein, 1992	Time as a resource and constraint for parents of young children with disabilities: implications for early intervention services	Focus groups	USA	21 parents: 18 mothers, 2 fathers, and 1 grandmother 19 professionals

Discipline of Professionals	Child's Difficulty	Age of Children	No. of Interviews	Major Themes
Physiotherapists and Occupational therapists	Cerebral palsy	2–5 years	Each parent interviewed twice	Themes: 1. What home programs? 2. If I only had a 25-hour day 3. We together 4. What does daddy do? 5. The long shadow 6. Therapy, therapy, therapy 7. The third parent 8. The roller coaster
Physiotherapists and Occupational therapists	Cerebral palsy	2–5 years	Each parent interviewed twice	Parents often found home programs difficult, adapted them to suit their daily routine
Therapists, case managers and administrators	Developmental delays, physical, intellectual and sensory impairments	0–5 years of age	—	Parents had concerns about improving service coordination. Parents involved in home-based programs more satisfied than parents whose children were involved in center-based programs.
Six disciplines represented including SLP	Nine types of handicapping conditions ranging from mild to severe	16 months –15 years	Each parent/ professional participated in one focus group	Support for parents' time Constraints on parents' time

continues

Table 3–1. *continued*

Study	Focus of Study	Type of Investigation	Country of Focus	No. of Participants
Rosenbaum, King, & Cadman, 1992	Identifying important components of care	Survey	Canada	88 professionals 213 parents
McBride, Brotherson, Joanning, Whiddon, & Demmitt, 1993	Family perception of the family-centeredness of services	Semi-structured interviews	USA	15 families: mostly mothers interviewed, some fathers and grandparents 14 professionals
Ross & Thomson, 1993	Parents' views about their involvement in home programs	Survey	UK	23 families
Case-Smith & Nastro, 1993	Mothers' perceptions of occupational therapy intervention	Interviews	USA	5 mothers

Discipline of Professionals	Child's Difficulty	Age of Children	No. of Interviews	Major Themes
Senior clinicians (including SLPs) and administrators at ambulatory treatment centers in Ontario	Children with a chronic physical disability	1–23 years	—	Parents identified parental involvement, information, treatment, available care, continuity, coordination, and family-centered care as important components of care
Special educators, social worker and an occupational therapist	Various disabilities including Down syndrome, cerebral palsy, hearing loss and brain damage Two children with language delay	Mean age: 16.2 months	Families interviewed twice	Families expressed satisfaction with services Different expectations of involvement
Physiotherapy	Cerebral palsy	Preschool age	—	Parents wish to be involved in intervention but have anxiety about the quality and quantity of their input. Some want more physio-therapist's input.
Occupational therapists	Cerebral palsy	Preschool age	Each parent interviewed twice	Themes: Just want to be mother Is anyone listening? More therapy is better Therapists—agents of change, source of information, and support

continues

Table 3–1. *continued*

Study	Focus of Study	Type of Investigation	Country of Focus	No. of Participants
McKenzie, 1994	Parents' perceptions of children's services and service professionals	Interviews	Australia	50 families: 38 mothers and 12 mother/ father dyads interviewed
McWilliam, Lang, Vandiviere, Angell, Collins, & Underdown, 1995	Family perceptions of early intervention services	Survey

Semistructured interviews | USA | 539 parents filled out survey

6 parents interviewed |
| Simeonsson, Edmonson, Smith, Carnahan, & Bucy, 1995 | Professional and parent perspectives of family involvement in assessment | Survey | USA | 39 parents
81 professionals |
| Washington & Schwartz, 1996 | Perceptions on the affect of physiotherapy and occupation therapy services on care giving competency | Semistructured interviews | USA | Two adoptive mothers |
| King, Law, King, & Rosenbaum, 1998 | Family and service provider's perceptions of family-centeredness of service | Survey | Canada | 436 parents
309 service providers |

Discipline of Professionals	Child's Difficulty	Age of Children	No. of Interviews	Major Themes
Staff of early intervention centers	Young children with disabilities —including autism, physical and intellectual impairment	3–5 years	Each family interviewed once	Aspects of staff perceived as helpful/unhelpful Parent-as-therapist aide
Staff of early intervention centers	Children had unspecified disabilities	0–6 years of age	Interviewed once	Overwhelming satisfaction with most services Difficulties accessing some services
Variety of service providers including SLPs	Known or suspected disabilities	10 months –16 years	—	Substantial variability in individual parents and professionals perceptions of their roles in child assessment.
Physiotherapists and occupational therapists	Cerebral palsy Meningo-myelocele	18 months and 3 years	Three interviews over a 5-week period	Themes: Knowledge is power Mother-therapist relationship— building a team to support the child Communication skills—an essential attribute
Service providers in early intervention center	Chronic, mostly neurodevelop-mental disorders	7 months– 20 years	—	Both parents and therapists identified information provision as an area of weakness in service provision

continues

83

Table 3–1. *continued*

Study	Focus of Study	Type of Investigation	Country of Focus	No. of Participants
Thompson, 1998	Mothers' perception of ideal vs. actual service provision	In-depth interviews	Australia	10 parents: 1 father and 9 mothers of 9 children
Crais & Belardi, 1999	Families' perceptions of their participation in their child's assessment	Survey	USA	23 family members (mostly mothers) 58 professionals
Van Riper, 1999	Perceptions of family-provider relationships	Survey	USA	94 parents
Glogowska & Campbell, 2000	Parental views of involvement in speech-language pathology	In-depth interviews	UK	16 parents: majority mothers

Discipline of Professionals	Child's Difficulty	Age of Children	No. of Interviews	Major Themes
Occupational therapists	Disabilities such as intellectual impairment and physical impairment	0–6 years	Each parent interviewed once	Themes: Doing the best for my child Helping the child develop skills I have to think of my whole family What does that do? —the place of services
Majority special educators, psychologists, SLPs' occupational therapists, social workers, and physiotherapists	Children with special needs	0–3 years	—	Gap between ideal and typical practices Families and professionals mostly agreed on ideal and actual practices Families and professionals feel many family-centered assessment practices are ideal
Health professionals	Down syndrome	0–22 years	—	Parents' perception of relationship with health professionals linked to satisfaction with care and emotional well-being
SLPs	Speech/ language delay	3;6–4;6 years	Interviewed once	Experiences centered around: Getting in Getting on Getting out of intervention experience

continues

Table 3–1. *continued*

Study	Focus of Study	Type of Investigation	Country of Focus	No. of Participants
Parette, Brotherson, & Huer, 2000	Parents' views of their involvement in decision making about alternative and augmentative communication (AAC) devices	Focus groups Individual interviews Surveys	USA	58 parents
McWilliam, Synder, Harbin, Porter, & Munn, 2000	Professionals' and families' perceptions of family-centered practices	Survey	USA	198 professionals 118 families
Glogowska & Roulstone, 2001	Parents' perceptions of speech-language pathology services	Survey	UK	147 parents
Baxendale, Frankham, & Heskert, 2001	Parents' perspective of a language program	In-depth interviews	UK	18 parents

Discipline of Professionals	Child's Difficulty	Age of Children	No. of Interviews	Major Themes
SLPs	Disabilities	Not specified	Participated in one interview or focus group Some parents also completed survey	Professionals should consider ethnic background of families Families want to be involved in decision-making process for the selection of an AAC device for their child
Teachers, administrators, and therapists	Developmental delays to severe disabilities	Average age: 24.9 months	—	Both families and professionals felt that services were family-centered Families would have liked more coordinated services
SLPs	Speech/ language delay	Not specified	—	Overall, parents satisfied with service Some parents dissatisfied with physical access to clinic, lack of information about home activities, appointment times, and number of appointments offered
SLPs	Speech/ language delay	2–3 years	Interviewed once	Parents expected 1:1 direct therapy with SLP; however, when exposed to a model of service including more parental involvement was satisfied with this model.

continues

Table 3–1. *continued*

Study	Focus of Study	Type of Investigation	Country of Focus	No. of Participants
Carrigan, Rodger, & Copely, 2001	Parent satisfaction with OT service	Interviews and focus groups	Australia	11 parents: 9 mothers and 2 fathers
King, Cathers, King, & Rosenbaum, 2001	Elements of parents satisfaction and dissatisfaction with services	Structured short interview	USA	231 parents
Piggot, Hocking, & Paterson, 2003	Parental perception of having a child with cerebral palsy and their involvement in their child's intervention	In-depth interviews and participant observations	New Zealand	8 parents, 1 father and 7 mothers of 7 children 4 occupational therapists
Law, Hanna, Hurley, King, Kertoy, & Rosenbaum, 2003	Factors affecting family-centered service delivery for children with disabilities.	Survey	Canada	494 parents 411 service providers 15 CEOs

Discipline of Professionals	Child's Difficulty	Age of Children	No. of Interviews	Major Themes
Occupational therapists	Children who received occupational therapy services from a university OT service	6–11 years	One interview or focus group	Parents' satisfaction linked to child's progress, aspects of professional, service delivery options and child's enjoyment of therapy
Early intervention professionals	Mostly cerebral palsy	Mean age 7 years	Identified from survey, interviewed once	Satisfaction associated with respectful and supportive care, dissatisfaction related to respectful and supportive care and service delivery issues (such as difficulty accessing intervention)
Physio-therapists and occupational therapists	Cerebral palsy	2–10 years of age	Interviewed 1–4 times each	Parents experience a compelling challenge to do all they can for their child. Coming to grips Striving to maximize their child's potential
Early intervention professionals, most frequent being occupational therapy, speech-language pathology, and physiotherapy	A variety of conditions, the most prevalent being cerebral palsy	Majority between 3–8 years of age	—	Satisfaction linked to parents' perception of the family-centeredness of the service

continues

Table 3–1. *continued*

Study	Focus of Study	Type of Investigation	Country of Focus	No. of Participants
Edwards, Millard, Praskac, & Wisniewski, 2003	Factors that encourage or inhibit family centered practice	Interviews	USA	6 mothers and 4 occupational therapists
Iversen, Poulin Shimmel, Ciacera, & Pabhakar, 2003	Perceptions of parents and professionals about the effectiveness of early intervention	Survey	USA	18 parents and 11 service providers
Leiter, 2004	Professionals and mothers' perceptions of parental involvement in their child's intervention	In-depth interviews and observation of home visits	USA	31 families: majority mothers interviewed
Goldbart & Marshall, 2004 (study also reported in Marshall & Goldbart, 2007)	Parents' perceptions of having a child who needs to use AAC	In-depth interviews	UK	Parents/ caregivers of 11 children
Keilmann, Braun, & Napiontek, 2004	Satisfaction of parents and SLP's with outcomes of intervention	Survey	Germany	169 parents 140 SLPs

Discipline of Professionals	Child's Difficulty	Age of Children	No. of Interviews	Major Themes
Occupational therapists	Special needs: cerebral palsy, micro-encephalitis, developmental delay	0–3 years	Interviewed once	Difficulty finding time to do home activities Adapting home activities to routine Importance of relationship with professional
Early intervention staff including SLPs	Developmental disabilities	Information not provided	—	Most parents satisfied, lesser scores related to ability to set goals, set limits for their child and be provided with info regarding other services
Early intervention staff including SLPs	May have established diagnosis or be biologically vulnerable	0–3 years of age	Interviewed once + home visit with professional observed	Professionals create a therapeutic imperative for parents. Parents not always compliant with this role.
SLPs	Cerebral palsy, intellectual impairment, hearing impairment, or epilepsy	3–11 years	Interviewed once	Three global themes: The child's communication or interaction Wider societal issues Parents' views and experiences
SLPs	Speech and language delays	2–9 years	—	Majority of parents satisfied with the outcome of SLP intervention Satisfaction not related to level of involvement

continues

Table 3–1. *continued*

Study	Focus of Study	Type of Investigation	Country of Focus	No. of Participants
Mirabito & Armstrong, 2005	Parents' perceptions involvement in speech-language pathology	Semistructured interviews	Australia	7 mothers
MacKean, Thurston, & Scott, 2005	Parents' and professionals' perceptions of their role in early intervention	Focus groups + semi-structured interviews	Canada	37 parents 16 health care providers
Brady, Skinner, Roberts, & Hennnon, 2006	Mother's perspectives of their child's communication	In-depth interviews	USA	55 mothers
Crais, Poston Roy, & Free, 2006	Professionals' and parents' perceptions of family-centered practices in child assessments	Survey	USA	134 professionals and 58 family members
Dyke, Buttigieg, Blackmore, & Ghose, 2006	Professionals and families' perceptions of the family-centeredness of an intervention service	Survey	Australia	43 professionals 158 families

Discipline of Professionals	Child's Difficulty	Age of Children	No. of Interviews	Major Themes
SLPs	Speech and language difficulties. Two children had "multiple disabilities"	3–7 years	Interviewed twice	Parents happy for therapist to take lead Participation at home (not session)
Health and allied health professionals including SLPs	19 autism 12 Down syndrome 6 developmental delay	Not specified	Interviewed once	Relational competency most important Parents want therapists to take lead
SLPs	Fragile X syndrome	Boys: mean age of 26.4 months Girls: mean age of 18.5 months	Each mother interviewed once	Concerns, challenges, stresses and frustrations regarding their child's communication Mothers' perceived roles
A range of disciplines with most prevalent being SLPs, special educators, and psychologists	Working at agency for "children with disabilities"	Mean age: 26.8 months	—	Parent/professional agreement re ideal and actual practices Implementation gap between ideal vs. actual family-centered practices
A range of disciplines including SLPs, occupational therapists, physio-therapists, and social workers	Cerebral palsy	Not specified	Not specified	Families rated respectful and supportive care as occurring most frequently and providing general information occurring least frequently

continues

Table 3–1. *continued*

Study	Focus of Study	Type of Investigation	Country of Focus	No. of Participants
Watts Pappas, McAllister, & McLeod, 2009	Parents' perceptions of their involvement in intervention for their child with speech impairment	Individual interviews	Australia	7 parents and 6 SLPs

SLPs = speech-language pathologists; UK = United Kingdom; USA = United States of America.

Parental Involvement in Intervention Provision

Expectations of Involvement

When parents are questioned about their expectations of involvement in their child's intervention they indicate that they had anticipated a mostly therapist-centered model of care in which the professional would work one-on-one with their child (Baxendale et al., 2001; Glogowska & Campbell, 2000; Leiter, 2004; Mirabito & Armstrong, 2004; Watts Pappas, 2007; Watts Pappas et al., 2009). Two studies (Mirabito & Armstrong, 2005; Watts Pappas et al., 2009b) found that some parents expected they would be asked to do home practice with their child but still anticipated that the bulk of the intervention would be provided by the professional. For example, parents in the Watts Pappas et al. (2009) study of children with speech impairment spoke about an expectation that their SLP would work with their child in the intervention sessions and formulate intervention goals and activities.

Discipline of Professionals	Child's Difficulty	Age of Children	No. of Interviews	Major Themes
SLPs	Speech impairment	Aged between 3;0–6;0 years	Each parent interviewed three times over the course of a period of intervention	Parents were motivated to do the right thing by their child. They were keen to be involved in homework activities but looked to their SLP to take the lead in the intervention provision and planning

Extent of Involvement

The way in which parents report that they are generally involved in their child's intervention is not discussed very often in research literature (see Table 3-1). The studies which do include this information indicate that parents usually attend and sometimes participate in assessment sessions (Crais & Belardi, 1999; Crais, Poston Roy, & Free, 2006; Watts Pappas et al., 2009). However, parental involvement in intervention seems to consist mostly of the completion of home activities (Hinojosa & Anderson, 1991; Mirabito & Armstrong, 2005). Parents often attend intervention sessions, or intervention sessions are conducted in their home; however, this is not always the case. For example, Keilmann and colleagues (2004) reported that 53.2% of parents surveyed did not attend speech-language pathology intervention sessions with their child; parents in a study conducted by Edwards, Millard, Praskac, and Wisniewski (2003) reported that they were not always able to attend occupational therapy intervention sessions for their child with cerebral palsy. Participation of parents in the intervention sessions is rarely discussed in research literature, but it appears that parents mostly observe rather than actively participate in the sessions (McBride et al., 1993; Mirabito & Armstrong,

2005; Watts Pappas et al., 2009). Occasionally, parents take on a coordinator role for their child's intervention, particularly when children are seeing a number of professionals (Mirabito & Armstrong, 2005).

Parents' Perceptions of Their Involvement in Their Child's Intervention Provision

When considering their involvement in their child's intervention, parents often speak about a desire to do the right thing by their child (Piggot et al., 2003; Thompson, 1998; Watts Pappas, 2007; Watts Pappas et al., 2009). Parents focus their energies on trying to help their child overcome their difficulties and accessing allied health intervention is seen as a major part of this process. In some instances, parents feel that their responsibility and role in the intervention is to be a professional or teacher for their child and to practise with them at home (Brady, Skinner, Roberts, & Hennon, 2006; Mirabito & Armstrong, 2005; Ross & Thompson, 1993; Watts Pappas et al., 2009). Many parents perceive that their involvement in this way is important to their child's progress (Andrews et al., 1989; Baxendale et al., 2001; Piggot et al., 2003; Thompson, 1998; Watts Pappas et al., 2009). However, for other parents, being involved in their child's intervention is perceived as a burden or unhelpful. Some parents speak about a need to have time to "just be a mother" (Brady et al., 2006, p. 359; Case-Smith & Nastro, 1993, p. 816) rather than constantly attending intervention sessions or doing home practice activities with their children (Brady et al., 2006; Case-Smith & Nastro, 1993; Hinojosa & Anderson, 1991; McKenzie, 1994). Particularly when a child has a pervasive disability, the long-term and possibly intensive nature of the intervention required may contribute to negative parental feelings about involvement in intervention.

Parents often struggle to do home activities with their children as prescribed by allied health professionals (Brotherson & Goldstein, 1992; Case-Smith & Nastro, 1993; Hinojosa & Anderson, 1991; Leiter, 2004; Piggot et al., 2003; Ross & Thompson, 1993) and speak of significant barriers to homework completion. Many parents have other children to care for and find that the time required to do the activities interferes with their care of other family members and their daily routine (Brotherson & Goldstein, 1992; Piggot et al., 2003; Ross & Thompson, 1993). In some cases, children are uncooperative with home activities (Hinojosa & Anderson, 1991; Piggot et al., 2003). Other parents feel that they are not qualified to do the activities at home with their child and are concerned about doing them incorrectly, especially if professionals fail to give adequate information to enable them to conduct the activities successfully (Case-Smith & Nastro, 1993; Glogowska & Roulstone, 2001; Goldbart & Marshall, 2004; Leiter, 2004; Parette et al., 2000; Ross & Thompson, 1993). For example, parents in a study conducted by Glogowska and Roulstone (2001) commented on the lack of information given to them about how to work with their children at home. Parents of children with speech impairment indicated that one of the most important components of a professional/parent partnership was the SLPs' ability to support them to do home activities with their child (Watts Pappas et al., 2009). Some studies revealed that parents were not always honest with professionals about the amount and type of home activities they had completed with their child, keeping up the appearance of doing the activities but in reality not completing them. This was particularly reported in the initial stages of intervention when parents were first coming to terms with their child's difficulties (Hinojosa & Anderson, 1991; Piggot et al., 2003).

Some parents have identified factors and strategies that facilitate their involvement in their children's intervention. Many parents manage the home activities by adapting them to incorporate them within their daily routine (Edwards et al., 2003; Hinojosa & Anderson, 1991; Piggot et al., 2003; Thompson, 1998; Watts Pappas et al., 2009). Additionally, parents have reported that observation of the professional working with their child increases their feelings of competence in doing the activities at home (Hinojosa & Anderson, 1991; Leiter, 2004; Mirabito & Armstrong, 2005). Parents have mentioned that they value the time the professional spends with their child during intervention sessions (Leiter, 2004; Mirabito & Armstrong, 2005; Watts Pappas et al., 2009) and see their role as an observer rather than as an active participant in the sessions (McBride et al., 1993; Mirabito & Armstrong, 2005; Watts Pappas et al., 2009).

Parental Involvement in Intervention Planning

Some parents report that they do not wish to be the primary decision-makers in their child's care (MacKean, Thurston, & Scott, 2005; McBride et al., 1993; Mirabito & Armstrong, 2005; Piggot et al., 2003; Thompson, 1998; Winton & Turnbull, 1981; Watts Pappas et al., 2009). For example, MacKean and colleagues (2005) described concern from parents about the expectation that they would take the lead in service planning for their child. This is contrary to the principles of family-centered practice, which promotes families as the final decision-makers for their child (Bailey, McWilliam, & Winton, 1992; Brown, Humphry, & Taylor, 1997). Researchers have theorized that parents may be reluctant to be involved in decision-making because of respect for the professionals' expertise (McBride et al., 1993; Watts Pappas et al., 2009), a perception of differentiation between professional versus parent roles (Thompson, 1998; Watts Pappas et al., 2009), lack of professional support for their involvement (Goldbart & Marshall, 2004), or a need to take a break from the responsibilities of being involved in intervention for their children (Winton & Turnbull, 1981). For example, some parents of children with disabilities in a study conducted by Thompson (1998) reported they felt that the occupational therapists were the experts and because of this perception were less involved in intervention planning and provision.

Some parents express a desire to collaborate with the professional in setting goals and feel that they can contribute unique information about their child and family (Crais & Belardi, 1999; McBride et al., 1993; Mirabito & Armstrong, 2005; Parette et al., 2000). However, even when parents value being part of the planning process they may still want the professional to take the leading role (Mirabito & Armstrong, 2005; Piggot et al., 2003; Thompson, 1998; Winton & Turnbull, 1981; Watts Pappas et al., 2009). In some studies, parents have been divided in their opinions about their involvement in decision-making, with different groups satisfied with more or less involvement (Goldbart & Marshall, 2004; McBride et al., 1993; Thompson, 1998).

Parental involvement in service planning and provision may increase over time, with parents of recently diagnosed children reporting an initial inability to be involved in their children's intervention and a reliance on professionals to guide them (MacKean et al., 1995; McBride et al., 1993; Piggot et al., 2003). In only two studies did parents report being satisfied with assuming the role of team leader for their child (Summers, Dell'Oliver, Turnbull, Benson, Santelli, Campbell, & Siegel-Causey, 1990; Washington & Schwartz, 1996). One of these studies was unique in that it involved two adoptive parents of children with cerebral palsy (Washington & Schwartz, 1996). As these parents knew of their child's diagnosis at the time of adoption they may have had different perceptions of the intervention process. It is not known why the parents in the second study (Summers et al., 1990) preferred this role.

Parent/Professional Relationships

Parents place great importance on the interpersonal skills of the allied health professionals working with their child. For example, in her study of maternal perceptions of professional-parent relationships, Van Riper (1999) found that if mothers were satisfied with the relationship they had with their child's health professional they were more satisfied with their overall care. Thompson (1998) reported that the perceived friendliness of their occupational therapist impacted on how motivated the parents were to be involved in their children's intervention. In some cases, the professionals' interpersonal skills seem to be more important to parents than their competency as a professional. For example, a survey conducted by Iversen and colleagues (2003) revealed that the relationship parents had with their health professional had a greater effect on their perception of the professional than the professionals' technical skills. Parents feel that these relationships take time to develop and that consistency in professionals helps more genuine relationships to emerge (Edwards et al., 2003; Piggot et al., 2003). Thus, both interpersonal skills and professional competency are facilitative when working with families.

Parents have spoken of interpersonal characteristics that can either build or block the parent/professional relationship. These can be summarized into six factors: professionals' responsiveness to the child, professionals' interpersonal skills, professionals' respect for parents' ideas and opinions, professionals' communication skills, professional competence, and the professional as a source of support and friendship. Examples of how these professional skills can be practically used to improve parent/professional relationships are outlined in the case studies of Chapters 4 through 11.

Professionals' Responsiveness to the Child

The professionals' relationship with and attitude toward the child can be an important aspect of parents' feelings toward that professional (Baxter, 1989; Carrigan et al., 2001; Case-Smith & Nastro, 1993; Mac-

Kean et al., 2005; McKenzie, 1994; Watts Pappas et al., 2009). Parents speak about the importance of the professionals' ability to establish rapport with their child as well as their perception of the professional caring about their child as a person. For example, the parents interviewed in a study of parent's perceptions of their involvement in intervention for their child's speech impairment (Watts Pappas et al., 2009) described the SLPs' relationship with their child as one of the most important elements in the formation of a parent/professional partnership. As one parent said: "You definitely have to win the child over to get the parent's trust" (Watts Pappas, 2007, p. 235).

Professionals' Interpersonal Skills

Parents speak of the importance of professionals being friendly, caring and sensitive to their feelings (Baxter, 1989; Dyke, Buttigieg, Blackmore, & Ghose, 2006; MacKean et al., 2005; McKenzie, 1994; Simeonsson, Edmonson, Smith, Carahan, & Bucy, 1995; Summers et al., 1990; Thompson, 1998; Watts Pappas et al. 2009). For example, "Respectful and supportive" care was a major factor in satisfaction and dissatisfaction with services in a survey study conducted by King and colleagues (2001, p. 127). Parents want professionals to be approachable and to treat them with respect and consideration. For example, a parent stated that she wanted her SLP to be "professional, but at the same time very personable, a real person, not condescending" (Watts Pappas, 2007, p. 237).

Professionals' Respect for Parents' Ideas and Opinions

Parents value professionals who ask for their input and respect the knowledge they can share (Brotherson & Goldstein, 1992; Dyke et al., 2006; Washington & Schwartz, 1996; Watts Pappas et al., 2009). When professionals disregard parents' ideas or fail to give them an opportunity to share their opinions, this blocks the establishment of a positive working relationship with that professional (Baxter, 1989; Case-Smith & Nastro, 1993; Glogowska & Campbell, 2000; Watts Pappas et al., 2009). For example, the five parents interviewed by Case-Smith and Nastro (1993) reported situations when they felt that their knowledge about their child was disregarded by professionals. These experiences were illustrated by their theme, "Is anybody listening?" (p. 813).

Professionals' Communication Skills

Parents also speak about professionals' communication skills as an important aspect of their satisfaction with the parent/professional relationship. Parents want professionals who are informative—providing practical information about their child's difficulties and the support they would need. For example, the parents of children with cerebral palsy interviewed by Case-Smith and Nastro (1993) saw one of the primary roles of their occupational therapist as a source of information. Parents value professionals who take the time to answer questions, explain aspects of their child's intervention and progress to them, and who can do this in a way that the parent can understand (Baxter, 1989; Carrigan et al., 2001; Dyke et al., 2006; King et al., 1998, 2001; MacKean et al., 2005; Ross & Thomson, 1993; Thompson, 1998; Washington & Schwartz, 1996; Watts Pappas et al., 2009).

Professional Competence

Parents expect that health professionals who work with their children are technically competent and able to fulfill a teaching role with both themselves and their children (Baxter, 1989; Goldbart & Marshall, 2004; MacKean et al., 2005; McKenzie, 1994; Parette et al., 2000; Watts Pappas et al., 2009; Winton & Turnbull, 1981). For instance, the major role that parents expected their SLP to play in the process of acquiring an alternative and augmentative communication (AAC) device was as a trainer/educator for their family (Parette et al., 2000). In another study, one of the major themes found in the analysis of a brief interview of 131 parents was "professional commitment" (Baxter, 1989, p. 267). These parents wanted professionals to be committed to increasing their professional knowledge and to providing services of a high standard. When parents felt that professionals were competent in facilitating their child's development they felt more comfortable about the intervention service (Winton & Turnbull, 1981).

Professional as a Source of Support and Friendship

Many parents consider professionals who work with their family not only as a change agents for their child, but also a source of support and friendship for them as parents (Edwards et al., 2003; Hinojosa & Anderson, 1990, 1991; Leiter, 2004; McKenzie, 1994; Summers et al., 1990; Thompson, 1998; Washington & Schwartz, 1996). Often parents describe relationships with their professionals that move beyond being friendly and approachable to the development of genuine friendships. For example, Leiter (2004, p. 840) reported parents speaking about professionals as "a member of the family" and Hinojosa and Anderson (1990, p. 154) summarized the feelings of parents about their child's physiotherapist with the theme "the third parent." This friendship was seen as a significant source of support for coping with a child with a disability. It is possible that this level of friendship does not develop when working with children on a short term basis. However, as SLPs and other health professionals can work with families for many years, this level of friendship can develop.

Focus of Intervention—Family or Child?

Parents' preference about whether intervention should focus on the child or the whole family varies. At odds with the usual model of family-centered practice, some parents speak about wanting services to focus on their child rather than their family (Leiter, 2004; McWilliam et al., 1995; Watts Pappas et al., 2009). For example, the seven parents of children with speech impairment interviewed by Watts Pappas et al. (2009) expressed a desire for the intervention sessions to focus on their child and considered the time the SLP spent with their child as more important than the time the SLP spent with the parent. For example, one parent said "You don't get involved in the session. She's there to do her job and if you step in you're only going to make it harder if you put your two bits in" (Watts Pappas, 2007, p. 226). This phenomenon caused Leiter (2004) to postulate that, for some parents, family-centered care is child-centered.

Conversely, other parents describe the time the professional spends with them in the intervention sessions as being just as important as the time the professional spends with their child (Hinojosa

& Anderson, 1991; Thompson, 1998) and appreciate the professional acting as a "sounding board" for day-to-day concerns not directly related to their child (Edwards et al., 2003, p. 247). These parents appear to be particularly alluding to the counselling/support role the professionals provide, which may be particularly important when children have lifetime diagnoses of cerebral palsy or other pervasive disabilities.

Service Delivery Issues

Service delivery issues often impact upon parents' experience of accessing and being involved in intervention services for their children. A lack of sufficient services has been commented on by many parents, leading to increased waiting times (Brady et al., 2006; King et al., 2001; Thompson, 1998; Watts Pappas et al., 2009) and less frequent intervention than parents would have preferred (Edwards et al., 2003, Glogowska & Campbell, 2000; Goldbart & Marshall, 2004; McWilliam et al., 1995, Piggot et al., 2003; Ross & Thompson, 1993). Many parents hold a belief that more intervention is better. This belief motivates some parents to access intervention from professionals in private practice when publicly funded services are not available (Case-Smith & Nastro, 1993; McWilliam et al., 1995; Thompson, 1998; Watts Pappas et al., 2009). Parents particularly believe that when the professional spends one-on-one time with their children, this facilitates the best results for the intervention and is preferable to other forms of intervention such as parent consultation with the professional (Baxendale et al., 2001; Glogowska & Campbell, 2000; McWilliam et al., 1995).

Due to the physical accessibility of services, attending intervention is difficult for some parents, particularly those living in rural locations or those who need to take public transport to get to appointments (Brotherson & Goldstein, 1992; Glogowska & Campbell, 2001; MacKenzie, 1994). Home visits are valued by parents and were associated with greater satisfaction in a survey study conducted by Able-Boone, Goodwin, Gordon, and Martin (1992). If professionals are able to accommodate siblings in sessions, this makes attendance easier and gives parents ideas about how siblings can be incorporated into home practice activities if necessary (Edwards et al., 2003; Thompson, 1998). The inclusion of siblings can also facilitate and support the role siblings play in the lives of children with communication impairment (Barr, McLeod, & Daniel, 2008).

A lack of coordination among professionals is often quoted as a cause for concern for parents, who sometimes feel it is left to them to transmit important information from professional to professional, a role they feel wastes time and for which they are not qualified (Brotherson & Goldstein, 1992; MacKean et al., 2005; McWilliam et al., 2000). Inconsistency of professionals is an additional negative service delivery issue that is mentioned by parents (Brotherson & Goldstein, 1992; Case-Smith & Nastro, 1993; King et al., 2001; McWilliam et al., 2000). For example, the parents in a study conducted by Brotherson and Goldstein (1992) indicated that the time required establishing a relationship with a new professional was frustrating and disruptive to their children's intervention.

Models of Practice

As highlighted in Chapter 1 there are three main models of practice: therapist-centered practice, parent-as-therapist aide practice and family-centered practice. The model of practice provided to the parents in the studies reviewed in Table 3–1 varied and could not always be determined by the information provided. In some studies, the service the parents reported receiving could be classified as a therapist-centered or parent-as-therapist aide model of practice (Leiter, 2004; Thompson, 1998). For example, only 10% of parents of children with disabilities interviewed by Thompson (1998) were involved in intervention planning; the majority of parents in the study perceived the occupational therapy services they received were focused on their child rather than the family. Parents in other studies appeared to be receiving predominantly family-centered models of care (Edwards et al., 2003; MacKean et al., 2005; McWilliam et al., 1995). However, not all parents were satisfied with this model. For example, the parents interviewed by MacKean and colleagues (2005) resisted the team leader role they were placed into by their family-centered professionals. In other studies, only certain elements of family-centered practice were used. For example, in the study by Piggot and colleagues (2003) in which both parents and professionals were interviewed, the service provided to the parents was family-centered in that the professionals attempted to build positive relationships with the parents and involved them in decision-making about their child's intervention. However, the study also highlighted that, although the professionals spoke about being in partnership with parents, they still made judgments about parents' compliance with their suggestions. Family-friendly practice, which has been introduced in this book, may represent a model of practice that is more acceptable to families.

Summary

Overall, parents seem satisfied with the allied health intervention services they receive for their child based on the review of studies in Table 3-1. This finding appeared to apply for parents of children receiving all types of allied health intervention, in a number of different countries and settings, and whether their children presented with mild to severe difficulties. Satisfaction with care appears to be significantly related to the parents' relationship with their child's allied health professional. Parents want these professionals to be friendly and caring, with good communication and technical skills. Service delivery issues such as wait-times, consistency of professionals, and coordination of services are also important in parents' experience of allied health intervention. Services that are easily accessible, sufficient for the children's needs, informative, coordinated, and consistent are associated with higher levels of parental satisfaction. Many of the aspects of care identified as desirable by parents are congruent with a family-centered model of service. However, other elements of family-centered practice are not as universally sought by parents.

Parents vary in their beliefs and feelings about their involvement in their children's allied health intervention. As Thomas (1998) noted, parents are a heterogeneous group and must be considered individually by professionals; however, some general trends in the parents' views are evident. One of these trends is a reluctance to take the lead role in intervention planning and provision for their child. Many parents continue to refer to the professional as the "expert," reinforcing the traditional hierarchy of parents and professionals. This is the case even in studies conducted recently (Leiter, 2004; MacKean et al., 2005; Mirabito & Armstrong, 2005; Watts Pappas et al., 2009). Although discussion in the literature about family-centered practice has increased in recent years, there appears to be little corresponding change in parents' perceptions of their relationship with their children's professionals and their role in the intervention process. Although parents want respectful and supportive care from their professionals, many want a more family-friendly model of practice in which intervention services focus on their children and the professional takes the lead role in the intervention.

References

Able-Boone, H., Goodwin, L. D., Sandall, S. R., Gordon, N., & Martin, D. G. (1992). Consumer based early intervention services. *Journal of Early Intervention, 16*, 201–209.

Andrews, J. R., Andrews, M. A., & Shearer, W. M. (1989). Parents' attitudes toward family involvement in speech-language services. *Language, Speech, and Hearing Services in Schools, 20*, 391–399.

Bailey, D. B., McWilliam, P., & Winton, P. J. (1992). Building family-centered practices in early intervention: A team-based model for change. *Infants and Young Children, 5*(1), 73–82.

Barr, J., McLeod, S., & Daniel, G. (2008). Siblings of children with speech impairment: Cavalry on the hill. *Language, Speech, and Hearing Services in Schools, 39*(1), 21–32.

Baxendale, J., Frankham, J., & Hesketh, A. (2001). The Hanen parent programme: A parent's perspective. *International Journal of Language and Communication Disorders, 36*(Suppl.), 511–516.

Baxter, C. (1989). Parent-perceived attitudes of professionals: Implications for service providers. *Disability, Handicap and Society, 4*(3), 259–269.

Brady, N., Skinner, D., Roberts, J., & Hennon, E. (2006). Communication in young children with Fragile X Syndrome: A qualitative study of mother's perspectives. *American Journal of Speech-Language Pathology, 15*, 353–364.

Brotherson, M., & Goldstein, B. (1992). Time as a resource and constraint for parents of young children with disabilities: implications for early intervention services. *Topics in Early Childhood Special Education, 12*(4), 508–527

Brown, S., Humphry, R., & Taylor, E. (1997). A model of the nature of family-therapist relationships: Implications for education. *American Journal of Occupational Therapy, 51*(7), 597–603.

Carrigan, N., Rodger, S., & Copley, J. (2001). Parent satisfaction with a paediatric occupational therapy service: A pilot investigation. *Physical and Occupational Therapy in Pediatrics, 21*(1), 51–76.

Case-Smith, J., & Nastro, M. (1993). The effect of occupational therapy intervention on mothers of children with cerebral palsy. *American Journal of Occupational Therapy, 47*(9), 811–817.

Crais, E., & Belardi, C. (1999). Family participation in child assessment: Perceptions of families and professionals. *Infant-Toddler Intervention: A Transdisciplinary Journal, 9,* 209–238.

Crais, E., Poston Roy, V., & Free, K. (2006). Parents' and professionals' perceptions of family-centered practices: What are actual practices vs. what are ideal practices? *American Journal of Speech-Language Pathology, 15,* 365–377.

Dyke, P. Buttigieg, P., Blackmore, A. M., & Ghose, A. (2006). Use of the Measure of Process of Care for families (MPOC-56) and service providers (MPOC-SP) to evaluate family-centered services in a paediatric disability setting. *Child: Care, Health and Development, 32*(2), 167–176.

Edwards, M., Millard, P., Praskac, L., & Wisniewski, P. (2003). Occupational therapy and early intervention: A family-centered approach. *Occupational Therapy International, 10*(4), 239–252.

Glogowska, M., & Campbell, R. (2000). Investigating parental views of involvement in pre-school speech and language therapy. *International Journal of Language and Communication Disorders, 35*(3), 391–405.

Glogowska, M., & Roulstone, S. (2001, Winter). Evidence-based practice: Seeking the whole truth. *Speech and Language Therapy in Practice,* pp. 8–10.

Goldbart, J., & Marshall, J. (2004). "Pushes and pulls" on the parents of children who use AAC. *Augmentative and Alternative Communication, 20*(4), 194–208.

Hinojosa, J. (1990). How mothers of preschool children with cerebral palsy perceive occupational and physical therapists and their influence on family life. *Occupational Therapy Journal of Research, 10*(3), 144–162.

Hinojosa, J., & Anderson, J. (1991). Mother's perceptions of home treatment programs for their preschool children with cerebral palsy. *American Journal of Occupational Therapy, 45,* 273–279.

Iversen, M., Poulin Shimmel, J., Ciacera, S., & Meenakshi, P. (2003). Creating a family-centered approach to early intervention services: Perceptions of parents and professionals. *Pediatric Physical Therapy, 15,* 23–31.

Keilmann, A., Braun, L., & Napiontek, U. (2004). Emotional satisfaction of parents and speech-language pathologists with outcome of training intervention in children with speech and language disorders. *Folia Phoniatrica et Logopaedica, 56*(1), 51–61.

King, G., Cathers, T., King, S., & Rosenbaum, P. (2001). Major elements of parents' satisfaction and dissatisfaction with pediatric rehabilitation services. *Children's Health Care, 30,* 111–134.

King, G., Law, M., King, S., & Rosenbaum, P. (1998). Parents' and service providers' perceptions of the family centeredness of children's rehabilitation services. *Physical and Occupational Therapy in Pediatrics, 18*(1), 21–40.

Law, M., Hanna, S., Hurley, P., King, S., Kertoy, M., & Rosenbaum, P. (2003). Factors affecting family-centered service delivery for children with disabilities. *Child: Care, Health and Development, 29*, 357–366.

Leiter, V. (2004). Dilemmas in sharing care: maternal provision of professionally driven therapy for children with disabilities. *Social Science and Medicine, 58*, 837–849.

MacKean, G., Thurston, W., & Scott, C. (2005). Bridging the divide between families and health professionals' perspectives on family-centered care. *Health Expectations, 8*, 74–85.

Marshall, J., & Goldbart, J. (2008). "Communication is everything I think" Parenting a child who needs Augmentative and Alternative Communication (AAC). *International Journal of Language and Communication Disorders, 43*(1), 77–98.

McBride, S., Brotherson, M., Joanning, H., Whiddon, D., & Demmitt, A. (1993). Implementation of family-centered services: Perceptions of families and professionals. *Journal of Early Intervention, 17*(4), 414–430.

McKenzie, S. (1994). Parents of young children with disabilities: Their perceptions of generic children's services and service professionals. *Australian Journal of Early Childhood, 19*(4), 12–17.

McWilliam, R. A., Lang, R. A., Vandiviere, P., Angell, R., Collins, L., & Underdown, G. (1995). Satisfaction and struggles: Family perceptions of early intervention services. *Journal of Early Intervention, 19*, 43–60.

McWilliam, R. A., Synder, P., Harbin, G., Porter, P., & Munn, D. (2000). Professionals' and families' perceptions of family-centered practices in infant-toddler services. *Early Education and Development, 11*(4), 519–538.

Mirabito, K., & Armstrong, E. (2005, May). *Parent reactions to speech therapy involvement.* Paper presented at the Speech Pathology Australia National Conference, Canberra.

Parette, H. P., Brotherson, M. J., & Huer, M. B. (2000). Giving families a voice in augmentative and alternative communication decision-making. *Education and Training of the Mentally Retarded, 35*(2), 177–190.

Piggot, J., Hocking, C., & Paterson, J. (2003). Parental adjustment to having a child with cerebral palsy and participation in home programs. *Physical and Occupational Therapy in Pediatrics, 23*(4), 5–29.

Rosenbaum, P., King, S., & Cadman, D. T. (1992). Measuring processes of caregiving to physically disabled children and their families. Part I: Identifying relevant components of care. *Developmental Medicine and Child Neurology, 34*, 103–114.

Ross, K., & Thomson, D. (1993). An evaluation of parents' involvement in the management of their cerebral palsy children. *Physiotherapy, 79*(8), 561–565.

Simeonsson, R. J., Edmonson, R., Smith, T. M., Carahan, S., & Bucy, J. E. (1995). Family involvement in multidisciplinary team evaluation: Professional and parent perspectives. *Child: Care, Health and Development, 21*(3), 199–215.

Summers, J., Dell'Oliver, C., Turnbull, A., Benson, H., Santelli, E., Campbell, M., & Siegel-Causey, E. (1990). Examining the individualized family service plan process: What are family and practitioner preferences? *Topics in Early Childhood Special Education, 10*, 78-99.

Thompson, K. (1998). Early intervention services in daily family life: Mothers' perceptions of 'ideal' versus 'actual' service provision. *Occupational Therapy International, 5*(3), 206-221.

Van Riper, M. (1999). Maternal perceptions of family-provider relationships and well-being in families of children with Down syndrome. *Research in Nursing and Health, 22*, 357-368.

Washington, K., & Schwartz, P. (1996). Maternal perceptions of the effects of physical and occupational therapy services on caregiving competency. *Physical and Occupational Therapy in Pediatrics, 16*(3), 33-54.

Watts Pappas, N. (2007). *Parental involvement in intervention for speech impairment*. Unpublished doctoral dissertation, Charles Sturt University, Bathurst, Australia.

Watts Pappas, N., McAllister, L., & McLeod, S. (2009). *Family involvement in paediatric speech intervention: What do parents think?* (manuscript in preparation).

Winton, P. J., & Turnbull, A. (1981). Parent involvement as viewed by parents of preschool handicapped children. *Topics in Early Childhood Special Education, 1*(3), 11-19.

Chapter 4

Working with Families of Young Children with Communication and Language Impairments: Identification and Assessment

Elizabeth R. Crais

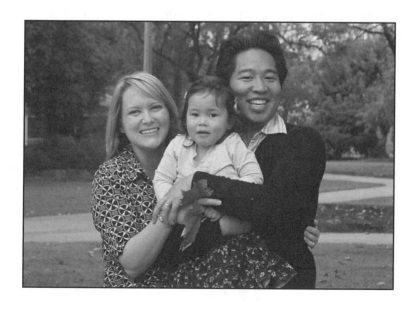

Introduction

Families can and should be offered a major role in the identification and assessment of communication skills in their young children who may be at risk for or have communication impairments. In recent years, families have been invited to take a more active role in intervention planning and implementation; however, their roles in the assessment process have been fairly limited and typically are not conducive to active participation or active decision-making. This chapter presents a brief overview of the historical role of families in the early identification and assessment of their young children with communication impairments, describes current practices and beliefs of families and professionals[1] about assessment, discusses current gaps between what could be viewed as actual and ideal practices in regard to family participation in assessment, and concludes with recommendations for the field and a case study to illustrate the recommendations.

Historical View of Family Participation in Identification and Assessment of Young Children

The roles of families within the assessment process in early intervention have been evolving over the last 30 years. Until the emergence of the theories, principles, legislation in the United States, and recommended practices surrounding family-centered care in the 1980s, families typically were offered limited roles in assessment (Bailey, 2004; McLean & Crais, 2004). The primary roles were of *informant* of the child's developmental and medical histories, sometime *observer* of the assessment process, and *recipient* of information provided by professionals. Thus, assessment was frequently performed within a very clinician-centered model with little input from the family. As family-centered principles and practices became more prominent in early

---

[1]The term "professional" is used throughout this chapter because most of the available literature on family participation in assessment has examined the practices and beliefs of professionals across a variety of disciplines in early intervention, with few studies (e.g., Watts Pappas, 2007) targeting speech-language pathologists specifically.

intervention services, additional roles such as *describer* of the child's daily routines, occasional *interpreter* of the child's behaviors, and *validator* of the child's performance on the day of testing began to be more prevalent (Crais, Roy, & Free, 2006; McLean & Crais, 2004). Furthermore, early interventionists routinely began to ask families to identify their primary concerns and priorities for their child and to take a greater role in the creation of intervention goals (Able-Boone, Goodwin, Sandall, Gordon, & Martin, 1992; Able-Boone, Sandall, Loughry, & Frederick, 1990; Boone & Crais, 1999). In addition, assessments that were performed within play-based and/or arena models also offered families the role of *participant* as families were asked to demonstrate certain behaviors or interactions with their child (Linder, 1993, 2008). Although these types of roles have become fairly common within assessments of young children, more active roles such as *evaluator*, *collaborator*, and *overall validator* of the assessment activities and results have not been routinely utilized (Crais et al., 2006). The following section provides further detail about current beliefs and practices of families and professionals regarding the roles families play in the assessment of their young children.

Current Beliefs and Practices of Families and Professionals About Family Roles in Assessment

The research evidence about family and professional beliefs and practices regarding assessment comes primarily from surveys or self-rating tools completed by professionals and/or families. Most of the studies were performed in the late 1990s with only a handful of studies within the last 10 years. There are several themes that emerge from these studies. First, despite the move toward the use of family-centered principles to guide practice, parents continue to be offered limited roles within the assessment process (Crais et al., 2006; McWilliam, Snyder, Porter, Harbin, & Munn, 2000). Second, despite these findings, a majority of families report that they are satisfied with the early intervention services they receive and feel they are generally family-centered in nature (Crais et al., 2006; Summers, Hoffman, Marquis, Turnbull, & Poston, 2005). Given their limited roles, however, several researchers have questioned the degree to which families are aware of their rights or the broad array of options available within the early intervention system (Crais et al., 2006; McWilliam et al., 2000). Furthermore, these researchers have hypothesized that when families are aware of additional options, they may choose more active roles. Indeed, the work of these two research groups has documented that when families are asked very specific questions about their participation in early intervention services, they indicate a preference for a greater role in the assessment of their child (Crais et al., 2006; McWilliam et al., 2000). These two studies are briefly described to provide specific information on the beliefs and practices of families and professionals in the assessment process.

To examine the extent to which professionals and families perceived early intervention services as family-centered, McWilliam et al. (2000) surveyed 198 professionals and 118 families using the *Family Orientation of Community and Agency Services* instrument (FOCAS, Bailey, 1991). The study participants were not receiving or providing services from or to each other; therefore, they were asked how practices they received or provided were implemented *typically*. Participants rated 12 service delivery practices as to how they actually occurred (i.e., actual practice) and how they might like them to occur (i.e., ideal practice). The results indicated that on average the parents' ratings tended to be lower than the professionals' on the same practices indicating that parents viewed these practices as happening less often and also not as ideal as professionals. Two of the items with the largest discrepancy between families and professionals were "family participation in the assessment process" and "participation in assessment decisions." In other words, families viewed these practices as occurring in a less family-centered manner than did the professionals. In addition, for two other practices related to assessment (e.g., family participation in assessment as well as team meetings; the family's role in the decision-making process), parents and professionals both believed the practices occurred less often than was ideal. Thus, for these practices, parents and professionals favored a more active role for parents in the assessment process.

The second study indicating that families (and to some extent professionals) preferred more active roles for families in assessment was conducted with families and professionals who were linked together in the delivery of services (Crais et al., 2006). Crais and colleagues surveyed 58 family members and 134 early intervention professionals (across a variety of disciplines) after they had participated together in a child assessment. For each assessment, two professionals from the team and one of the family members of the child assessed were surveyed. The families and professionals were asked to reflect on 42 family-centered assessment practices and to indicate whether each practice was implemented in the just completed assessment (i.e., actual practice) and whether the family/professional would like to have/offer this choice in future assessments (i.e., ideal practice). The results indicated that a number of the 42 family-centered practices were implemented within the assessments. The 10 practices that were used most frequently according to family/professional perceptions are listed in Table 4–1. For these practices, 75% or more of the

Table 4–1. Top 10 Most Frequently Occurring Practices and Percent of Family/Professional Pairs Who Agreed the Practice Occurred

Rank Order[+]	% of Pairs*	Family-Centered Practice
1	93	Time was spent finding out the family's most important concerns.
2	91	All assessment results were described or explained to the family.
3	89	Time was spent identifying the next steps for both family and professionals.
4	89	Conclusions were summarized after sharing assessment results with the family.
5	83	Family was asked if behaviors observed in the assessment were typical of child.
6	83	Family was given the choice to be present for all assessment activities.
7	81	Family was asked about the child's strengths.
8	81	During the assessment, professionals made positive comments about the child.
9	79	Family was given the choice to describe their child's daily routine.
10	79	Family was given the choice to sit beside their child during assessment.

[+] Rank order of practices (from most often to least often occurring) according to respondent pairs.
*Percent of pairs where both respondents said "Yes" a practice actually occurred during the assessment.
Source: Crais, Roy, and Free (2006).

family/professional pairs agreed that they had occurred in the assessment. In addition, 90% or more of the pairs viewed these practices as "ideal." Thus not only were these practices occurring fairly frequently, they were also valued by both families and professionals. When looking at the 10 most frequently occurring practices, however, the limited roles that were offered to the families within these practices is quite apparent. For example, families had primarily *recipient, observer,* and *describer* roles. In contrast when looking at the 10 least frequently used practices (Table 4–2), the roles available to families within them offer greater opportunities for participation, however as indicated, these practices were seldom utilized. Thus roles that could have been offered to families (e.g., *collaborator* in planning or *overall validator* of the assessment activities; *observer, reporter, or evaluator* of child behaviors) were offered infrequently (or not at all).

A further issue raised in both studies was the apparent implementation gap between what practices actually occurred in the assessments and the degree to which these practices were viewed as ideal by families and professionals. Specifically in the Crais et al. (2006) study, 20 out of 42 practices evidenced this type of implementation gap. Across these 20 practices, the mean agreement that they were ideal was over 80% of family/professional pairs with some individual variations across the practices. Thus, in most cases the families and professionals agreed that these practices would be good to include in future assessments. If this is the case, then why are these practices not included in routine assessments of young children? Some of the reasons that have been suggested for the lack of active parent participation in assessments include the belief that testing can only be administered in a standard manner in order to ensure reliability, professionals' general hesitancies to give up the role of primary decision-maker, concerns over time constraints, and the belief that parents lack the knowledge and expertise to adequately assess their child (Bruder, 2000; Crais et al., 2006). In addition, there is increasing evidence that the type of preparation that students receive in their graduate programs is associated with the practices that they utilize in their job settings after graduation (Crais, Boone, Harrison, Freund, Downing, & West, 2004; Mellon & Winton, 2003). Unfortunately, little information is available regarding the degree to which family-centered practices in child assessment (or overall in early intervention) are currently discussed and modeled in coursework and practica at the graduate level. An additional reason for the limited roles families are offered in assess-

Table 4–2. Ten Least Frequently Occurring Practices and Percent of Family/Professional Pairs Who Agreed the Practice Occurred

Rank Order[+]	% of Pairs[*]	*Family-Centered Practice*
33	30	If a diagnosis was made, the family was asked whether they agreed with the diagnosis.
34	29	Family was given the choice to choose the location of the assessment.
35	25	Family was asked to identify strategies to use in the assessment.
36	23	Family was asked to observe or write down observations of the child before the assessment.
37	10	Family was given the choice to complete an assessment tool or checklist.
38	7	Family was asked what activities or techniques in the previous assessment were the most/least successful.
39	6	If the family completed an assessment tool/checklist, they were asked to talk about what they noticed.
40	6	If the family wrote down observations before the assessment, they were asked to describe what they saw.
41	6	Family met with whole team before the assessment.
42	0	Family was given choice to write down observations of the child during the assessment.

[+]Rank order of practices (from most often to least often occurring) according to respondent pairs.
[*]Percent of pairs where both respondents said "Yes" a practice actually occurred during the assessment.
Source: Crais, Roy, and Free (2006).

ment may be the current orientation of many inservice activities. For example, just think back over the last few inservice activities you have encountered. Most likely they were focused on the participation of families in the goal setting and implementation of intervention services, with less or no emphasize on the role of families in the assessment process. Thus, neither our preservice nor inservice arenas are focused on reshaping the assessment process to provide maximal opportunities for participation and decision making by families.

Recommendations for Increasing Family (and Other Caregiver) Participation in Child Assessment

The recommendations provided focus on three sets of strategies related to child assessment. They include broadening the view of who takes part in the assessment process, considerations for how to enhance family (and other caregiver) decision-making related to assessment, and ways to increase the number of roles that parents and other caregivers are offered in the assessment process. Many people use the African proverb "It takes a village to raise a child" and the same principle can be applied to using a "village" in the process of assessing young children. The village could be made up of anyone the family felt would be important to the assessment process, anyone who could either contribute to or learn from the process. Furthermore, professionals may have ideas about who might be important to include. With this type of ecological approach, others who are important in the child and family's life such as grandparents, siblings, or early education and care providers can be included (with the family's approval) in the information gathering and assessment of the child. This type of approach is particularly valuable in gaining a broad picture of the child across settings and interactants, and can be especially helpful during the intervention planning, implementation, and monitoring phases of service delivery. In this way, the family's natural partners in their lives and in any intervention that is planned and implemented can be "on board" from the very beginning. In addition, if there are disagreements or differences of opinion among the partners on whether the child has a deficit, the nature of it, and what is to be done about it, there can be a forum for discussion and further investigation if needed.

Practical strategies to broaden the village could include asking the family about the people who are most important to the child and family and who spend a good deal of time with the child. If the parents feel that including these partners is valuable, then they could be invited to be a part of the assessment process by completing checklists or routines-based questionnaires or interviews, observing, and commenting on how the child interacts with them and others, or describing the child's strengths and challenges from their perspective in their setting (e.g., grandparents' home, early care program). Over the years, the author has found this type of collaboration extremely beneficial to the validity of the assessment process, the child and family, and to the participating partners. If we believe in the importance of the child's natural environments, especially the relationships surrounding the child and family, it only makes sense to consider these important partners during the assessment and intervention planning process.

The second strategy involves enhancing parental decision making by first examining who maintains the control over the decisions made during the assessment process and then by finding out the family's preferences. Historically in assessment, professionals have made most of the decisions (and recommendations) and families were left to agree, just go along and not say very much, not fully understand the information provided, or disagree and choose not to follow through with the assessment results or recommendations. In contrast, as suggested by a number of professionals (Beukelman & Mirenda, 2005; Boone & Crais, 1999; Dunst, Trivette, & Deal, 1988; McLean & Crais, 2004), the assessment process should be viewed as a series of *consensus building* activities. Indeed, Beukelman and Mirenda (2005) argue that a major goal of initial assessment should be the development of long-term consensus building and management. Dunst et al. (1988) in their early work on family empowerment, focused on the lack of consensus building by professionals as a major reason for parent and professional conflict regarding early intervention services and for some families' lack of follow through on professional recommendations. Dunst and his colleagues suggested that consensus building needs to take place around three critical points: the nature of the presenting concern, the need for treatment, and the course of action. A major premise of the current chapter is that the assessment process can provide rich opportunities for consensus building with families. Through active enhancement of the family's decision-making in assessment, we may not only improve the immediate assessment and our current interactions with families, but we may also facilitate collaborative interactions and relationships in the future.

Practical strategies for enhancing decision-making by families throughout the assessment process include first laying the groundwork for collaboration in all conversations and activities that involve the family and professionals. From the first phone call or the first time professionals communicate with the family, it is important to use words or phrases that indicate collaboration such as:

- "We value what you know about your child,"
- "We want to gather information from you and others important to your child,"

▧ "We know that you know your child best so we need your help," or

▧ "We will try to figure out together what's best for your child."

These types of communications can set the stage for families to feel that they are important to the assessment process and may further encourage their participation.

One strategy that has worked well for the author is to utilize a preassessment planning approach where one or more team members meet with the family (and their other key partners) to gather information from the family and plan the assessment. In addition to information about the child's background, birth and medical history, current skills, and family concerns, time is spent discussing options for assessment. Decision-making in planning the assessment could include asking families (if these choices are possible in a particular work setting):

▧ when/where the assessment should take place,

▧ who would you like to include,

▧ how can we see the best in your child,

▧ how can we see the challenges your child faces,

▧ what types of toys/materials would work best for your child (e.g., pictures or objects used to examine your child's sound productions),

▧ do you prefer a more formal (e.g., describing properties of typical standardized tests) or informal (e.g., describing more informal measures) assessment approach, and

▧ what are your concerns and what do you want to get out of the assessment?

These are just a few of the many possible opportunities for decision making that professionals can offer families in the assessment process. It is important to remember that families can only be informed decision makers and actively help plan their child's assessment when they know all the options available to them. For additional ideas and strategies for using a preassessment planning approach, see Crais (1996a, 1996b) and Boone and Crais (1999).

The final strategy to enhancing the participation of families in child assessment is to offer families the option of taking a variety of roles. Clearly, families will vary as to the types of roles they may choose in assessment and professionals must respect the family's choice about those roles. It has also been my experience that as families see that professionals truly want to hear about their ideas, perceptions, and beliefs about their child and then use these ideas to collaboratively plan and implement the assessment, family members typically become more active in the process. Choice making is again vital to this process. Choices such as:

- asking families if they would like to observe and write down their thoughts/comments about the child before and/or during the assessment (e.g., providing a pad and pen to the family during the assessment);
- asking families (and others important to the child) if they would like to complete a checklist, developmental assessment, or inventory about the child's skills and daily routines;
- if the child has been assessed previously, asking (a) the family to talk about what techniques/materials worked well/did not work well with the child, (b) if they agreed with the findings and recommendations, and (c) what information/recommendations were most useful/least useful;
- asking the family to help elicit particular child behaviors or skills, or to demonstrate typical interactions (e.g., feeding, dressing, playing, communicating);
- generating with the family the child's strengths and challenges within and outside of the assessment;
- planning together the next steps for the child and family;
- asking the family if they would like to review a draft of the report before it is finalized; and
- asking if the family is willing to give follow-up feedback to the professionals about the assessment process in person or in writing.

These recommended practices have been utilized within child assessments in our clinic over the last 10 to 15 years with increased success in enhancing the role of families in the assessment process. In the beginning, we started with one aspect of the assessment (interviewing) and then with time began to modify other components (e.g., assessing the child, sharing assessment results) as we became more comfortable with inviting parents to be more active participants. As families began to see how important they were to the assessment process and they understood fully the kinds of options available to them, their participation (and satisfaction) increased. For families who had experienced more traditional assessments in other settings, their enthusiasm and appreciation of the "newer" model was particularly noteworthy. Moreover, with the changing populations of children and families seen in our clinic in recent years and the mismatch that can occur in sociocultural characteristics between service providers and families, identifying and respecting each family's beliefs, values, and customs becomes increasingly important throughout the early intervention process (Barrera & Corso, 2002). Moreover, the assessment itself is an opportunity to introduce families to a model of family/professional collaboration and to set the stage for increased participation across other aspects of early intervention (e.g., intervention planning, implementation, and monitoring). Finally, the key to enhancing the family's role in the assessment process is not to identify a particular set of practices to use with all families, but to recognize the family's role in helping decide on the practices and activities that are best for their child and their family.

Case Study Illustrating Active Participation by Family Members and Other Caregivers

Elijah was a 28-month-old boy who lived with his mother, Maria, who was 18 years old, his maternal grandmother, Beba, and his mother's younger teenage sister, Eva. Elijah spent his mornings at the community early care center and his grandmother took care of him the rest of the day while his mother worked and his aunt went to school.

First Contacts

Maria referred Elijah to the early intervention (EI) team because of her concerns (and those of his teacher) that he was not talking and not very interested in playing with toys. Because the EI team believed in making strong and early connections with the family, one of the team members, Felicia, contacted Elijah's mother. Felicia was chosen because of her expertise in speech-language pathology and the fact that language was one of Maria's major concerns. After talking briefly with Maria, it was clear that Maria was interested in having Elijah assessed by the EI team. Felicia explained that the team's approach included having a preassessment planning meeting the first week with her and an assessment of Elijah the next week. She told Felicia about the purpose of the planning meeting and said that it could also include Elijah and that Maria could identify any others she wanted to attend (e.g., family/friends close to her, other professionals). Felicia told Maria about the various disciplines represented in their EI program and gave Maria the choice of meeting with one professional or the whole team. Maria said she would like to meet with the whole team because she wanted to see what the others thought of Elijah's delays. She also seemed pleased that she could ask her mother and sister to be there because she said both were important in her and Elijah's lives. Felicia asked Maria whether she would like the team to come to her house or meet at the EI center. Maria indicated that their house was rather small and that it might be more comfortable at the EI center. Once they had agreed on a date, Felicia asked Maria if she would complete a developmental and medical history form about Elijah that would come in the mail. Felicia also said that she would send Maria a list of the professionals who would be at the meeting and their disciplines so that Maria, Beba, Eva, and Elijah would know who to expect. She also told Maria about what they would talk about in the upcoming meeting (e.g., Elijah's medical and developmental history, Maria's and others' concerns and what they wanted to get from the assessment, what Elijah could do well and liked, his challenges, and planning for the assessment) and said she would send a brief overview of these questions to Maria.

Preassessment Meeting

On the day of the preassessment planning meeting, the team met Elijah, Maria, Beba, and Eva in a room in the EI center that was set up as a small living area (e.g., carpeted room with couch, chairs, coffee table, book and toy shelf). After introductions and settling Elijah on the floor with some toys near Maria and Beba (Eva sat on the floor with him), Felicia began the information gathering part of the meeting focusing on Elijah's birth, medical, and developmental histories and current skills across all domains. During the meeting, a couple of the professionals also joined into the play with Elijah to help him become more familiar with them and they with him. Felicia then began to find out the family's perceptions of Elijah's strengths, likes, dislikes, challenges, and their concerns and priorities.

Throughout the preassessment meeting, the team gathered information from all three of Elijah's caregivers, being sure to acknowledge Maria as the key decision-maker, but also to make sure that Beba and Eva felt fully part of the process. For example, when asking questions about Elijah (e.g., "What do you think his greatest strengths/challenges are"? "What kinds of things would you like to see him be able to do that he isn't doing now?"), the team typically asked Maria first and then would address Beba and Eva and ask their thoughts as well. As with most families, although there were many similarities in their ideas and opinions, there were sometimes differences. For example, whereas Maria felt that Elijah's talking was the most important thing he needed to learn to do, his grandmother felt strongly that he needed to be better behaved and be able to do what she asked him to do without having to tell him or show him what to do. Eva, on the other hand, was most worried about Elijah's play skills compared to their little cousin who was the same age.

For the next phase of the meeting, Richard, the early childhood special educator, described to the family the options for the assessment such as using formal versus informal or a combination of approaches, whether including a hearing testing was something they wanted, whether Maria, Beba, and Eva would be willing to play with Elijah to show the team how best to interact with him, whether they would like to complete a parent report tool related to Elijah's skills (and/or ask the teacher to do the same), and were there other locations that would be best for the team to observe Elijah (e.g., early care center, home). Maria and Beba thought that Elijah might do best in the more informal approach the team offered. All three family members said they would be happy to play with Elijah during the assessment and help in any way they could. They liked the idea of taking home a tool to use to observe Elijah's behaviors and think of how he gets along in daily routines, and they welcomed the ideas of having the early care teacher be a part of the assessment process and someone from the team meeting with her and observing Elijah. They also said that having Elijah's hearing tested would be a good idea and something they hadn't thought of having done.

After everyone had talked about the options for the assessment and had created a list of what would take place, Elizabeth, the psychologist, asked the family's advice about the order of the activities for the day. At first, Maria said she was willing to go along with whatever the professionals thought, but when Elizabeth followed up by asking which of the listed items would make Elijah initially feel more comfortable, Maria immediately said playing with her. She suggested she begin playing with Elijah to "warm him up" and then the professionals could ease into the picture and begin some of their assessments. When asked about when to do the hearing testing, Maria suggested that it might go better a little later in the morning so that Elijah would be more comfortable with them. Maria agreed to bring a snack for Elijah and a few of his favorite toys. She also said she would talk to the director and Elijah's teachers of his early care center about the upcoming classroom observation and discussion.

Toward the end of the meeting, the professionals reiterated the order of the activities, indicated the approximate amount of time the process would take, and talked about what the "sharing" meeting after the assessment would entail. They closed by asking the family if there was anything else they had not had a chance to talk about. Overall, all three family members were concerned that it may be hard to assess Elijah as "he doesn't like sitting in one place and doesn't follow directions very well." Indeed, the professionals had noticed that Elijah spent most of the time moving about the room, mouthing and banging the toys, and making sing-song vocalizations to himself. Eva was only able to engage him on a few occasions with some blocks and a pop-up toy, and similarly the professionals had difficulty maintaining his engagement. He enjoyed peek-a-boo and several toys with lights or sounds, but became frustrated easily when others tried to take turns with him. The team members assured all three family members that they were primarily interested in knowing more about Elijah and they were used to tailoring the assessment process to each child.

Benefits of Preassessment Planning

For Elijah, meeting the team and becoming familiar with them, their center, and their toys before the assessment, potentially increased the likelihood that he would be more comfortable the next week when he returned for the assessment. For his family, it gave them an opportunity to meet and talk with the team in an informal setting and to be a central part of the planning and decision making for his assessment. In addition, it allowed them time between the preassessment and assessment to document Elijah's behaviors and performance in daily routines and to think about some of the questions raised in the planning meeting (e.g., what are Elijah's major strengths and challenges, what are their priorities for Elijah). For the team, having a week between gave them time to gather additional information needed (e.g., get reports from the social services caseworker the family had seen, perform observations of Elijah in his early care classroom, talk with his teachers). Furthermore, it facilitated building a relationship with Elijah and his family. Seeing what skills Elijah demonstrated in this "low pressure" setting, was a big help in knowing what types of activities to include and in what ways the team members could get the best from him (and observe his challenges) in the assessment. Finally, this preassessment approach also allowed the team to see two families each morning (i.e., 8:00–9:15 AM preassessment with one child and family, 9:30–11:30 AM assessment with the child and family from the previous week's preassessment planning meeting) and thus make effective use of their time together each week.

A few days after the meeting, Felicia observed Elijah in his early care center during snack time, free play, and story time. She also had a chance to talk with Elijah's primary teacher. The teacher reported that Elijah rarely communicated with the teachers or children; he often wandered around the room (even during story time) and only played with toys for short periods of time. Felicia observed that the only times that he seemed engaged were when one of the teachers played a chase game with him or when she changed his diapers and sang to him and tickled him. During snack time, he typically "grazed" by walking by the table and picking up cookies and later some juice, but generally roamed about the room. The teacher indicated that she was very concerned about his seeming lack of comprehension of the classroom routines or what others were saying to him.

The Assessment

On the day of the assessment, once everyone was settled in the assessment room, the team asked the family to talk about their observations during the week and the parent-report tool they had completed. Maria noted that after last week's discussions, completing the forms, and watching Elijah at home this week, all three of them were much more aware of how little he seemed to understand what was said to him. They indicated that they generally have to lead him by the hand to perform tasks, but when they show him what to do, he is more cooperative. When Maria played with Elijah she said that she had tried some of the things she had seen one of the team members doing such as giving him choices between two things or holding objects up a bit higher and closer to her face so that he would reach for them and look at her. She said that she already felt that she was better at interacting with him just from watching the professionals the week before. Because the professionals had spent time with Elijah the week before and had read Felicia's and the teachers' observations of Elijah in his classroom, they were able to tailor the assessment to his special needs and challenges. A good part of their interactions with him were to find out what things he did understand and could indicate, and to try to identify what activities and materials might engage him. Throughout the activities, Maria, Beba, and Eva were invited to participate and to try out some new strategies to engage Elijah. Although they were more hesitant in the beginning, especially Beba, by the later part of the assessment they had each tried out one to two new strategies with Elijah and seen some success.

After the assessment phase was completed, the family was reminded that the professionals would take some time to each compile their individual thoughts and the family could take a break and have the snack Maria had brought. During the sharing meeting, one of the team members played with Elijah in another room so that his family members could be free to focus on the information and generation of ideas. The discussion began with the suggestion that everyone contribute their ideas about Elijah's skills and behaviors, his strengths, and later his challenges. Felicia made sure to seek Maria, Beba, and Eva's perceptions of how they viewed Elijah during these discussions. As different behaviors were raised across domains, the professionals added in their comments and observations about his skills and challenges. Thus, although each team member talked briefly about Elijah's skills related to their specific domain, they only covered the high points without going into great detail about the tests utilized or all the individual scores. As the professionals talked about Elijah's skills across domains, each team member made sure to check out the family members' perceptions about what they had said using clarification questions such as "Does that information fit with how you see Elijah?" or "Did any of that information surprise you?" They also used example behaviors from what the family had reported and what had been seen during the assessment to illustrate their comments. Finally, the group began to discuss options for Elijah and to identify what his family preferred. The team then began to plan with the family for the next steps for Elijah and them. Maria was also given the choice of looking over a draft of the written report before it was finalized and although she initially said that wasn't necessary, Eva spoke up and said "Yes, I think all three of us would like to see it, so why don't you send it to us." Felicia said she would contact Maria a week or so after the report was sent out to see if there were any additions/modifications that she, Beba, or Eva felt were important to include.

Conclusion

As indicated throughout this chapter, the assessment of young children is a prime opportunity to set the stage for upcoming interactions and relationships with families. It is a time to gather broad input to the assessment process, to engage family members and other caregivers to the degree they feel comfortable and supported, and, most importantly, to provide families with the kinds of information necessary for them to be effective decision-makers regarding their child's best interests. The principles of family-centered practices can only be realized fully when families have the choices and the information to make those choices in partnership with the professionals who serve them. The assessment process can be an excellent starting point on that path.

References

Able-Boone, H., Goodwin, L., Sandall, S., Gordon, N., & Martin, D. (1992). Consumer based early intervention services. *Journal of Early Intervention, 16*(3), 201–209.

Able-Boone, H., Sandall, S. R., Loughry, A., & Frederick, L. L. (1990). An informed, family-centered approach to public law 99-457: Parental views. *Topics in Early Childhood Special Education, 10*(1), 100–111.

Bailey, D. B. (1991). *Family orientation of community and agency services.* Chapel Hill: University of North Carolina at Chapel Hill.

Bailey, D. B. (2004). Assessing family resources, priorities, and concerns. In M. McLean, M. Wolery, & D. Bailey (Eds.), *Assessing infants and preschoolers with special needs* (3rd ed., pp. 172-203). Upper Saddle River, NJ: Pearson Merrill Prentice-Hall.

Barrera, I. & Corso, R. (2002). Cultural competency as skilled dialogue. *Topics in Early Childhood Special Education, 22*(20), 103-113.

Beukelman, D. & Mirenda, P. (2005). *Augmentative and alternative communication: Supporting children and adults with complex communication needs* (3rd ed.). Baltimore: Paul H. Brookes.

Boone, H., & Crais, E. (1999). Strategies for achieving family-driven assessment and intervention planning. *Young Exceptional Children, 3*(1), 2-12.

Bruder, M. B. (2000). Family-centered early intervention: Clarifying our values for the new millennium. *Topics in Early Childhood Special Education, 20*(2), 105-115.

Crais, E. (1996a). Applying family-centered principles to child assessment. In P. McWilliam, P. Winton, & E. Crais (Eds.), *Practical strategies for family-centered early intervention* (pp. 69-96). Baltimore: Paul H. Brookes.

Crais, E. (1996b). Preassessment planning with caregivers. *Asha, 34,* 38-39.

Crais, E., Boone, H., Harrison, M., Freund, P., Downing, K., & West, T. (2004). Interdisciplinary personnel preparation: Graduates' use of targeted practices. *Infants and Young Children, 17*(2), 82-92.

Crais, E., Poston Roy, V., & Free, K. (2006). Parents' and professionals' perceptions of the implementation of family-centered practices in child assessments. *American Journal of Speech-Language Pathology, 15*(4), 365-377.

Dunst, C., Trivette, C., & Deal, A. (1988). *Enabling and empowering families.* Cambridge, MA: Brookline Books.

Linder, T. (1993). *Transdisciplinary play-based assessment* (rev. ed.). Baltimore: Paul H. Brookes.

Linder, T. (2008). *Transdisciplinary play-based assessment* (2nd ed.). Baltimore: Paul H. Brookes.

McLean, M., & Crais, E. (2004). Procedural considerations in assessing infants and toddlers with disabilities. In M. McLean, M. Wolery, & D. Bailey (Eds.), *Assessing infants and preschoolers with special needs* (3rd ed., pp. 45-70). Upper Saddle River, NJ: Pearson Merrill Prentice-Hall.

McWilliam, R. A., Synder, P., Harbin, G., Porter, P., & Munn, D. (2000). Professionals' and families' perceptions of family-centered practices in infant-toddler services. *Early Education and Development, 11*(4), 519-538.

Mellon, A. & Winton, P. (2003). Interdisciplinary collaboration among early intervention faculty members. *Journal of Early Intervention, 25*(3), 173-188.

Summers, J., Hoffman, L., Marquis, J., Turnbull, A., & Poston, D. (2005). Relationship between parent satisfaction regarding partnerships with professionals and age of child. *Topics in Early Childhood Special Education, 25*(1), 48-58.

Watts Pappas, N. (2007). *Parental involvement in intervention for speech impairment.* Unpublished doctoral dissertation, Charles Sturt University, Bathurst, Australia.

Chapter 5

Working with Families of Young Children with Communication and Language Impairments: Intervention

Luigi Girolametto and Elaine Weitzman

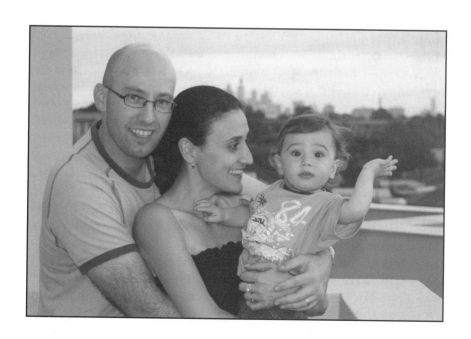

Research: Historical Overview of Family Involvement in Young Children with Communication and Language Impairments

Language is the most important developmental skill children must master in the preschool years. Developmental language disorders can be defined as overall delay in receptive and/or expressive language development relative to other developmental areas, and is the most common single difficulty in the preschool years, affecting approximately 7% of children at the age of 4 years. Language disorders place children at risk for long-term social, emotional, and academic difficulties (Beitchman et al., 2001; Johnson et al., 1999). Many types of language intervention programs exist to prevent or ameliorate the symptoms of this condition. These programs vary considerably in terms of the service delivery method and may include direct intervention by a speech-language pathologist (for individual children or groups of children) or indirect intervention in which the speech-language pathologist trains a caregiver to conduct intervention (e.g., parents, early childhood educators). As services for children have shifted to earlier identification and treatment, parental involvement has become a key component of all early language intervention programs for young children. On a practical level, parental involvement provides continuity of intervention from the school/clinic into the home environment, generalization of communication and language skills learned in the school/clinic setting to the home environment, motivation for the child to communicate in naturalistic activities, and ongoing intervention once direct therapy has ended. Recent legislation in the United States has mandated the involvement of parents in the decision-making processes about intervention in the Individuals with Disabilities Education Act (IDEA) Amendments of 2004, which prescribes the provision of prevention and intervention programs in the child's natural environment (Paul-Brown & Caperton, 2001). IDEA has the following goals: (a) to improve the development of infants and toddlers with disabilities; (b) to reduce educational costs by minimizing the need for special education through early intervention; and (c) to enhance the capacity of families to meet their child's needs, and "to the maximum extent appropriate, provide early intervention services in the natural environments" (IDEA Part C Section 635). This chapter focuses on parent-focused intervention for children with language disorders in which parents' involvement in the intervention process is designed to equip them to become the primary change agents for their children. A range of parent-administered intervention approaches are briefly summarized. In the latter section of this chapter, the content and focus of It Takes Two to Talk®—The Hanen Program® for Parents (Pepper & Weitzman, 2004) is described, along with the research evidence supporting this parent-focused intervention approach.

Historical Overview

In the 1970s, there were few reports of parent programs for children with language disorders. The programs that were published, and included outcome data, ranged from behavioral interventions that taught parents to use stimulus-response-reinforcement techniques to social-interactive programs that taught parents to model communication and language in naturalistic activities. One behavioral program was the Environmental Language Intervention Strategy (ELI) (MacDonald, Blott, Gordon, Spiegel, & Hartmann, 1974; MacDonald & Presser Blott, 1974). The ELI program taught parents to use behavioral techniques to promote receptive language, expressive vocabulary, and two-word utterances in young children with developmental and language disorders. The outcome data indicated that children participating in this program increased their expressive language skills in the areas targeted (i.e., 2- and 3-word semantic relations). However, interpretation of the data is limited by the small sample size (i.e., three children in the experimental group). The 1970s also witnessed several published reports of parent programs for children with developmental disorders that ascribed to a social-interactionist perspective. These naturalistic interventions taught parents to use a greater frequency of responsive language input and the results for children included increased talkativeness and mean length of utterance (Cheseldine & McConkey, 1979; Seitz, 1975). In this latter approach, parents were taught to engage their children in conversation and model language at their level during these interactions. Unfortunately, these studies used pretest-posttest designs and the lack of stringent methodologies, such as randomization or control groups, precluded the conclusion that the treatments played a causal role in accelerating the children's language development. Nonetheless, growing awareness of the potential for parents to become therapeutic agents in language intervention gained momentum.

The 1980s saw a proliferation of published reports about parent involvement in language intervention for children with developmental and/or language disorders. Concurrently, psychologists were examining the effectiveness of teaching parents behavioral strategies to ameliorate the behaviors of children with conduct problems (e.g., McMahon & Forehand, 1983), thereby providing collateral support for parent-administered interventions in related disciplines. Model parent programs designed to facilitate language intervention included the Transactional Intervention Program (Mahoney & Powell, 1988), the Conversational Engineering Program (MacDonald & Gillette, 1984), It Takes Two to Talk (Manolson, 1985), and the Language Interaction Intervention Program (Weistuch & Brown, 1987; Weistuch & Lewis, 1985). Most of these aforementioned programs adhered to a naturalistic model of intervention that taught parents to (a) use everyday contexts for promoting language development, (b) model language that is highly responsive to the children's interests, and (c) reduce directive interactions. One exception was the Milieu Teaching approach (for a review, see Warren & Kaiser, 1986), which maintained its focus on behavioral strategies, instructing parents how to capitalize on children's communicative initiations to elicit language using mand-model, shaping, and reinforcement procedures. Some reports of children's outcomes were still plagued with methodological issues that did not permit causal interpretation (e.g., Mahoney & Powell, 1988; McConkey & O'Connor, 1982). However, more stringent methodologies (e.g., control groups, single-subject designs) appeared in some published reports, permitting researchers to conclude that parent-administered language intervention resulted in positive changes in children's language development. For example, Weistuch and colleagues reported increases in the mean length of utterance and use of multiword utterances in children with language disorders relative to an untreated control group (Weistuch & Brown, 1987; Weistuch, Lewis, & Sullivan, 1991). Girolametto and colleagues (Girolametto, 1988; Tannock et al., 1992) reported increases in social-communication skills and social participation in interaction for children with developmental disorders relative to a waiting list control group. Table 5–1 provides a brief description of parent programs and children's outcomes.

Table 5–1. Description of Parent-Administered Language Intervention Programs

Description of Program	Author/Year	Target Children	Results
Early Parent Programs—1970s			
Environmental Language Intervention (ELI) Strategy Phase 1 = 7 week individual training period, twice weekly with clinicians and parents working together with the child. Phase 2 = 6 months of home sessions by parents, 3 times per week; with monthly follow-up meetings with clinicians	MacDonald et al. (1974)	Children with developmental disabilities, 3–5 years of age	Children increased their MLU (words), frequency of multiword utterances, and use of semantic-grammatical rules relative to a control group.
Parent-Child Language Intervention Program One hour a day, 3 days per week for 8 weeks; during the first 6 sessions, the parents observed graduate students modeling strategies with their children	Seitz (1975)	Children had MLUs of 1.0 to 1.5 words and were between 27 to 41 months of age	Children increased the total number of utterances, MLU from pretest to post-test. The lack of a control group makes interpretation of findings difficult.
Putting Two Words Together Training occurred once a week for 7 weeks	Cheseldine & McConkey (1979)[1] McConkey, Jeffree, & Hewson (1979)[2]	Used with children who have developmental disabilities (e.g., Down syndrome) and are beginning to combine words into two word phrases	[1,2]Children increased their frequency of word combinations and vocabulary diversity from pre- to post-test. The lack of a control group makes interpretation of findings difficult.

continues

Table 5–1. *continued*

Description of Program	Author/Year	Target Children	Results
	Later Parent Programs—1980s		
Putting Two Words Together Training occurred once a week for 7 weeks	McConkey & O'Connor (1982)	Used with children who have developmental disabilities (e.g., Down syndrome) and are beginning to combine words into two word phrases	Children increased their frequency of word combinations and vocabulary diversity from pre- to post-test, replicating previous results. The lack of a control group makes interpretation of findings difficult.
Language Interaction Intervention Project Option 1: weekly 2-hour parent group workshops for a total of 8 weeks Option 2: 20 1-hour workshops (held 2–4 times per week); during parent workshops, children participated in groups lead by a speech-language pathologist; workshops ended with a 1-hour parent-child practice session.	Weistuch & Lewis (1985)[1] Weistuch, & Brown (1987)[2] Weistuch, Lewis, & Sullivan (1991)[3]	Designed for preschoolers aged 2-5 years with language disorders and an MLU of 1.0–3.0	[1]No changes were noted in the language and communication of children with handicaps relative to controls; authors hypothesize that an intervention longer than 8 weeks is required. [2,3]Children in a 20-session program increased their MLU and multiword utterances relative to controls.
It Takes Two to Talk® *(ITTT— General Stimulation Model* Training occurred once a week for 11 weeks groups of up to 8 families; included 8 evening sessions and 3 video-feedback sessions; sessions were 2.5 hours long and video-feedback was 1 hour	Girolametto (1988)[1] Tannock et al. (1992)[2] Girolametto et al. (1993)[3]	Used with preschool-aged children with various etiologies: developmental delay	[1,2]Parent training using a "general stimulation model" promoted social conversational skills relative to untreated control groups, but did not promote language development. [3]Parents who received intervention gave a positive consumer evaluation of the program format and content.

Table 5–1. *continued*

Description of Program	Author/Year	Target Children	Results
Transactional Intervention Program Weekly home visits from teacher consultants. The intervention period ranged from 5 to 24 months	Mahoney & Powell (1988)	Children were between 2 and 32 months of age and had developmental disabilities	Gain was measured using the Bayley Scales of Infant Development. The overall gain of the children was equivalent to their rate of development prior to the intervention. The lack of a control group makes interpretation of findings difficult.
Later Parent Programs with Supportive Research—1990s			
It Takes Two to Talk® *(ITTT)—Focused Stimulation Model* Training occurred once a week for 11 weeks groups of up to 8 families; included 8 evening sessions and 3 video-feedback sessions; sessions were 2.5 hours long and video-feedback was one hour	Baxendale & Hesketh (2003)[1] Girolametto et al. (1998)[2] Girolametto et al. (1996a, 1996b, 1997)[3]	Used with preschool-aged children with various etiologies: developmental delay[4], Down syndrome[2], language disorders of no known etiology[1], late talking toddlers[3]	[1]Parent training was as effective as direct treatment from a clinician; no untreated controls. [2,3]Parent training using focused stimulation promoted children's vocabulary, speech sound development, and utterance length in comparison to untreated control groups.
Focused Stimulation Training occurred once a week for 12 weeks and once a month for another 2 months; sessions were 2 hours long; each family received three home visits during the 12 weeks and two individual clinic visits during the last 2 months	Fey et al. (1993)	Used with preschool children with a focus on morpho-syntactic targets	Parent training was as effective as direct treatment from a clinician and both were more effective than untreated controls. However, treatment effects were more consistent in the clinician-administered treatment. Children made gains in syntax as measured by DSS total score and DSS subcategories (main verb, sentence score).

continues

Table 5–1. *continued*

Description of Program	Author/Year	Target Children	Results
Parent Group Language Intervention 11 sessions of group language training, once every 2 weeks for 6 months	Gibbard (1994)	Children were between 2;3 and 3;3 years of age and had a 30-word vocabulary size or less; no developmental delay	Children in the experimental group made significant changes in expressive language relative to controls; parent-administered intervention was as effective as clinician-administered intervention; children were matched across groups for gender, birth order, socioeconomic status, and parent and child age.
Enhanced Milieu Teaching (EMT) Parent training ranged from 20 to 36 individual parent sessions in order for parents to reach criterion on all components of EMT; sessions were ¾ to 1 hour long	Hemmeter & Kaiser (1994)[1] Kaiser & Hancock (2000)[2]	Used with preschool-aged children who are (a) verbally imitative, (b) produce at least 10 productive words, and (c) have MLUs between 1.0 and 3.5.	[1]Parent training had positive effects on spontaneous word use, receptive language, and target use in a multiple baseline subject design. [2]Parent training was as effective as therapist-administered intervention for teaching language targets (MLU, productive syntax, receptive vocabulary). However, at the 6-month follow-up, parent training yielded better results for expressive language.

Table 5–1. *continued*

Description of Program	Author/Year	Target Children	Results
Ecological Communication Organization (ECO) Program Biweekly, individual sessions of 1.5 hours for 6 months; followed by 3 monthly post-treatment sessions	MacDonald & Wilkening (1994)	Children were from 23–64 months of age and had developmental disabilities; communication skills were delayed by at least 1 year with significant delays in one other area of development	Children improved in their turn-taking skills and overall ability to communicate with others. The lack of control makes interpretation of findings difficult.
Responsive Teaching Weekly 1-hour individual parent-child sessions over a 1-year period (average 33 sessions per year)	Mahoney & Perales (2005)	Children were approximately 2 years old and had delays in cognitive and/or language development. Mean expressive language age was 12 months.	Children with developmental disorders increased their rates of cognitive, language, and socioemotional development over baseline. The lack of control makes interpretation of findings difficult.
Responsivity Education and Prelinguistic Milieu Teaching Parents were taught to use responsive interaction techniques from It Takes Two to Talk; 12 sessions: 4 were group sessions and 8 were individual sessions Children received direct treatment from clinicians using prelinguistic milieu teaching procedures	Yoder & Warren (2002)	Toddlers with intellectual disabilities who used fewer than 10 nonimitative words	Treatment accelerated growth of child-initiated comments, child-initiated requests, and lexical density in subgroups of children (namely children with low frequency of comments and canonical vocal communication at entry and children without Down syndrome).

The 1990s witnessed three distinct trends in the parent training literature. First, there was a move toward increasing the naturalness of language intervention strategies in many program packages. For example, Mahoney and colleagues developed the Relationship-focused Intervention Program for parents (Mahoney, Wiggers, & Lash, 1996). This parent program was based on the Transactional Intervention Program but extended the naturalness further by (a) increasing the repertoire of parental responsive behaviors it taught and (b) linking specific responsive strategies to pivotal child development behaviors, thus making intervention targets for parents and children clearer and more cohesive (Mahoney & Perales, 2005). Kaiser and Hester (1994) redeveloped Milieu Teaching into an innovative model called Enhanced Milieu Teaching that included responsive interaction strategies within the intervention package. Concurrently, Yoder and Warren (2002) included responsive interaction strategies in the original Milieu Teaching approach that they used with prelinguistic children. The aim of adding responsive strategies to the behavioral teaching techniques of Enhanced Milieu Teaching and Milieu Teaching (e.g., mand-model, elicitative imitation) was to maximize the child's language learning in naturalistic interactions across the day. Both milieu treatments were found to be effective in increasing children's communication skills (Kaiser & Hester, 1994; Yoder & Warren, 2002), but the independent contribution of responsive interaction on the children's outcomes could not be determined. A second trend was seen in the increasing stringency of evaluation studies. Consistent with the prevailing demands of clinical services to adopt evidence-based practices, there was a greater interest in submitting parent programs to stringent methodologies that permitted causal conclusions about the effects of intervention on language development. Consequently, there was an escalation in research studies that used stringent methodologies with sufficient experimental control to conclude that parent training was an effective treatment for children with language disorders (e.g., Fey, Cleave, Long, & Hughes, 1993; Girolametto, Pearce, & Weitzman, 1996b; Kaiser & Hester, 1994). The third trend observed in the literature was a move beyond questions of simple efficacy. Some research reports began to question the differential efficiency of parent training versus traditional clinician-administered therapy (Baxendale & Hesketh, 2003; Fey et al., 1993; Gibbard, 1994). Taken together, the findings of these latter studies reported that parent-focused intervention produced higher gains in language development compared to untreated control groups and was at least as effective as clinician-centered treatment. Indeed, Gibbard's study illustrated that the effects of parent-administered intervention produced better results than clinician-administered treatment. Other research groups examined the effects of program modifications designed to increase the effectiveness of parent programs while seeking to add to the evidence-base of support for parent involvement. Girolametto et al. (1997) added a focused stimulation strategy to It Takes Two to Talk® (Manolson, 1992), building on previous research suggesting that this model did not produce changes in language development. The addition of focused stimulation resulted in highly significant differences in vocabulary, morphosyntax, and phonology in a group of late talkers relative to an untreated control group (Girolametto et al., 1996b, 1997). Moreover, as mentioned previously, the Milieu Teaching model was enhanced by the addition of responsive interaction strategies within the treatment package. The results of studies on milieu teaching indicated that prelinguistic children increased their use of requests and lexical density (Yoder & Warren, 2002) and linguistic children increased their use of language targets, word use, and receptive language skills (Hemmeter & Kaiser, 1994). Finally, consistent with the trend to go beyond accounts of efficacy, the collateral benefits associated with parent training were beginning to be reported, such as decreased parenting stress, satisfaction with services, and more synchronous parent-child relationships (Girolametto, Tannock, & Siegel, 1993; Tannock, Girolametto, & Siegel, 1992).

At present, parent-focused intervention programs are considered to be conventional approaches for the provision of indirect speech and language services. A recent review of mainstream language interventions by McCauley and Fey (2006) included many parent-administered intervention programs as viable models of treatment for young children with language disorders (e.g., It Takes Two to Talk®, Enhanced Milieu Teaching, Responsivity Education/Prelinguistic Milieu Teaching). Unfortunately, none of the studies reviewed above included information about the longer term effects of intervention on the children's communication and language abilities. Nonetheless, parent training is viewed by increasing numbers of clinicians and administrators as a feasible, practical, and family-centered model of intervention. As evidence, approximately 15,000 speech-language pathologists worldwide have been certified by The Hanen Centre to provide It Takes Two to Talk®—The Hanen Program® for Parents; approximately 1,200 additional clinicians receive this training on an annual basis.

Therapist-Centered Approaches

Therapist-centered approaches to language intervention are commonly used in speech-language pathology settings (Paul, 2007). In therapist-centered approaches, the speech-language pathologist assumes the major responsibility for assessment and intervention planning. The clinician is responsible for selecting and implementing goals, strategies, and activities and for communicating these to parents. However, parents are not regarded as the primary change agents and there is limited opportunity for them to (a) provide input into the assessment and treatment planning process and (b) learn and practice intervention strategies 95 the majority of therapy time is taken up by the clinician providing direct treatment for the child. Clinicians seeking evidence for treatment efficacy often find that therapist-centered approaches are commonly used in research reports. In such cases, researchers utilize clinicians as intervention agents to provide a consistent treatment regimen (Warren, 1992; Wilcox, Kouri, & Caswell, 1991; Yoder & Warren, 1998) and measure child change following a standard treatment protocol. Typically, parents are not involved in the intervention. For example, in a study by Best, Melvin, and Williams (1993), the efficacy of group intervention was examined in a nursery school setting where the intervention was provided by clinicians; parents were not involved. The results indicated that children in the experimental group performed better on language measures than untreated controls at post-test. In a second example (Robertson & Ellis Weismer, 1999), toddlers were seen in groups of four for script-based therapy that focused on enhancing vocabulary and word-combining skills. In comparison to a no-intervention control group, children in the experimental group made gains in oral language as well as in social development (e.g., participating in games with others, imitating others, sharing toys, taking turns in games). Once again, parents were uninvolved in this intervention, which was administered by a clinician. Such reports provide a trial of the intervention techniques and are an important first step before intervention is tested with parents as the intervention agent. Unfortunately, they do not provide guidance regarding the role of parents or if parents can successfully implement the procedures themselves.

In other studies, parents may not be involved in the intervention but may be utilized to provide a measure of generalization of newly learned skills within the home environment. Wilcox et al. (1991) examined the efficacy of a clinician-administered intervention in the context of parent-child interaction in the home. In this study, group language intervention was compared to individual intervention for preschool children at the one-word stage of language development. Both interventions were equally effective in promoting vocabulary development, but the group intervention program yielded better rates of generalization to the home environment, presumably because group practice facilitated carryover to other conversation partners. A second example is a study by Yoder and Warren (1998) in which the intervention was offered by research staff and child outcomes were examined within the context of mother-child interactions to determine if children's gains were associated with higher rates of responsive interaction from their mothers. This study indicated that increases in intentional communication generalized from training sessions and trainers to mothers in naturalistic environments. Moreover, mothers who were highly responsive at pretreatment had children who made the greatest gains in intentional communication in milieu teaching sessions.

As discussed above, several studies compare outcomes of therapist-centered treatment with parent-centred treatment (Baxendale & Hesketh, 2003; Fey et al., 1993; Gibbard, 1994). In these studies, children in both types of interventions made equivalent gains in language development. However, Fey et al. (1993) concluded that more consistent treatment effects were displayed by children in the clinician-administered intervention than in the parent-administered intervention. Baxendale and Hesketh (2003) reported that children with receptive *and* expressive language disorders made greater changes in the parent-administered intervention than children with expressive language disorders. The latter group of children had better language outcomes in the clinician-administered intervention. Finally, Gibbard noted that children receiving parent-administered treatment made greater changes than those receiving clinician-administered treatment. Clearly, more research is needed in this area to delineate the families and contexts for which parent-focused approaches may be most beneficial.

In summary, it appears that therapist-centered interventions continue play an important role in the provision of services to children with language disorders. They are useful in research program and may necessary for families who are unable or unwilling to participate.

However, given recent philosophical trends towards family-centered treatment, it would appear that parental involvement in some form should be a key feature of treatment (Paul, 2007).

Parent-as-Aide Approaches

In interventions that utilize parents as aides, children receive direct intervention from the speech-language pathologist and parents may play a secondary or supportive role. Parental involvement may consist of observation of all or part of the therapy session, participation in conducting activities during the session, verbal and/or written guidance regarding how to facilitate generalization of the child's newly learned skills, or the completion of home practice assignments. Clinically, the use of parents as aides extends the "dosage" of language intervention within the treatment session or in the home environment. For example, in some cases, the parent may be required to conduct activities alongside the clinician with the expectation that the parent will eventually continue to conduct the activity in a similar way in the home. Alternatively, at the end of a session, parents may be prescribed home practice activities that extend the therapy into the child's home and daily activities. There are no extant studies that have examined the impact of parent home practice versus no home practice on the child's language development. Indeed, an important research agenda would be to determine the extent to which home programs are utilized by parents and whether they are effective.

Family-Centered Approaches

Family-centered intervention recognizes the child as part of a dynamic social system and the family as the most important element in a child's life. This philosophical orientation recognizes the interrelatedness of the family system in that any action or event affecting one member of the family unit affects them all (e.g., Donahue-Kilburg, 1992). The family is a critical part of any early intervention as it is widely recognized that without family involvement, intervention is unlikely to be successful and any short-term positive effects erode quite rapidly (Bronfenbrenner, 1974). Thus, family-centered practice provides the support and resources families need to create culturally appropriate learning opportunities and promote the child's development (Dunst, Leet, & Trivette, 1988; Dunst, 2002). Family-centered approaches for language intervention may differ widely in terms of the family's involvement in the intervention program. Negotiation with the family regarding the child's goals, the format, frequency, and location of the intervention program, and the family's level of involvement are important hallmarks of family-centered approaches. Ultimately, the family's needs and goals are essential to the decision-making process. One family-centered model for intervention with young children is parent-focused intervention in which parents become the primary change agents for their children. In this model, the parents themselves are the direct recipients of the speech-language pathologist's efforts and their children do not normally receive therapy from the speech-language pathologist concurrently.

The intervention described in the remainder of this chapter is an indirect service delivery program in which the speech-language pathologist teaches parents of children with language disorders to facilitate language development in naturalistic contexts. Specifically, this report focuses on It Takes Two to Talk®—The Hanen Program® for Parents (Pepper & Weitzman, 2004). This parent-focused intervention program is offered by a Hanen certified speech-language pathologist to groups of eight families and consists of a preprogram assessment, a minimum of 16 hours of group training for parents, and three individual consultations, which include videotaping and feedback. The purpose of this intervention program is to promote adult behaviors that are thought to influence children's developmental progress in prelinguistic aspects of communication (e.g., joint attention/action, intentional communication acts), vocabulary, and early word combinations (including early morphologic development). To accomplish this, parents are taught to use three clusters of responsive strategies: (a) child-centered strategies (e.g., observe, wait, and listen; follow the child's lead), (b) interaction-promoting strategies (e.g., match your child's turn; ask questions that continue the conversation), and (c) language-modeling strategies (e.g., label; expand). In addition to these language facilitation strategies, parents also target specific interaction and communication goals (e.g., prelinguistic skills, vocabulary, two-word phrases) using a focused stimulation procedure in which the target is repeated several times within an interaction (Ellis Weismer & Robertson, 2006; Fey, 1986).

It Takes Two to Talk® reflects a family-centered model of intervention that places intervention within a naturalistic context of the home and daily routines with family members. In the It Takes Two to Talk® Program, the family is considered to be the client and a collaborative, respectful partnership is built with parents, who are acknowledged as knowing their child best. Empowerment of parents involves supporting and strengthening their capacity to access knowledge and gain practical skills, which in turn, bolsters their sense of self-efficacy in relation to fostering their child's development (Dempsey & Dunst, 2004). Therefore, one of the program's aims is to help parents feel more competent in their roles as responsive communication partners and language facilitators. Initially, families are invited to attend an orientation session to learn more about the program's format and content and to obtain information about the required time commitment. Those families who do not wish to be involved may receive regular services, if the agency provides alternative programs (e.g., individual or group language therapy, consultation visits to the child care center, home programs). Parent group sessions are generally held in the evenings to permit working parents to attend. The 2.5-hour group sessions are held weekly and are interspersed with individual home/center visits for videotaping and feedback that are scheduled at the parents' convenience. Children do not attend the group sessions but must be present for the individual home/center consultations.

Theoretically, It Takes Two to Talk® adheres to social interactionist perspectives of language acquisition (Bohannon & Bonvillian, 1997). Instructors apply principles of adult education to teach parents how to use responsive interaction strategies in naturalistic interactions. The parent training sessions are designed to be user friendly, experiential in format, and accommodate a variety of learning styles (e.g., interactive learning, discussion, coaching, and practice). The following description of the content relates program strategies to their base of support in the literature.

Week 1. In the first group session, parents learn about the stages of communication development, which includes information on the importance of nonverbal communication as a developmental precursor to verbal communication. They also learn that positive, reciprocal interactions in everyday conversation and routines provide the content for language learning. In order to facilitate the child's active participation in interactions, the session focuses on facilitating child initiations through heightened sensitivity to all his/her attempts to communicate, both verbal and nonverbal. Strategies taught include: (a) get face to face and (b) observe, wait, and listen to your child.

Strategies such as waiting for the child to initiate set the stage for conversational interactions that are centered on the child's plan-of-the-moment. By increasing their focus on the child's agenda, parents avoid controlling the interaction. Social interactionist theory maintains that children use fewer cognitive resources to attend to child-selected topics, thus making the language input easier to process (e.g., Rocissano & Yatchmink, 1983). The resulting match between the child's interests and the language input permits the child to devote more cognitive resources (e.g., attention, motivation, memory) to the task of language learning.

Week 2. In the second group session, parents learn to follow the child's lead by using responsive strategies, such as: (a) respond immediately with interest, (b) join in and play, (c) imitate what the child says/does, (d) interpret the child's message; and (e) comment on the child's focus. The strategy of following the child's lead by responding immediately with interest is drawn from the literature on contingent responding, which has been shown to increase child initiations (e.g., Rocissano & Yatchmink, 1983) and is inconsistent with intrusive, directive interaction (e.g., Girolametto & Tannock, 1994; Tannock, 1988). Another way to follow the child's lead, imitation, is a strategy that is associated with children's own use of imitation. Chapman found that parents who imitated their children's vocalizations had children who, in turn, were more likely to imitate them (Chapman, 2000; Folger & Chapman, 1978). The value of imitation as a language teaching strategy has long been utilized to promote children's language productivity and grammar in trialled intervention approaches (Connell, 1987; Haley, Camarata, & Nelson, 1994; Tager-Flusberg & Calkins, 1990). The strategy of interpreting has also been used in intervention approaches for prelinguistic children (Yoder, Warren, Kim, & Gazdag, 1994). Interpreting a child's vocal or gestural acts as meaningful provides the child with a word or words that model vocabulary and language that matches his or her focus. Finally, using comments that reflect the child's interests increases responsive language input. Simplified, responsive language input provided by caregivers helps children make comparisons between the nonlinguistic and linguistic contexts and induce the relationships between objects, actions, external events, and words (e.g., Bohannon & Bonvillian, 1997; Bruner, 1975).

Week 3. Following the second group session, parents receive an individual video feedback session that is conducted in the clinic or the family's home. The aim of this session is to give parents an opportunity to practice the strategies they have learned and to receive coaching from the speech-language pathologist to ensure appropriate strategy application. This is the first of three video feedback sessions and the format of all three sessions is similar. Parent-child interaction is video-taped and, during the interaction, the speech-language pathologist provides coaching to help the parent modify her or his interactive behaviour so strategies are applied successfully. It is important for the parent to see a positive impact on the child through successful mod-ification of his/her behavior because a key factor in behavior change is the learner's perception of demonstrable results in relation to change (Guskey, 1986). Once the videotaping is complete, the clinician reviews the videotaped interaction with the parents to identify instances when the strategies were used well and the consequent impact on the child's interactive behaviour, as well as opportunities that were missed.

During this process, the speech-language pathologist aims to build parents' self-awareness and ability to self-evaluate with a view to promoting their ability to integrate newly learned skills into their behavioural repertoire. The approach taken to feedback is adapted to the parents' current level of self-awareness and ability to self-evaluate. For example, a parent may be unaware of exactly what she did differ-ently and what the impact was on the child, despite being coached to use a specific interactive strategy. In this case, it is helpful for the speech-language pathologist to juxtapose the two segments of the videotape (when the parent did not use the strategy versus when she did) and to facilitate an analysis of the differences, with a focus on the differential impact on the child. The speech-language pathologist pauses the videotape frequently, using a process of questioning and reflective listening to facilitate learning. Once parents can clearly see the different in the children's interaction and communication as a result of their own interactive behaviour, their motivation to apply the strategy is far stronger. Seeing the pleasure their child derives from interaction within a simple social routine or how repeated use of labelling enables the child to imitate a word for the first time is a pow-erful reinforcer for parents.

Sometimes, however, long-standing patterns of behavior are hard to change and parents express frustration at how difficult it is to replace old habits with new ones. To help parents self-monitor their interactive behavior, the speech-language pathologist explores the use of metacognitive strategies with them. These strategies, used as mental reminders, are designed to help parents monitor and adapt their interactive behavior. For example, a parent may decide to use the mental reminder, "turn a question into a comment" if he or she finds it difficult to reduce the number of test questions. The speech-language pathologist and parent plan how the parent will remember to use this strategy and how she or he will evaluate whether it was used successfully. By the end of each video feedback session, parents should experience an increased sense of self-awareness and competence in relation to their ability to implement new strategies.

Week 4. In the third group session, parents learn interaction-promoting strategies that prolong conversations, such as (a) using routines to promote conversational turn-taking; (b) matching their turns to the child's turns in terms of topic, length, and number of turns; (c) using cues to encourage the child to take a turn; and (d) asking questions to encourage extended conversations. The aim of these four strategies is to keep the child engaged in conversational interaction and provide multiple opportunities for the child's participation. Questions play a key role in promoting conversational participation because rising question intonation solicits children's attention and explicitly invites young children to take speaker turns. Although the role of the first of these strategies has not been previously investigated, the impact of questions on children's ensuing responses has been examined. For example, Yoder, Davies, Bishop, and Munson (1994) reported that preschool-aged children with developmental delays were more likely to respond to topic-continuing Wh-questions than to topic-continuing comments. Within the ensuing adult-child exchanges, children have opportunities to practice using language, acquire the rules of conversational discourse, and learn from the adult's advanced linguistic models (e.g., Bohannon & Bonvillian, 1997).

Week 5. In the next group session, parents learn to model language at their child's stage of communication by: (a) labeling a shared referent or action, (b) expanding the child's words (by adding a syntactic or semantic element), and (c) highlighting their language by slowing down and using short utterances with exaggerated intonation and visual cues. Labeling is a strategy that provides the child with a referent for an object or action that is within his or her focus. It is an important strategy for teaching children expressive vocabulary (Mervis & Bertrand, 1993; Ninio & Bruner, 1978) and especially powerful when utilized to label objects the child is interested in (Tomasello & Farrar, 1986; Tomasello & Todd, 1983). Expansions (also called recasts) utilize the child's words to create grammatically complete utterances that model the next steps for the child. The Vygotskian concept of the child's "zone of proximal development" (Vygotsky, 1978) suggests that children's learning is optimized when adults start with language models that are at the child's level and progressively model and scaffold language at higher levels as the child's skills improve. Expansions or recasts have been used successfully in previous studies to promote language acquisition in typically developing children as well as children with language disorders (Camarata, Nelson, & Camarata, 1994; Nelson, Camarata, Welsh, Butkovsky, & Camarata, 1996). Highlighting language involves using features of child-directed speech, such as high pitch, slower tempo, and exaggerated intonation (Owens, 2008) that are thought to provide the child with important cues to linguistic boundaries, grammatical classes of words, and even the meanings of novel words (e.g., Bedore & Leonard, 1995).

Week 6. In this group session, parents learn how to promote the child's receptive language skills. For children who are verbal and whose receptive language skills are not significantly delayed, there is instruction on how to model language that extends the conversation beyond the "here and now" by using decontextualized language. Decontextualized language includes talk about the past or future, abstract events, and objects that are removed from the immediate context (Westby, 1991). Linguistic interactions centered on past or future events provide opportunities for adults to model abstract language that links the current conversation to past events, make inferences about others' emotions, or offer predictions about future events. As children's language and thinking skills develop, adults may scaffold their verbal participation at increasingly higher levels of abstraction, withdrawing support when children are able to make decontextualized observations on their own. Such ability has been linked to advanced language skills (van Kleeck, Gillam, Hamilton, & McGrath, 1997; van Kleeck, Vander Woude, & Hammett, 2006). Parents also learn to "add language in two ways," first by providing a model to extend the child's expessive language skills and then adding information designed to foster receptive language, the latter involving use of longer and more complex sentences. For example, if a child is dragging a heavy bag along the ground and says, "Evi," the parent responds, "Heavy. Yes, that bag is very heavy (expanding). You have to be strong to carry such a heavy bag" (adds information to foster receptive language).

Week 7. In the seventh week, receive a second video feedback session that is similar to the first in terms of format. The videotaped interaction is reviewed with the aim of providing parents feedback on the strategies learned in the preceding two group sessions.

Weeks 8 through 11. The remaining three evening sessions and individual video feedback session include information on books, play, and music. In each session, the key intervention strategies are reviewed to emphasize how they are used in each of these three contexts. The focus is on developing a conversational interaction during books, play, and music so that the child is participating fully as a partner and exposed to increased opportunities to practice conversational interaction and learn language. A video feedback session is provided in the second last session to help parents consolidate the skills they have learned.

Evidence Base of Effectiveness of Family Involvement

It Takes Two to Talk® has been the focus of numerous evaluations that have demonstrated the efficacy of parent-focused intervention on children's communication and language outcomes. This intervention program has been used effectively with late-talking toddlers, preschool-aged children with cognitive and developmental delays (e.g., Down syndrome), and children with receptive and expressive language disorders. All of these studies are pretest-post-test control group designs, with random assignment to groups. Following the experimental, all families in the control groups received the experimental intervention following the post-tests.

Children with Cognitive and Developmental Disorders

Three studies using It Takes Two to Talk® have been conducted with 32, 20, and 12 children with cognitive and developmental disorders (Girolametto, 1988; Girolametto, Weitzman, & Clements-Baartman, 1998; Tannock et al., 1992). The children were between 22 and 62 months of age, their etiologies were mixed (e.g., Down syndrome, chromosomal abnormalities, mild cerebral palsy, general delays in development), and their language levels ranged from prelinguistic, intentional communication to two-word utterances. In each study, families were randomly assigned to experimental or delayed treatment control groups. Taken together, the results indicated that parent-focused language intervention exerted significant effects on conversational skills (joint engagement, greater responsiveness and assertiveness), vocabulary acquisition, and language productivity, in comparison to a control group.

Late-Talking Toddlers

Two studies using It Takes Two to Talk® have been conducted with 25 and 16 late talking toddlers with expressive vocabulary delays (Girolametto, Pearce, & Weitzman, 1996a; 1996b). All children were between 2;0 and 3;6 years of age, had IQs in the normal range, no known sensory, motor, or social-emotional problems, and were still at the single word stage of language development. The families were randomly assigned to experimental and waiting list control groups. In comparison to the control group, treatment effects were found for vocabulary acquisition, development of multiword sentences, and speech sound development.

Children with Receptive and/or Expressive Language Disorders

Thirty-seven children with a diagnosis of language impairment aged 30 to 42 months were assigned on a geographic basis to receive parent-focused intervention (using It Takes Two to Talk®) or direct individual intervention (Baxendale & Hesketh, 2003). All children had normal hearing and nonverbal cognitive development. Significant gains in language outcomes were observed in both groups of children; however, children with receptive and expressive language disorders made greater changes with the parent-focused intervention, whereas children with expressive disorders only made greater changes in individual intervention. Because the interventions were not randomly assigned, it was not possible to determine whether intervention was effective overall.

There are several limitations with all of these studies that are important to acknowledge. First, the participants have generally been well-educated, middle-income parents who are English speaking and self-refer to the program in response to recommendations by professionals or physicians, raising the issue of selection bias. Second, the numbers of participants in these studies have been small (8–12 per group). Third, few studies include long-term follow-up beyond 4 months. Fourth, there are no studies evaluating whether parent-focused intervention, in combination with other service delivery models (e.g., parent involvement plus individual treatment) produces better outcomes than any one service delivery model alone. Finally, given the emphasis on parent-child interaction, there is no research to demonstrate the efficacy of this approach for (a) families from lower socioeconomic and educational backgrounds and (b) families from different cultural groups (for whom parent-child interactions differ from the mainstream culture).

Overall, research on the efficacy of It Takes Two to Talk® suggests positive effects for a wide range of children with language disorders. Less is known about its usefulness for families from different linguistic and cultural groups. Replication studies to confirm and extend the findings with children who have diverse etiologies and disorders would further contribute to our knowledge of this program's effects on language development. Longitudinal findings to determine longer term outcomes are also needed. Presently, the available data indicate a positive effect of parent-focused intervention on children's language development, a result that theoretically should impact positively on language acquisition, socioemotional development, and academic achievement.

In summary, It Takes Two to Talk® is a parent-focused program that has three objectives. First, it provides parent education concerning language development and their child's language learning style. Second, it provides social support for families raising a child with a disability. Finally, it provides intervention strategies that parents can use to improve their child's communication development. The research data on this parent program indicate that it is effective in promoting children's language skills and enhancing overall family functioning.

Families' Views of Involvement in SLP for Children with Language Disorders

Parental satisfaction with the usefulness of a program's format and content offers a perspective that may provide insights into whether the interactive model of language intervention is socially acceptable, or makes inappropriate or unreasonable demands on the child and family, resulting in unexpected negative consequences (Baker, 1988; Dunst et al., 1988). There are few studies that describe the extent and nature of family involvement in interventions for young children with language disorders from the speech-language pathologist's point of view. However, there are several studies that have used survey methods to describe the parents' involvement in and satisfaction with speech-language therapy services. Two of the studies included parents as aides to the therapy program. A survey of 40 families of preschoolers (3–5 years) who were receiving therapy at the Mayo Clinic revealed that approximately 48% of the parents did not know what the goals of treatment were for their child (Stoeckel & Strand, 2007). Thirty-one percent of the parents reported that they had not been asked to conduct home activities. The authors concluded that home practice activities were limited, even among the parents who were asked to complete homework. Furthermore, meetings between the speech-language pathologist and the parent were infrequent.

Glogowska and colleagues (2002) reported that many parents in a large RCT anticipated that the clinician would provide direct treatment to their preschool-aged child and did not expect that they would play a large role in the intervention program. Moreover, parents in this program felt that they were not given sufficient information about activities to help their children. The combined findings from these two studies suggest that parents' role in speech and language services is not clearly delineated and when parents do participate, the extent of their involvement is vague.

Limited information is available on the social acceptability of parent-focused intervention where the parent is taught to be the primary change agent. In a study by Girolametto et al. (1993), parents involved in It Takes Two to Talk® exhibited a high rate of program completion and assigned positive ratings to program techniques, organization, and instructional components (e.g., group sessions, instructional activities, video feedback sessions). Mothers rated the usefulness of small group activities lower than ratings of individualized instruction and home visits. These data suggest that information that is specific to the parent and/or child are perceived as more useful by the parents. The ratings also provided insights into three areas requiring fine-tuning, such as reducing the requirements for home assignments, minimizing small group work, and introducing regular follow-up consultations. The parents were overwhelmingly positive about the parent and child changes made following intervention, providing evidence for the acceptability of the program's content and format. Moreover, parents' comments revealed that there were no adverse consequences resulting from participation in the program.

Cultural Issues

Our understanding of how parent-administered language intervention applies to different linguistic and cultural groups is still in its infancy. Future research is needed to disentangle the influences of linguistic structure and culture on parental language input before we advocate wholesale adoption of this service delivery model to other cultural groups. Until such research is available, translated versions of any of the parent programs in Table 5–1 should be used cautiously and only if the clinician and parent both understand and accept that this intervention promotes linguistic and cultural values that may not be consistent with the language and culture of the target child. van Kleeck (1994) recommends that a mainstream program can be altered to fit a family from a different cultural background through frequent and frank discussions of the interaction strategy being recommended and the cultural beliefs from which it is derived. In this way, parents may be freer to select the strategies that work best in their family context. When providing early language intervention to children whose home language is a minority language, Kohnert and colleagues (2005) recommend parent training in the minority language to support the acquisition of the home language. They recommend that the training reflect features of successful parent training programs, such as adopting a systematic approach to instruction, focusing on specific strategies, incorporating varied instructional methods, and individualizing the intervention for each child and family. Such an approach requires many sessions and must include time to allow parents to change their interactive behavior and maintain these changes over time.

Nexus Between Research, Clinical Practice, and Families' Views

As clinicians move to evidence-based clinical approaches, the adoption of effective therapies has become an important concern. In general, the research on parent-administered language intervention discussed above provides clinicians with supportive evidence for the efficacy of parent training. Moreover, evidence exists to substantiate the view that parents, on the whole, do not experience adverse reactions to participation in parent programs (Girolametto et al., 1993; Glogowska et al., 2002). However, there is still much more to be learned in providing parents with services that are family-centered and meet their needs. Despite positive reports of treatment outcomes, some parents may not adopt responsive language strategies (or other teaching strategies) and parental commitment may decrease over time. Moreover, some parents may elect not to participate in parent training programs, requiring flexible, alternative models of service delivery to meet the needs of these families and their children. Attrition and nonattendance at sessions are rarely examined in studies of language intervention (McConkey & McEvoy, 1984). Insights from the field of behavioral interventions reveal that parents' education and income have been positively related to attendance, with more highly educated parents and high income parents being more likely to attend a greater number of training sessions (Snow, Frey, & Kern, 2002). In contrast, gender, age, race, and marital status did not predict attrition rates.

Many of the parent programs in Table 5–1 combine elements of home-based instruction, center-based instruction, or both. For example, It Takes Two to Talk® contains individual videotaping consultations that may take place in the home and group sessions that take place in a classroom setting. The suitability of classroom-based learning needs to be examined in the context of parent education levels and research is needed to determine if this context may be more accessible to parents who have the learning skills consistent with higher educational achievement. Extant research suggests that providing flexible parent training (e.g., experiential learning using home based or centre-based instruction with children present), shorter sessions, and adjusting the language level/amount of information taught may increase parents' access to services (Snow et al., 2002). Nevertheless, Kohnert et al. (2005) caution against brief interventions and those that rely heavily on written materials when working with families who speak minority languages.

Little is known about the dosage and frequency of intervention sessions that are necessary to create meaningful change. As Warren, Fey, and Yoder (2007) point out, interventions in language have focused on trialing short-term programs and/or procedures. A necessary next step is the investigation of the effects of differential dosage or intensity of treatment on child language development. On this issue, it appears that clinician-administered interventions at a low dosage (8 clinical contacts and 6 hours of therapy in an 8-month period) may be insufficient for preschool-age children with speech and/or language disorders (Glogowska, Roulstone, Enderby, & Peters, 2000). However, for children with very mild delays in language development, a parent program of shorter duration (e.g., 6 weeks) may be appropriate. In the field of parent training for behavior disorders, shorter programs as well as print-based programs have been found to be effective for children with mild conduct disorders (Long, 2007). Justice and Ezell (2000) used a brief instructional videotape to train parents to use print referencing strategies successfully. In our experience, however, parents still need the same learning components currently included in It Takes Two to Talk®, such as opportunities for discussion, multimedia examples, coaching, and feedback.

Therefore, extant research evidence on parent-administered intervention suggests that parents can learn to use responsive strategies that have a positive impact on children's communication and language skills. Although emerging research and federal legislation (e.g., IDEA) support the use of parent-administered interventions in clinical practice, there are still many unknown issues. Currently, there is no research to guide clinicians on how to select a parent training program that is suitable for a particular child's characteristics and language level. In the absence of such research, the clinician may proceed with parent involvement but must carefully monitor the child's development and the family's progress.

Case Study of Family Involvement

Background

Dana was born with Down syndrome. Dana's parents enrolled in a parent program when Dana was 24 months old. Dana is the youngest of three children and lives with her biological mother and father. Dana and her parents were involved in a home visiting program since birth. At 2 years of age, Dana entered a special preschool program for children with disabilities. The speech-language pathologist employed by the preschool center offered It Takes Two to Talk® to all families of children enrolled in the center.

Details About the Child's Impairment

The speech-language pathologist noted that her oral motor development appeared to be adequate for eating and drinking. She had good lip seal for swallowing and chews her food appropriately. There was no evidence of drooling, although her tongue sat forward in her mouth and she generally had open mouth posture. According to parental report as well as direct observation during testing, Dana was able to produce approximately 8 speech sounds, including: /m/, /h/, /n/, /b/, /g/, /k/, /d/, and /t/.

Dana's mother completed a vocabulary checklist, the MacArthur-Bates Communicative Development Inventory: Words and Gestures (Fenson et al., 1993). Her mother reported that Dana comprehended 85 words in a variety of classes (including household objects, animals, food, toys, people, places, action words and locations) and spoke 6 different words (including *mom, dad, bubbles, bye, hi,* and *no*), usually pronouncing only the first portion of the word. According to parent report, Dana had only acquired one new word (*bubbles*) in the last 6 months.

Dana's mother reported that her vision is fine and her general health is excellent. Her hearing has been tested and is within normal limits. Although she has had many ear infections, her otolaryngologist has not recommended tubes and she has been treated with antibiotics. Dana enjoys simple interaction games with others, uses common household objects for play, imitates simple adult movements like clapping, and shows interest in the activities of others. She does not yet imitate words or engage in make-believe play. The speech-language pathologist's observation of Dana's interactions at preschool nursery revealed that Dana plays alongside other children by playing side by side but infrequently initiates verbal interaction with other children. On one occasion, Dana used a whole hand (but did not extend her index finger) to point to a toy she wanted.

How/Why the Family Accessed SLP Services

Dana's parents attended an orientation session at which the speech-language pathologist described the parent program, played a videotape illustrating the program strategies, and outlined the expectations for attendance at all eight evening group sessions and three home visits. Following the orientation session, parents were asked to confirm their interest. Dana's mother and father both attended the orientation session and agreed to participate in the parent program. Seven other parents signed up during the orientation session and the speech-language pathologist scheduled the program to start 2 weeks later.

Family Involvement in Assessment

A full speech and language assessment was not conducted because Dana was enrolled in a special treatment preschool program for children with disabilities and previous assessments were available. Therefore, the speech-language pathologist scheduled a preprogram consultation session to discuss parents' concerns, to conduct an informal communication assessment, and to videotape a 5-minute mother-child play interaction. Because Dana's father had also agreed to participate, a 5-minute father-child play interaction with a different set of toys was also filmed. During these two videotaped interactions, the speech-language pathologist noted that Dana frequently shared joint attention with her parents, smiled in response to their utterances, and responded to their questions using a combination of gestures and vocalizations. She did not initiate interaction, her responses were generally uninterpretable, and she did not take conversational turns. Her mother monitored her play carefully, commented on her ongoing actions, and displayed positive affect. However, her strategies to engage Dana in interaction included (a) asking many yes/no questions that went unanswered and (b) using long and complex utterances. The father's input to Dana included (a) many commands to direct her play behavior and (b) long and complex utterances to describe her actions. Neither parent interpreted her gestures and sounds as meaningful words, nor did they use responsive labeling effectively to capture the focus of her interest. At the end of the assessment, the speech-language pathologist asked Dana's parents what they wanted Dana to learn. Both parents expressed frustration with her lack of progress in word learning and agreed that they wanted her to use more words. The speech-language pathologist agreed with their goal and suggested that that Dana might be more likely to learn new words if she was exposed to sign language at the same time. Dana's father was reluctant to consider this alternative because he feared that Dana would "get stuck" and never learn to express words orally. However, he agreed to try it on it a trial basis for the duration of the 11-week program. This was consistent with the philosophy of the preschool, which encouraged multimodal communication for all children.

Family Involvement in Intervention

Dana's parents attended seven of the eight evening group sessions and all three video feedback sessions that were conducted in the home. They missed one evening session because both Dana and her father were ill. The content of the missed evening session was reviewed at the next home visit.

Home Visits

During the first two evening sessions the parents learned how to follow the child's lead and to imitate, interpret, or comment on the child's topic. Therefore, in the first video feedback session, Dana's parents were encouraged to (a) observe and wait without speaking to give Dana time to show an interest or initiate interaction (e.g., a play activity) with them and (b) respond to Dana's initiations by interpreting her vocalizations as meaningful or using short comments on the topic of her activity. Dana's parents were videotaped separately for five minutes each. Dana did not use any words during this video feedback session, but she vocalized frequently while looking at her parents' face, presumably to comment. During filming, the speech-language pathologist paused the video camera and coached the parents to respond to Dana's vocalizations by interpreting them as meaningful or making comments. At the end of the home visit, Dana's father commented that he was surprised to find that pausing and waiting often resulted in a vocalization on Dana's part that gave him a clue as to how to respond. They then discussed when they would make an effort to wait for her to initiate and agreed that the father would focus on assisting Dana with dressing and the mother would focus on play time.

During sessions 4 and 5 of the parent group, the speech-language pathologist taught strategies to promote conversational turn-taking and to provide language input, including focused stimulation of labels and expansions. During the following video feedback session, the speech-language pathologist and Dana's parents selected five target words/signs to use. The objective was to use focused repetition of these words/signs during social routines and play interactions. With some coaching, Dana's father successfully emphasized the words "shoe" and "on" repetitively during dressing. Her mother used "cookie" and "eat" during playtime with dolls. During the doll play, the speech-language pathologist paused the camera and coached Dana's mother to replace yes/no questions with comments. Later, while observing their videotapes Dana's parents stated that they understood the focused stimulation strategy better and realized that they could also interpret many of her sounds as words. Dana attempted the sign for "eat" during the doll play and this encouraged both parents to continue using focused repetitions of words paired with signs. Moreover, Dana's mother effectively reduced her yes/no questions and replaced them with comments on Dana's play.

During the next three group evening sessions, the speech-language pathologist taught parents how to generalize the strategies learned thus far to play and books. Parents also learned to use language to talk about past events, feelings, and so forth. The third video feedback was used to consolidate the main strategies that Dana's parents had learned, that is, follow Dana's lead, interpret her sounds and gestures using words or short comments, and use focused stimulation of words/signs. They were also encouraged to keep Dana in an interaction for more turns on topic. In reviewing the parents' videotapes, the speech-language pathologist and Dana's parents noted that Dana was attempting more signs and had started to accompany the sign for "cookie" with the first sound in the word. By engaging her in more turns on topic, they had many more opportunities to interpret her sounds using labels and use short comments to describe her actions. Both parents notably reduced their use of yes/no questions and commands to direct her play.

Family Involvement in Discharge Planning

Because Dana was enrolled in a treatment preschool center, the speech-language pathologist was able to integrate the parents' communication goals into her preschool program. The preschool was structured to include parent consultations on a monthly basis so that the speech-language pathologist could help parents select additional vocabulary goals as Dana learned new words/signs. Thus, when Dana was ready to transition to two-word/sign combinations, the speech-language pathologist would be in a position to help them focus on expansions, which is a strategy found useful for promoting this stage of language development.

Family Involvement in Evaluation of Service

At the end of the parent program, both parents completed an evaluation form that asked their perceptions of the program format and content. In addition, the evaluation asked parents' opinions about child
and self change. Both parents noted that Dana's communication had
improved (i.e., that her vocalizations and vocabulary had increased)
and that their interactions with Dana had become more responsive as
a result of their involvement in It Takes Two to Talk®. Dana's mother
observed that, following the program, she listened more, commented
and interpreted more often, and spent more time playing with Dana.
She stated that she liked the duration and number of home visits, the
group size, sharing with others in the group, and the home visits.
Dana's father noted that, after the program, he waited and listened
more often and repeated or expanded on Dana's communication
attempts. He also rated the following aspects of the program positively: the duration of the program, number of home visits, group sharing, and evaluating videotapes in the evening sessions.

Facilitators and Barriers in Family Involvement

Dana's parents were initially reluctant to use signs with words. They
wanted Dana to be a verbal communicator and felt that if she was
exposed to sign language she would be further delayed in her use of
speech to communicate. Dana's father cited a number of cases of children with Down syndrome for whom sign was not used and the
children learned to talk. Although there were several previous meetings with the preschool educators who had explained the advantages
of using sign language to assist verbal communication development,
Dana's parents had not followed through on home programming to
introduce signs in the home setting.

   The speech-language pathologist was able to suggest attempting
signs for a trial period by citing the results of recent research (for a
review, see Robertson, 2007). In addition, the support of the group
was instrumental in showing them that other parents of children with
disabilities were incorporating words and signs with success. This is
one case where the group feedback and support made a difference to
the parents' beliefs about sign language.

Summary and Conclusions

Parent-administered language intervention is a widely used, viable, and highly important mode of service delivery for preschool children with language disorders. Regardless of the parent program utilized, research studies support the efficacy of parent training for improving a variety of communication and language skills (e.g., pragmatic functions, vocabulary, mean length of utterance, morphosyntax). The length of parent training programs (number of weeks/months), intensity (number of times per week) and dosage (in terms of input to the child) varies considerably across the parent programs reviewed in this chapter (e.g., from 8 weeks to 33 weekly sessions in 1 year). One consideration that may dictate the treatment regimen is the disability of the child; longer interventions were offered to children with developmental disabilities whereas less intensive programs were offered to late talkers and children with language disorders. In general, it appears that programs longer than 8 weeks may show more promise of yielding unequivocal child gains as the one program that was 8 weeks long did not produce encouraging results (Weistuch & Lewis, 1985). Although there are few studies that compare parent training to clinician-administered treatment, the extant research indicates that parent training is at least as effective as direct treatment offered by a speech-language pathologist. Given the philosophical, legislative, and theoretical reasons for involving parents in their children's intervention programs, it is important for future research to address questions of program intensity, added value of parent and clinician-administered treatments, and longer term effects of treatment.

References

Baker, B. (1988). Evaluating parent training. *Irish Journal of Psychology, 9,* 324–345.

Baxendale, J., & Hesketh, A. (2003). Comparison of the effectiveness of the Hanen Parent Programme and traditional clinic therapy. *International Journal of Language and Communication Disorders, 38,* 397–415.

Bedore, L., & Leonard, L. (1995). Prosodic and syntactic bootstrapping and their clinical applications. *American Journal of Speech-Language Pathology, 4,* 66–72.

Beitchman, J., Wilson, B., Johnson, C., Atkinson, L., Young, A., Adlaf, E., Escobar, M., & Douglas, L. (2001). Fourteen-year follow-up of speech/language impaired and control children: Psychiatric outcome. *Journal of the American Academy of Child and Adolescent Psychiatry, 40*, 75-82.

Best, W., Melvin, D., & Williams, S. (1993). The effectiveness of communication groups in day nurseries. *European Journal of Disorders of Communication, 28*, 187-212.

Bohannon, J., & Bonvillian, J. (1997). Theoretical approaches to language acquisition. In J. Berko Gleason (Ed.), *The development of language* (4th ed., pp. 259-316). Needham Heights, MA: Allyn & Bacon.

Bronfenbrenner, U. (1974). *Is early intervention effective?* (No. (CDH) 74-25). Washington, DC: Office of Child Development.

Bruner, J. (1975). From communication to language: A psychological perspective. *Cognition, 3*, 255-287.

Camarata, S., Nelson, K., & Camarata, M. (1994). Comparison of conversational-recasting and imitative procedures for training grammatical structures in children with specific language impairment. *Journal of Speech and Hearing Research, 37*, 1414-1423.

Chapman, R. (2000). Children's language learning: An interactionist perspective. *Journal of Child Psychology and Psychiatry and Allied Disciplines, 41*, 33-54.

Cheseldine, S., & McConkey, R. (1979). Parental speech to young Down's syndrome children: An intervention study. *American Journal of Mental Deficiency, 83*, 612-620.

Connell, P. (1987). An effect of modelling and imitation teaching procedures on children with and without specific language impairment. *Journal of Speech and Hearing Research, 30*, 105-113.

Dempsey, I., & Dunst, C. (2004). Helpgiving styles and parent empowerment in families with a young child with a disability. *Journal of Intellectual and Developmental Disability, 29*, 40-51.

Donahue-Kilburg, G. (1992). *Family-centered early intervention for communication disorders*. Gaithersburg, MD: Aspen.

Dunst, C., Leet, H., & Trivette, C. (1988). Family resources, personal well-being and early intervention. *Journal of Special Education, 22*, 108-116.

Dunst, C. J. (2002). Family-centered practices: Birth through high school. *Journal of Special Education, 36*, 139-147.

Ellis Weismer, S., & Robertson, S. (2006). Focused stimulation approach to language intervention. In R. McCauley & M. Fey (Eds.), *Treatment of language disorders in children* (pp. 175-202). Baltimore: Paul H. Brookes.

Fenson, L., Dale, P., Reznick, S., Thal, D., Bates, E., Hartung, J., et al. (1993). *MacArthur-Bates Communicative Development Inventory*. San Diego, CA: Singular.

Fey, M. (1986). *Language intervention with young children*. Austin, TX: Pro-Ed.

Fey, M., Cleave, P., Long, S., & Hughes, D. (1993). Two approaches to the facilitation of grammar in children with language impairment: An experimental evaluation. *Journal of Speech and Hearing Research, 36,* 141-157.

Folger, J., & Chapman, R. (1978). A pragmatic analysis of spontaneous imitations. *Journal of Child Language, 5,* 25-38.

Gibbard, D. (1994). Parental-based intervention with pre-school language-delayed children. *European Journal of Disorders of Communication, 29,* 131-150.

Girolametto, L. (1988). Improving the social-conversational skills of developmentally delayed children: An intervention study. *Journal of Speech and Hearing Disorders, 53,* 156-167.

Girolametto, L., Pearce, P., & Weitzman, E. (1996a). The effects of focused stimulation for promoting vocabulary in children with delays: A pilot study. *Journal of Childhood Communication Development, 17,* 39-49.

Girolametto, L., Pearce, P., & Weitzman, E. (1996b). Interactive focused stimulation for toddlers with expressive vocabulary delays. *Journal of Speech and Hearing Research, 39,* 1274-1283.

Girolametto, L., Pearce, P., & Weitzman, E. (1997). Effects of lexical intervention on the phonology of late talkers. *Journal of Speech, Language, and Hearing Research, 40,* 338-348.

Girolametto, L., & Tannock, R. (1994). Correlates of directiveness in the interactions of fathers and mothers of children with developmental delays. *Journal of Speech and Hearing Research, 37,* 1178-1192.

Girolametto, L., Tannock, R., & Siegel, L. (1993). Consumer-oriented evaluation of interactive language intervention. *American Journal of Speech-Language Pathology, 2,* 41-51.

Girolametto, L., Weitzman, E., & Clements-Baartman, J. (1998). Vocabulary intervention for children with Down syndrome: Parent training using focused stimulation. *Infant-Toddler Intervention: A Transdisciplinary Journal, 8,* 109-126.

Glogowska, M., Campbell, R., Peters, T., Roulstone, S., & Enderby, P. (2002). A multimethod approach to the evaluation of community preschool speech and language therapy provision. *Child: Care, Health and Development, 28,* 513-521.

Glogowska, M., Roulstone, S., Enderby, P., & Peters, T. (2000). Randomised controlled trial of community based speech and language therapy in preschool children. *British Medical Journal, 321,* 923-927.

Guskey, T. (1986, May). Staff development and the process of teacher change. *Educational Researcher,* pp. 5-12.

Haley, K., Camarata, S., & Nelson, K. (1994). Social valence in children with specific language impairment during imitation-based and conversation-based language intervention. *Journal of Speech and Hearing Research, 37,* 378-388.

Hemmeter, L., & Kaiser, A. (1994). Enhanced milieu teaching: Effects of parent-implemented language intervention. *Journal of Early Intervention, 187,* 269–289.

Johnson, C., Beitchman, J., Young, A., Escobar, M., Atkinson, L., Wilson, B., et al. (1999). Fourteen-year follow-up of children with and without speech/language impairments: Speech/language stability and outcomes. *Journal of Speech, Language, and Hearing Research, 42,* 744–760.

Justice, L., & Ezell, H. (2000). Enhancing children's print and word awareness through home-based parent intervention. *American Journal of Speech-Language Pathology, 9,* 257–269.

Kaiser, A., Hancock, T., Solomon, N., Windsor, K., & Howard, F. (2000, Nov.). *Project III: Generalized effects of parent- and therapist-implemented enhanced milieu teaching.* Paper presented at the American Speech-Language-Hearing Association Annual Convention, Washington, DC.

Kaiser, A., & Hester, P. (1994). Generalized effects of enhanced milieu teaching. *Journal of Speech and Hearing Research, 37,* 1320–1340.

Kohnert, K., Yim, D., Nett, K., Kan, P., & Duran, L. (2005). Intervention with linguistically diverse preschool children: A focus on developing home language(s). *Language, Speech, and Hearing Services in Schools, 36,* 251–263.

Long, N. (2007). Learning from experience: Shifting from clinical parent training to broader parent education. *Clinical Child Psychology and Psychiatry, 12,* 385–392.

MacDonald, J., Blott, P., Gordon, K., Spiegel, B., & Hartmann, M. (1974). An experimental parent-assisted treatment program for preschool language-delayed children. *Journal of Speech and Hearing Disorders, 39,* 395–415.

MacDonald, J., & Gillette, Y. (1984). Conversation engineering: A pragmatic approach to early social competence. *Seminars in Speech and Language, 5,* 171–184.

MacDonald, J., & Presser Blott, J. (1974). Environmental language intervention: The rationale for a diagnostic and training strategy through rules, context and generalization. *Journal of Speech and Hearing Disorders, 39,* 244–256.

MacDonald, J., & Wilkening, P. (1994, May). *Parent-child relationships for communicative development: An intervention study.* Paper presented at the Annual Meeting of the American Association of Mental Retardation, Boston.

Mahoney, G., & Perales, F. (2005). Relationship-focused early intervention with children with pervasive developmental disorders and other disabilities: A comparative study. *Journal of Developmental and Behavioral Pediatrics, 26,* 77–85.

Mahoney, G., & Powell, A. (1988). Modifying parent-child interaction: Enhancing the development of handicapped children. *Journal of Special Education, 22,* 82–96.

Mahoney, G., Wiggers, B., & Lash, S. (1996). Using a relationship-focused intervention program to enhance father involvement. *Infant-Toddler Intervention, 6,* 295-308.

Manolson, H. (1985). *It takes two to talk: A parent's guide to helping children communicate* (2nd ed.). Toronto, ON: The Hanen Centre.

Manolson, H. (1992). *It takes two to talk: A parent's guide to helping children communicate* (3rd ed.). Toronto, ON: The Hanen Centre.

McCauley, R., & Fey, M. (2006). *Treatment of language disorders in children.* Baltimore: Paul H. Brookes.

McConkey, R., Jeffree, D., & Hewson, S. (1979). Involving parents in extending the language development of their young mentally handicapped children. *British Journal of Disorders of Communication, 14,* 203-218.

McConkey, R., & McEvoy, J. (1984). Parental involvement courses: Contrasts between mothers who enroll and those who do not. *Perspectives and Progress in Mental Retardation, 1,* 435-442.

McConkey, R., & O'Connor, M. (1982). A new approach to parental involvement in language intervention programmes. *Child: Care, Health and Development, 8,* 163-176.

McMahon, R., & Forehand, R. (1983). Consumer satisfaction in behavioral treatment of children: Types, issues and recommendations. *Behavior Therapy, 14,* 209-225.

Mervis, C., & Bertrand, J. (1993). Acquisition of early object labels: The roles of operating principles and input. In A. P. Kaiser & D. B. Gray (Eds.), *Enhancing children's communication: Research foundations for intervention* (Vol. 2, pp. 287-316). Baltimore: Paul H. Brookes.

Nelson, K., Camarata, S., Welsh, J., Butkovsky, L., & Camarata, M. (1996). Effects of conversational recasting treatment on the acquisition of grammar in children with specific language impairment and younger language-normal children. *Journal of Speech and Hearing Research, 39,* 850-859.

Ninio, A., & Bruner, J. (1978). The achievement and antecedents of labelling. *Journal of Child Language, 5,* 1-15.

Owens, R., Jr. (2008). *Language development: An introduction* (7th ed.). Boston: Allyn and Bacon.

Paul, R. (2007). *Language disorders from infancy through adolescence* (3rd ed.). St Louis, MO: Mosby Elsevier.

Paul-Brown, D., & Caperton, C. (2001). Inclusive practices for preschool-age children with specific language impairment. In M. Guralnick (Ed.), *Early childhood inclusion: Focus on change* (pp. 433-464). Baltimore: Paul H. Brookes.

Pepper, J., & Weitzman, E. (2004). *It takes two to talk: A practical guide for parents of children with language delays* (2nd ed.). Toronto, ON: The Hanen Centre.

Robertson, S. (2007, November). *Using sign to facilitate oral language: Building a case with parents.* Paper presented at the American Speech-Language-Hearing Association Convention, Boston.

Robertson, S., & Ellis Weismer, S. (1999). Effects of treatment on linguistic and social skills in toddlers with delayed language development. *Journal of Speech, Language, and Hearing Research, 42,* 1234-1248.

Rocissano, L., & Yatchmink, Y. (1983). Joint attention in mother-toddler interaction: A study of individual variation. *Merrill-Palmer Quarterly, 30,* 11-31.

Seitz, S. (1975). Language intervention—Changing the language environment of the retarded child. In R. Koch, F. de la Cruz, & F. Menolascino (Eds.), *Down's syndrome: Research, prevention and management.* New York: Bruner/Mazel.

Snow, J., Frey, M., & Kern, R. (2002). Attrition, financial incentives, and parent education. *Family Journal: Counselling and Therapy for Couples and Families, 10,* 373-378.

Stoeckel, R., & Strand, E. (2007, November). *Parental involvement in speech therapy: A review.* Paper presented at the American Speech-Language-Hearing Association Convention, Boston.

Tager-Flusberg, H., & Calkins, S. (1990). Does imitation facilitate the acquisition of grammar? Evidence from a study of autistic, Down's syndrome and normal children. *Journal of Child Language, 17,* 591-606.

Tannock, R. (1988). Mothers' directiveness in their interactions with their children with and without Down syndrome. *American Journal on Mental Retardation, 93,* 154-165.

Tannock, R., Girolametto, L., & Siegel, L. (1992). Language intervention with children who have developmental delays: Effects of an interactive approach. *American Journal on Mental Retardation, 97,* 145-160.

Tomasello, M., & Farrar, M. (1986). Joint attention and early language. *Child Development, 57,* 1454-1463.

Tomasello, M., & Todd, J. (1983). Joint attention and lexical acquisition style. *First Language, 4,* 197-212.

van Kleeck, A. (1994). Potential cultural bias in training parents as conversational partners with their children who have delays in language development. *American Journal of Speech-Language Pathology, 3,* 67-78.

van Kleeck, A., Gillam, R., Hamilton, L., & McGrath, C. (1997). The relationship between middle-class parents' book-sharing discussion and their preschoolers' abstract language development. *Journal of Speech, Language, and Hearing Research, 40,* 1261-1271.

van Kleeck, A., Vander Woude, J., & Hammett, L. (2006). Fostering literal and inferential language skills in Head Start preschoolers with language impairment using scripted book-sharing discussions. *American Journal of Speech-Language Pathology, 15,* 85-95.

Vygotsky, L. (1978). *Mind in society*. Cambridge, MA: Harvard University Press.

Warren, S. (1992). Facilitating basic vocabulary acquisition with milieu teaching procedures. *Journal of Early Intervention, 16*, 235-251.

Warren, S., Fey, M., & Yoder, P. (2007). Differential treatment intensity research: A missing link to creating optimally effective communication interventions. *Mental Retardation and Developmental Disabilities, 13*, 70-77.

Warren, S., & Kaiser, A. (1986). Incidental language teaching: A critical review. *Journal of Speech and Hearing Disorders, 51*, 291-299.

Weistuch, L., & Brown, B. (1987). Motherese as therapy: A program and its dissemination. *Child Language: Teaching and Therapy, 3*, 58-71.

Weistuch, L., & Lewis, M. (1985). The language interaction intervention project. *Analysis and Intervention in Developmental Disabilities, 5*, 97-106.

Weistuch, L., Lewis, M., & Sullivan, M. (1991). Project profile: Use of a language interaction intervention in the preschools. *Journal of Early Intervention, 15*, 278-287.

Westby, C. (1991). Learning to talk, talking to learn: Oral-literate language differences. In C. Simon (Ed.), *Communication skills and classroom success* (pp. 334-357). Eau Claire, WI: Thinking Publications.

Wilcox, M., Kouri, T., & Caswell, S. (1991). Early language intervention: A comparison of classroom and individual treatment. *American Journal of Speech-Language Pathology, 1*, 49-62.

Yoder, P., Davies, B., Bishop, K., & Munson, L. (1994). Effect of adult continuing wh-questions on conversational participation in children with developmental disabilities. *Journal of Speech and Hearing Research, 37*, 193-204.

Yoder, P., & Warren, S. (1998). Maternal responsivity predicts the prelinguistic communication intervention that facilitates generalized intentional communication. *Journal of Speech-Language-Hearing Research, 41*, 1207-1219.

Yoder, P., & Warren, S. (2002). Effects of prelinguistic Milieu Teaching and parent responsivity education on dyads involving children with intellectual disabilities. *Journal of Speech, Language, and Hearing Research, 45*, 1158-1174.

Yoder, P., Warren, S., Kim, K., & Gazdag, G. (1994). Facilitating prelinguistic communication skills in young children with developmental delay II: Systematic replication and extension. *Journal of Speech and Hearing Research, 37*, 841-851.

Chapter 6
Working with Families of Children Who Stutter

Ann Packman and Marilyn Langevin

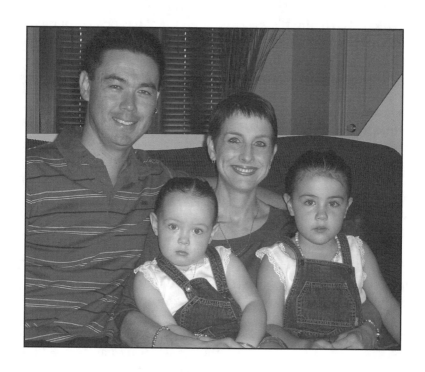

Research: Historical Overview of Family Involvement in Stuttering

Historical Overview

Stuttering is perhaps unique among the communication disorders in that it has prompted an enormous number and range of treatment approaches. Yairi, for example, reported that as a child and young adult during the 1940s and 1950s he received no fewer than 16 different interventions for his stuttering (Yairi & Ambrose, 2005). Even today, there is little consensus about what should be considered "best practice" for the treatment of stuttering in children. In a recent handbook of early stuttering intervention (Onslow & Packman, 1999), 8 treatments were proposed by their proponents as being viable, and that list is not conclusive.

It seems to us that there are two main reasons for this lack of consensus. The first is that, although there has been a burgeoning of behavioral and brain research into the nature and cause of stuttering over the last 20 to 30 years, its cause remains unknown. This has given rise, over the decades, to the development of many causal theories, most of which are untestable (Packman & Attanasio, 2004). Given the propensity in the field of stuttering to have theory driven treatment (for discussions of this see Packman & Attanasio, 2004; Siegel, 1998; Yairi & Ambrose, 2005), this has resulted in a plethora of treatments, developed from widely varying theoretical positions.

Stemming from the work of Freud, early in the 20th century parents were thought to have caused their child's stuttering because of a disturbed parent-child relationship (Glauber, 1943). Later, Johnson (1959) proposed his diagnosogenic theory, which said that parents caused stuttering by labelling their child's normal disfluencies "stuttering": in other words, stuttering was caused by its diagnosis. Thus, the object of intervention was not the child but the parent. This would seem to be an extreme example of the *family-centered approach* for early stuttering!

Although the diagnosogenic theory is no longer considered viable, the notion that parents either cause or partially cause stuttering, or that they contribute to its persistence, remains today (see Yairi & Ambrose, 2005). This is encapsulated in a recent theoretical perspective that stuttering is multifactorial; namely, that many factors contribute to the cause of stuttering and that the cause of stuttering is different in each person (for an overview see Packman & Attanasio, 2004). Consequently, treatments driven by this perspective are also multifactorial. They incorporate a number of direct and indirect strategies, targeting parent communicative behaviors, various features of the environment, and children's speech behavior. The Demands and Capacities is a well-known and widely accepted multifactorial model, which has driven treatment now for around a decade and a half (Starkweather, 1989).

It should be said that it is not exactly counterintuitive that parents cause stuttering. Again, stuttering is unique among the developmental disorders of communication because it starts after a period of apparently normal speech development. Children are typically at the 2- to 3-word level before stuttering becomes apparent. Although some neural processing explanations have been put forward for this in recent times (e.g., see Packman, Code, & Onslow, 2007), it is not surprising that parents feel that they must have contributed to the appearance of stuttering in some way. Stuttering also tends to run in families and although current genetic research is now starting to explain this, this does nothing to assuage a parent's guilt if there is a history of stuttering in the family. And, of course, there is a long history of parents, particularly mothers, being blamed for other childhood disorders, such as autism.

Not all treatments for childhood stuttering are theory driven, however. With the rise in popularity of behavior therapy and it application to the treatment of stuttering in the 1960s (see Ingham, 1982), the emergence of operant procedures and programmed instruction shifted the focus from the parent to the child.

The second reason for the wide range of interventions for childhood stuttering relates to the changing course of stuttering during the childhood years. It has been known for decades that although around 5% of children start to stutter between the ages of 2 to 4 years, 74 to 80% will recover within the first few years without professional intervention (see Yairi & Ambrose, 2005). This has led to different treatment approaches according to age. As a legacy of the diagnosogenic theory, it was thought for many decades that drawing attention to stuttering in the first years after onset would make it worse. This resulted in the adoption of largely indirect interventions that focused on instructing parents to change the child's environment, while hoping the child would "grow out of" the stuttering. Once a child moved into the school age years and was still stuttering, and the chances of natural recovery greatly diminished, more direct interventions were considered more appropriate.

We now go on to look at some of the more widely used current interventions, according to the extent to which they involve the family. For relevance, we confine these to treatments that have been reported in the last 15 years. It must be said, however, that many of these treatments are eclectic (Guitar, 2006; Shapiro, 1999; Wall & Myers, 1995; Yairi & Ambrose, 2005). Thus, categorizing them is not always straightforward.

Therapist-Centered Approaches

Current approaches that could be categorized as therapist-centered are primarily behavioral in nature, wherein treatment is delivered by the speech-language pathologist (SLP) in the clinic and the focus is on modifying the child's speech.

Speech Motor Training (Riley & Riley, 1999) is an example. The aim of this treatment is to establish fluency through having children drill correct syllable production in response to a model. This starts at a slow speech rate and, with programmed instruction, the child moves through a series of steps until four-syllable chains of various vowel-consonant combinations are produced correctly. There is no parent involvement in the program.

Two other examples are Extended Length of Utterance (ELU) (Costello, 1983), which is used primarily with preschoolers, and Gradual Increase in Length and Complexity of Utterances (GILCU), which is part of the Monterey Fluency Program (Ryan & Ryan, 1999). This is used primarily with school-aged children. These treatments are based on operant principles and programmed instruction, in that children move systematically from single words to connected speech, with reinforcement for stutter-free speech and some sort of penalty for stuttering. A penalty may consist of the SLP saying "stop" and/or the child moving to a lower level. There is typically little involvement of parents in these treatments. However, subsequent to initial publications of ELU parents were reported to carry out some of this treatment at home. In this case, then, the parent could be considered as a therapy aide.

Shine (1984) described a treatment for children age 3 to 12 years, in which children are taught, in the clinic, to reduce speech rate, pitch, vocal fold tension, hard glottal attacks, and airflow rate.

Parent-as-Aide Approaches

The Fluency Rules Program (Runyan & Runyan, 1999) was developed for preschoolers and early school-aged children. The program focuses on having children learn rules for fluent speech production, which include, "speak slowly," "say one word at a time," "say it short," and "use speech breathing." Treatment is conducted in the clinic and the SLP uses hand signals to indicate to the child when the rules are, or are not, being followed. Parents are taught the hand signals and use them to facilitate "carryover" in the home environment (p. 167).

A recent report (Laiho & Klippi, 2007) described an intensive group therapy program for school-aged-children based on the traditional stuttering control techniques of cancellation, pull-outs, and preparatory set. Parents were included in the program to the extent that they attended information-giving groups and acted as aides in the SLP-delivered treatment.

Family-Centered Approaches

This is by far the most widely used family model for the management of childhood stuttering. Approaches known loosely as child-family (parent) interaction include the Parent-Child Group Approach (Conture & Melnick, 1999), the Differential Strategies Intervention (Gregory, 1999), the Stuttering Intervention Program (Pindzola, 1999), Parent-Child Interaction (Rustin, Botterill, & Kelman, 1996), and Family Focused Treatment (Yaruss, Coleman, & Hammer, 2006). A similar intervention, the Multiprocess Approach (Gottwald & Starkweather, 1999), is driven by the multifactorial Demands and Capacities model mentioned above. In all these approaches, the child is considered within the context of the family, and treatment focuses primarily on having parents modify the way they talk with their children and make changes to the child's home environment. Although direct manipulation of the child's speech may occur in these interventions, the direct manipulation of parental behaviors and the child's environment is typically the first and primary focus of intervention.

Family-Friendly Approaches

The Lidcombe Program of Early Stuttering Intervention (Onslow, Packman, & Harrison, 2003) has been included as a family-friendly approach, as it appears to meet all except the criteria of variable family involvement outlined in Chapter 1. The treatment was developed for preschoolers who stutter and is operant in nature, with the parent delivering treatment in the child's everyday environment. This is done for prescribed periods each day. The parent gives verbal contingencies (comments) for stutter-free speech and for moments of stuttering. The schedule of contingencies, and the ratio of contingencies for stuttering and stutter-free speech, vary according to the severity of the child's stuttering and the child's response to them. The parent learns how to deliver the treatment during weekly visits with the child to the SLP, and all decision-making is done jointly by the SLP and the parent. Although one parent usually takes the role of therapist, others in the family may be recruited if it seems appropriate. As well as delivering the treatment, the parent measures the child's stuttering severity each day on a 10-point scale and reports these to the SLP at the weekly clinic visit. They are taken into account in adjusting the treatment from week to week. Problem-solving is also a critical activity during the clinic visits, so that together the parent and SLP find ways to overcome everyday obstacles to treatment delivery such as the presence of younger siblings, parental work schedules, and child factors such as sensitivity to contingencies, garrulousness, etc. Thus, it can be seen that the parent is not simply a therapy aide but is essential to the successful delivery of the program.

Another family-friendly approach for preschoolers is the Westmead program, which is still in the early stages of development (see Trajkowski, Andrews, O'Brian, Onslow, & Packman, 2006). The treatment relies on the use of syllable-timed speech, which involves the child speaking in time to a rhythm. The model of service delivery and involvement of family is the same as for Lidcombe Program; it is only the treatment agents that differ.

An example of a family-friendly treatment approach for school-aged children is the Comprehensive Stuttering Program for School-Age Children (Langevin, Kully, & Ross-Harold, 2007), a 4-week intensive treatment program for children 7 to 12 years of age. The program addresses stuttering through the use of fluency enhancing skills (e.g. prolongation, gentle starts, pull-outs, and self-corrections of moments of stuttering, etc.) and addresses the attitudinal-emotional consequences of stuttering, including teasing and bullying, through discussion and a variety of activities.

In the early stages of development, this treatment would have been described as a *parent as aide* approach (Kully & Boberg, 1991), in that parents observed sessions, completed home assignments with their children to aid carryover, participated in acquisition and transfer when suitable, and attended parent education meetings. At that time the SLP was the primary decision-maker. However, since then the developers of the program responded to a growing awareness and understanding of the child within the context of the family over time, and now parents are joint decision-makers with the SLP. During the treatment program parents participate in and learn to deliver treatment. They learn the fluency enhancing skills alongside their children and they learn to give verbal contingencies for (a) accurate use and need for correction of fluency skills, and (b) moments of stuttering. Drawing from the Lidcombe Program (Onslow et al., 2003), parents also learn to give contingencies for fluent speech that is naturally achieved and they make daily severity ratings that provide the bases for making adjustments to treatment. Parents continue to participate in meetings; however, in addition to education about stuttering and learning how to help their child with the emotional-attitudinal consequences of stuttering, meetings provide a forum in which parents can freely share their feelings and their concerns. When possible, discussions with siblings and other family members are conducted to help them understand stuttering and what they can do to help the child who stutters.

Evidence Base of Effectiveness of Family Involvement

One of the major obstacles to evidence-based practice in intervention for children who stutter is the lack of clinical trials evidence (see Onslow, Packman, O'Brian & Menzies, 2007). Because of this, it is not possible to conduct meta-analyses of family-oriented interventions, or to even compare interventions that include families with those that do not. In terms of looking at family involvement in therapy, the only intervention for which there is evidence of efficacy from randomized controlled trials is the family-friendly Lidcombe Program (for reviews of the levels of evidence for stuttering interventions see reviews in Onslow et al., 2007). In a phase III randomized control trial Jones, Onslow, Packman, et al. (2005) compared a group of preschool children who received the Lidcombe Program with a no-treatment control group. Nine months after randomization, stuttering frequency (percent syllables stuttered) was significantly lower in the treatment group. Long-term follow-up indicated that stuttering may return in some children after some years (Jones, Onslow, Packman, et al. 2008), and that parents need to re-introduce treatment if this occurs.

Lewis, Packman, Onslow, Simpson, and Jones (2008) reported the results of a phase II randomized control trial of a telehealth adaptation of the Lidcombe Program. In this delivery model, there is no face-to-face contact and communication between the SLP and family is conducted via the telephone, E-mail and/or the Internet. The Lidcombe Program is ideally suited to this delivery model, given that it is conducted by parents in the child's everyday environment. Results showed that, again, 9 months after randomization, stuttering frequency was significantly lower in the treatment group than in the no-treatment group. It was clear, however, that telehealth delivery of the program takes about three times as long as standard clinic-based delivery.

Clinical Practice: SLP's Involvement of Families in Stuttering Treatments

Despite the claims of a number of authors that families are included in their interventions, very little is known about the extent to which this actually occurs. That is, there have been virtually no treatment fidelity studies. Again, the only clear evidence of this relates to the Lidcombe Program, in that research into the program now typically includes a treatment fidelity check. However, a survey of SLPs in Australia (Rousseau, Packman, Onslow, Robinson, & Harrison, 2002) on their actual use of the Lidcombe Program yielded some rather sobering results. Of SLPs who were treating preschoolers who stutter, around 85% were using the Lidcombe Program, while less than half of them were actually using it according to the treatment manual. That is, more than half were not using the program as it had been researched. Workplace restrictions was the main reason for this finding, and this situation raises serious concerns about the extent to which families are actually participating in the Lidcombe Program, and indeed in other programs that purport to involve families. Informal discussions with SLPs in Australia indicate that, in some instances, SLPs see themselves as delivering the treatment in the clinic, rather than the parent delivering it outside the clinic. This is not consistent with the way the program is designed; as described above, the treatment is meant to be delivered by a parent in the child's naturalistic environment. The purpose of clinic visits is to train the parent, to monitor progress, to engage in problem solving with the parent, and to ensure the treatment is an enjoyable experience for child and family. Clearly, further research is needed to see whether SLPs are actually conducting other treatments for children who stutter as outlined in publications.

Families' Views of Involvement in Treatment for Stuttering

Again, the only reports we have of families' views on their involvement in treatment for childhood stuttering relate to the Lidcombe Program (Francken, Kielstra-van der Schalk, & Boelens, 2005; Hansen, Herland, & Packman, 2004; Hayhow, Enderby, & Kingston, 2000; Packman, Hansen, & Herland, 2007).

Hayhow et al. (2000) developed the Bristol Stammering Questionnaire, which they administered to 59 parents in the United Kingdom who had completed the Lidcombe Program (response rate 88%). Francken et al. (2005) administered the same questionnaire to 11 parents in The Netherlands who had conducted part of the Lidcombe Program (response rate 100%). There are five statements in this questionnaire, to which parents respond with *Agree (1)*, *Mostly agree (2)*, *Not sure (3)*, *Mostly disagree (4)*, or *Disagree (5)*. The five statements and the responses for both studies are shown in Table 6-1. Each statement is scored out of 5. Respondents also rate the overall acceptability of the treatment out of 5. Clearly, the parents in both studies registered high levels of satisfaction with the Lidcombe Program.

Hansen et al. (2004) and Packman et al. (2007) reported the results of a survey that they developed and administered to parents who had conducted the Lidcombe Program. Authors Hansen and Herland wanted to ascertain Australian parents' perceptions of the program before introducing it to Norway. They reported anecdotally that response to the program in Norway to that point had been quite negative. The survey was given to 37 parents who had participated in the Lidcombe Program in Sydney, Australia (response rate 94%). They responded to 24 closed and open-ended questions about their experiences with the program, their perceptions of their children's experiences with the program, and their perceptions of the effectiveness of the program. They

Table 6–1. The Five Statements in the Bristol Stammering Questionnaire and the Responses of 52 Parents in the United Kingdom and 11 Parents in the Netherlands

	Hayhow et al. (2000) The United Kingdom (N = 52)	Francken et al. (2005) The Netherlands (N = 11)
1. Therapy sessions in the clinic were well structured*	1.2	1.5
2. This approach expects too much from parents+	4.5	3.9
3. This approach is disruptive for the rest of the family+	4.5	4.2
4. I would recommend this approach to other parents whose young children stammer*	1.2	1.9
5. I was pleased to be able to help my child myself*	1.1	1.3
Overall acceptability (out of 5)	4.7	4.3

*1 = "Agree" and 5 = "Disagree" (see text) for these statements.
+1 = "Disagree" and 5 = "Agree" (see text) for these statements.

were recruited from two clinics, a generalist clinic in an upper socioeconomic area of the city and a specialist stuttering clinic in a lower socioeconomic area, which was culturally and linguistically diverse.

Parents were asked about their experiences with various aspect of conducting the program. Responses were positive: 91% agreed that the severity rating scale was easy to use, 100% agreed that the SLPs feedback was helpful, 89% agreed that they felt free to ring the SLP between clinic visits if they felt they needed to, and 86% agreed that the program suited their family. However, interestingly, 66% agreed that they found it hard to find time for the treatment sessions each day. Parents were asked how easy they found the program to administer. Most reported that they found it easy, but only 23% said they found it easy to keep the required ratio of contingencies for stuttering and stutter-free speech. In response to questions about how they felt "being the therapist," over half said they felt positively about it.

Only two reported feeling uncomfortable with that role. The results of these three studies, conducted independently in three different countries, suggest that involvement in the Lidcombe Program is a positive experience for parents. To get a more personal feel for parents' reactions to the Lidcombe program, readers are referred to Chapter 16 in the Onslow et al. (2003) Lidcombe text, where parents' descriptions of their experiences with the program are reported verbatim. None had participated in the research reported above.

Nexus Between Research, Clinical Practice, and Families' Views

Again, limited to the Lidcombe Program, research shows that this family-friendly intervention is efficacious and parents are largely satisfied and believe that the program suits their family. However, some parents reported that it is hard to find time for the treatment sessions each day. Of concern is the finding that less than half of Australian SLPs are implementing the program in the way it is described in the manual and there is a perception among some that the program can be delivered by the SLP in the clinic.

Case Study of Family Involvement in Stuttering

This case study of the involvement of a parent and child in the Lidcombe Program is fictional. To illustrate the involvement of the family in the program, it has been written from the perspective of the parent. However, it is stressed that all aspects of this fictional case are empirically based; that is, we have drawn on what we know about the program and parents' experiences of it, and about how stuttering impacts on parents and children. This knowledge comes from publications such as the three studies of parents' experiences reported above and also from some groundbreaking research that we have conducted into the social and psychological impact of stuttering on preschoolers and their families (Langevin, Packman, & Onslow, 2008a, 2008b). Langevin et al. (2008a) reported the results of a survey of 77 parents of preschoolers, which investigated the impact of stuttering on their children and on themselves, and Langevin et al. (2008b) reported the findings of the first ever observational field study of preschool stuttering children in a naturalistic setting. As would be expected, the description of how the program is conducted draws from the clinical text (Onslow et al., 2003).

Background

Jay was 3 years, 6 months when his mother Karen took him to an SLP. Jay had been stuttering for 8 months. Karen had been told by her local medical practitioner that she should wait for a year or so before taking action, to see if Jay recovered naturally. She had also been advised by other mothers she knew that Jay would grow out of it. However, Jay's grandfather stuttered and Karen was starting to feel quite distressed. She did not know what to do to help Jay when he stuttered. She was also worried that Jay might never get over the stuttering and that it would limit his educational and vocational potential. She was also worried that the stuttering was affecting how Jay related to his peers at preschool. The preschool teacher had noticed his stuttering, but had not detected any signs of teasing by his peers.

Karen was also feeling guilty that she was not spending enough time with Jay and that this could be harmful. Jay had two sisters, one older and one younger, and Karen often felt "stretched." Jay's father worked long hours in a stressful job, and did not have much free time to spend with the children. Karen found she sometimes became impatient with Jay and wished he would just stop talking so that she would not be reminded of his stuttering, just for a moment or two. She would immediately feel ashamed of harboring such thoughts. Jay had also recently started indicating that he was aware of his stuttering. He had started slapping his mouth and asking Karen why he couldn't talk properly. As the stuttering was quite severe, and showing no signs of abating after 8 months, Karen decided it was time to seek professional help.

The Program

Karen was relieved to find that the SLP, Poppy, had completed a Lidcombe Program workshop (for details of workshops see the Web site of the Australian Stuttering Research Centre, http://www.fhs.usyd

.edu.au/asrc) and had treated many stuttering preschoolers with the program. She was reassured when Poppy told her that the program was supported by extensive research and that she had every confidence that it would be effective with Jay. Karen was surprised to hear that the evidence suggests that, all things being equal, children may respond better if treatment is delayed for a year or so after the onset of the stuttering. However, when Kay told Poppy how fearful she was, and that Jay was now frustrated and distressed by his stuttering, and when she told Poppy that Jay's grandfather had stuttered all his life, Poppy reassured her that in Jay's case they would start the program immediately.

Karen was somewhat taken aback to learn that she was to be Jay's therapist, rather than Poppy. What's more, she would be doing the therapy each day, at home and in other everyday situations, rather than in the clinic. "How will I ever be able to do it without upsetting him?" she wondered. "How will I ever find the time?" However, Poppy reassured her that they would work it out together, on the basis that she, Poppy, was the expert in stuttering and Karen was the expert on her own child. Karen learned that Poppy would train her how to do the treatment during weekly visits to the clinic. She would also learn how to measure the severity of Jay's stuttering each day. At each visit they together would look at Poppy's clinic stuttering measures and Karen's outside stuttering measures, and together ascertain whether the treatment was working and determine how it should be adjusted for the following week. Poppy also reassured Karen that they would together work out how Karen could adjust her daily schedule in order to find the time to sit and talk with Jay for 15 minutes or so, in order to conduct structured treatment sessions. Poppy informed her that at an appropriate stage, Karen would do the treatment in more natural conversational exchanges, for example, in the car driving to preschool, or at bath time. She also learned that once Jay's stuttering reached low levels both inside and outside the clinic, with Poppy's guidance and support they would move from stage 1 of the program to stage 2, which would involve Karen systematically withdrawing the treatment and a decrease in frequency of the clinic visits.

Karen felt both daunted and elated on hearing how the program worked. She was daunted by the prospect of conducting the treatment herself, but was elated at the thought that the program was likely to be effective and that she was finally going to be able to something to help her son.

At each clinic visit Karen demonstrated for Poppy how she had been doing therapy the previous week, and Poppy gave her feedback and suggested how she could modify it for the next week, in order to maximize effectiveness. To her surprise, Karen found that with Poppy's input she was quite capable of conducting the therapy sessions at home. However, at first Jay did not like his mother commenting on his stuttering. When Karen reported this to Poppy, Poppy immediately suggested that she terminate the contingencies for stuttering until Jay's stuttering severity decreased. Karen was relieved to find that the overriding principle of the program is that it must be an enjoyable experience for the child and family. She was relieved that, together, she and Poppy were always able to find ways to make it so.

Jay met the low stuttering criteria both inside and outside the clinic after 17 weeks, and so moved to stage 2. Jay's stuttering remained at a very low level and the frequency of visits to Poppy decreased. Every now and again Karen would hear a stutter but she knew just what to do when that happened, without having to consult Poppy. This was empowering. After a year, at Karen and Jay's final visit to Poppy, Poppy advised Karen to remain vigilant for stuttering, just in case it should return. Kay was relieved to know that she could contact Poppy again at any time in the future if she had any concerns about Jay.

Summary and Conclusions

In this chapter, we have concentrated to a large extent on the Lidcombe Program (Onslow et al., 2003), which was developed for preschoolers who stutter. The reason for this is that the Lidcombe Program is the only intervention for childhood stuttering that has been investigated with randomized controlled trials. In other words, it is the only intervention for which efficacy can be claimed. The research to date indicates that, although the treatment manual outlines the necessary components of the program, it can be delivered in ways that suit individual families. One of the strengths of this family-friendly program is that it translates across cultures. Parents can present the program in ways that accord not only with their own parenting styles but that are also culturally appropriate. Although the program was developed in Australia, it is now used widely around the world, including non-English speaking countries such as The Netherlands, Denmark, Germany, and Iran.

References

Conture, E. G., & Melnick, K. S. (1999). Parent-child group approach to stuttering in preschool children. In M. Onslow & A. Packman (Eds.), *The handbook of early stuttering intervention* (pp. 17–51). San Diego, CA: Singular.

Costello, J. (1983). Current behavioral treatments for stuttering. In D. Prins & R. J. Ingham (Eds.), *Treatment of stuttering in early childhood: Methods and issues.* (pp. 69–112). San Diego, CA: College-Hill Press.

Franken, M-C. J., Kielstra-van der Schalk, J., & Boelens, H. (2005). Experimental treatment of early stuttering: A preliminary study. *Journal of Fluency Disorders, 30,* 189–199.

Glauber, I. P. (1943). Psychoanalytic concepts of the stutterer. *Nervous Child, 2,* 172–180.

Gottwald, S. R., & Starkweather, C. W. (1999). Stuttering prevention and early intervention: A multiprocess approach. In M. Onslow & A. Packman (Eds.), *The handbook of early stuttering intervention* (pp. 53–82). San Diego, CA: Singular.

Gregory, H. G. (1999). Developmental intervention: Differential strategies. In M. Onslow & A. Packman (Eds.), *The handbook of early stuttering intervention* (pp. 83–101). San Diego, CA: Singular.

Guitar, B. (2006). *Stuttering: An integrated approach to its nature and treatment.* Philadelphia: Lippincott Williams & Williams.

Hansen, E., Herland, M., & Packman, A. (2004). Lidcombe-Programmet: Foreldre som hovedaktorer I direkte stammebehandling. *Spesialpedagogikk, 9,* 28–35.

Hayhow, R., Enderby, P., & Kingston, M. (2000). Parental satisfaction with stammering therapy. The development of a questionnaire. In H. G. Bosshardt, J. S. Yaruss, & H. F. M. Peters, (Eds.), *Proceedings of the Third World Congress on Fluency Disorders,* (pp. 322–325). Nijmegen: University Press Nijmegen.

Ingham, R. J. (1982). *Stuttering and behavior therapy.* San Diego, CA: College-Hill Press.

Johnson, W., & Associates (1959). *The onset of stuttering.* Minneapolis: University of Minnesota Press.

Jones, M., Onslow, M., Packman, A., O'Brian, S., Hearne, A., Williams, S., Ormond, T., & Schwarz, I. (2008). Extended follow-up of a randomised controlled trial of the Lidcombe Program of Early Stuttering Intervention. *International Journal of Language and Communication Disorders.* Online version ahead of print available at http://www.informaworld.com/smpp/content~content=a792963525~db=all~jumptype=rss

Jones, M., Onslow, M., Packman, A., Williams, S., Ormond, T., Schwarz, I., et al. (2005). Randomised controlled trial of the Lidcombe Program for early stuttering intervention. *British Medical Journal, 331*(7518), 659–663.

Kully, D., & Boberg, E. (1991). Therapy for school-age children. *Seminars in Speech and Language, 12,* 291–300.

Laiho, A. & Klippi, A. (2007). Long- and short-term results of children's and adolescents' therapy courses for stuttering. *International Journal of Language and Communication Disorders, 42,* 367–382.

Langevin, M., Kully, D. A., & Ross-Harold, B. (2007). The Comprehensive Stuttering Program for School-age Children with strategies for managing teasing and bullying. In E. G. Conture & R. F. Curlee (Eds.), *Stuttering and related disorders of fluency* (3rd ed., pp. 131–149). New York: Thieme.

Langevin, M., Packman, A., & Onslow, M. (2008a). The impact of stuttering on preschool children and their parents (Manuscript submitted for publication).

Langevin, M., Packman, A., & Onslow, M. (2008b). Peer responses to stuttered utterances of in the preschool setting (Manuscript submitted for publication).

Lewis, C., Packman, A., Onslow, M.,, Simpson, J. A., & Jones, M. (2008). Phase II trial of telehealth delivery of the Lidcombe Program of Early Stuttering Intervention. *American Journal of Speech-Language Pathology, 17,* 139–149.

Onslow, M., & Packman, A. (1999). *The handbook of early stuttering intervention.* San Diego, CA: Singular.

Onslow, M., Packman, A., & Harrison, E. (2003). *The Lidcombe Program of early stuttering intervention: A clinician's guide.* Austin TX: Pro-Ed.

Onslow, M., Packman, A., O'Brian, S., & Menzies, R. G. (2007). *Evidence based practice in the management of stuttering* (Under contract). Austin, TX: Pro-Ed.

Packman, A., & Attanasio, J. S. (2004). *Theoretical issues in stuttering.* London: Psychology Press.

Packman, A., Code, C., & Onslow, M. (2007). On the cause of stuttering: Integrating theory with brain and behavioural research. *Journal of Neurolinguistics, 20,* 353–362.

Packman, A., Hansen, E. J., & Herland, M. (2007). Parents' experiences of the Lidcombe Program: The Norway-Australia connection. In J. Au-Yeung & M. M. Leahy (Eds.), *Research, treatment, and self-help in fluency disorders: New horizons. Proceedings of the Fifth World Congress on Fluency*

Disorders, Dublin, Ireland (pp. 418-422). Dublin: International Fluency Association.

Pindzola, R. H. (1999). The Stuttering Intervention Program. In M. Onslow & A. Packman (Eds.), *The handbook of early stuttering intervention* (pp. 119-138). San Diego, CA: Singular.

Riley, J., & Riley, G. (1999). Speech motor training. In M. Onslow & A. Packman (Eds.), *The handbook of early stuttering intervention* (pp. 139-158). San Diego, CA: Singular.

Rousseau, I., Packman, A., Onslow, M., Robinson, R., & Harrison, E. (2002). Australian speech pathologists' use of the Lidcombe Program of Early Stuttering Intervention. *ACQuiring Knowledge in Speech, Language and Hearing, 4*, 67-71.

Runyan, C. M., & Runyan, S. E. (1999). In M. Onslow & A. Packman (Eds.), The Fluency Rules Program. In M. Onslow, & A. Packman (Eds.) *The handbook of early stuttering intervention* (pp. 159-169). San Diego, CA: Singular.

Rustin, L., Botterill, W., & Kelman, E. (1996). *Assessment and therapy for young dysfluent children: Family interaction.* London: Whurr.

Ryan, B. P., & Ryan, B. V. (1999). The Monterey Fluency Program. In M. Onslow & A. Packman (Eds.), *The handbook of early stuttering intervention* (pp. 170-188). San Diego, CA: Singular.

Shapiro, D. A. (1999). *Stuttering intervention: A collaborative journey to fluency freedom.* Austin, TX: Pro-Ed.

Shine, R. E. (1984). Assessment and fluency training with the young stutterer. In M. Peins (Ed.), *Contemporary approaches in stuttering therapy* (pp. 173-216). Boston: Little, Brown & Company.

Siegel, G. (1998). Stuttering: Theory, research and therapy. In A. Cordes & R. J. Ingham, (Eds.), *Treatment efficacy for stuttering: A search for empirical bases* (pp. 103-114). San Diego, CA: Singular.

Starkweather, C. W. (1989). The Demands and Capacities model of stuttering development and the treatment of young children. *Folia Phoniatrica, 41*, 5-4.

Trajkovski, N., Andrews, C., O'Brian, S., Onslow, M., & Packman, A. (2006). Treating stuttering in a preschool child with syllable-timed speech: A case report. *Behaviour Change, 23*, 270-277.

Wall, M. J., & Myers, F. L. (1995). *Clinical management of childhood stuttering* (2nd ed.). Austin TX: Pro-Ed.

Yairi, E., & Ambrose, N. G. (2005). *Early childhood stuttering.* Austin, TX: Pro-Ed.

Yaruss, J. S., Coleman, C., & Hammer, D. (2006). Treating preschool children who stutter: Description and preliminary evaluation of a family-focused treatment approach. *Language, Speech, and Hearing Services in Schools, 37*, 1-19.

Chapter 7
Working with Families of Children with Speech Impairment

Nicole Watts Pappas and Sharynne McLeod

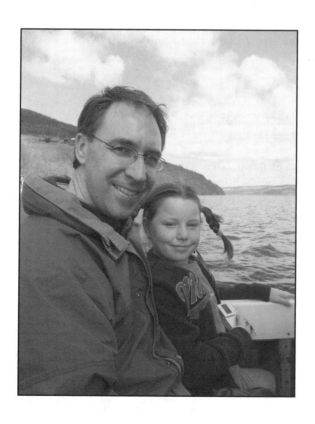

Introduction

Children with speech impairment form a large component of pediatric SLPs' clinical caseloads (Watts Pappas, McLeod, McAllister, & McKinnon, 2008). Prevalence rates for children with speech impairment are higher for younger children (McKinnon, McLeod, & Reilly, 2007), increasing the likelihood that speech-language pathologists (SLPs) may be required to work with the child's family as part of the intervention. SLPs' confidence and expertise in working with families is therefore of vital importance when providing intervention to this common clinical population. In this chapter, we review the history of family involvement in intervention for speech impairment, consider how families are involved in current recommended intervention approaches, review the literature on the impact of family involvement in speech intervention, and discuss studies that have explored parents' and SLPs' perceptions of family involvement in intervention for speech impairment. The nexus between the findings of efficacy research and parents' and SLPs' perceptions is then considered in a case study of working with a family of a child with speech impairment.

Defining Speech Impairment

A speech impairment is defined as a difficulty producing speech sounds that is of unknown origin (Shriberg & Kwiatkowski, 1994). It may also be referred to as speech-sound disorder/delay, articulation disorder/delay, or phonological disorder/delay. Across studies, the prevalence of children with speech impairment has been reported as ranging from 2.3% to 24.6% (Law, Boyle, Harris, Harkness, & Nye, 2000; McKinnon et al., 2007). Children with speech impairment may be difficult to understand by both familiar and unfamiliar listeners (Dodd, 1985). Some studies have reported that children with speech impairment are at greater risk of literacy difficulties when they begin school, especially children whose speech impairment persists beyond 5;6 years of age (Bird, Bishop, & Freeman, 1995). Speech impairment can be associated with long-term academic, social, and occupational difficulties

(Felsenfeld, Broen, & McGue, 1992, 1994). Effective and timely intervention therefore is important for these children. The possible impact of involving families in their child's intervention and the influence of individual family/professional relationships is an important consideration in determining the most effective way to provide intervention to this clinical population.

Research: Historical Overview of Family Involvement in Intervention for Speech Impairment

Historical Overview

Recommended parent and family involvement in intervention for speech impairment has undergone many changes in the past 50 years (see Table 7-1 on p. 195). As with intervention for other developmental delays, SLPs traditionally gave families limited opportunity to be involved in intervention for their child's speech impairment. In fact, a belief which persisted to the 1960s was that the family (particularly the mother) could be the cause of speech impairment in children (Moll & Darley, 1960; Solomon, 1961; Sommers et al., 1964; Wood, 1946). For example Sommers and colleagues stated that "Some investigators have found that attitudes toward child-rearing practices tend to be less desirable in parents of children with functional misarticulations" (1964, pp. 126–127) Similar to some of the forms of early intervention for stuttering described in Chapter 6, this belief gave rise to intervention that could be described as radically family-centered in which psychological treatment for "paternal maladjustment" was suggested to form part of the speech intervention (Wood, 1946, p. 255).

In the 1970s, 1980s, and early 1990s there was an increased interest in the effects of parental involvement in the speech intervention provided to the child. This interest mainly focused on parental provision of home activities that either supplemented or replaced the intervention provided by the SLP (McPherson, Morris, & Ferguson, 1987). Parental involvement was seen as a method of increasing the effectiveness of the intervention and decreasing the time the SLP was required to spend with the child. Parental provision of home programs for speech impairment was the focus of many experimental studies during this period (Broen & Westman, 1990; Costello & Bosler, 1976; Dodd & Barker, 1990; Shelton, Johnson, & Arndt, 1972; Shelton, Johnson, Willis, & Arndt, 1975; Wing & Heimgartner, 1973). More recently, interest in family involvement in speech intervention appears to have decreased with the majority of experimental studies making limited mention of parental involvement in the descriptions of their intervention approaches (Watts Pappas, McLeod, McAllister, & Simpson, 2005). A number of recent textbooks on intervention for speech impairment and related disorders also make few references to working with families (Bauman-Waengler, 2004; Bernthal & Bankson, 2004; Pascoe, Stackhouse, & Wells, 2006). There are some notable exceptions to this trend. For example, the relatively recent PACT (Parents and Children Together) approach which incorporates considerable family involvement in intervention (Bowen & Cupples, 1998). Using the models of practice described in Chapter 1 as a reference, we now consider some of the most common contemporary approaches to speech intervention with regard to the extent and type of family involvement incorporated in the intervention approach.

Therapist-Centered Approaches

Most intervention approaches for speech impairment incorporate some form of parental involvement. However, as noted above, several experimental studies of intervention approaches for speech impairment have been conducted without mention of parental involvement in the intervention planning or provision. For example, the minimal pairs (Blanche, Parsons, & Humphreys 1981; Elbert, Powell, & Swartzlander, 1991), maximal pairs (Gierut, 1989; Gierut & Champion, 2000), and multiple opposition (Williams, 2000) approaches to speech intervention have all been demonstrated to be effective without any mention of parental involvement. In therapist-centered approaches parents may not be required or given an opportunity to be involved in the intervention. The SLP assesses the child, determines the intervention goals, carries out the intervention, and evaluates the child's progress. Therapist-centered approaches may be acceptable to some families who do not wish to be involved in their child's intervention. It is important to consider here that research versions of intervention may be different from clinical application of these interventions that may include families.

Parent-as-Therapist Aide Approaches

Many intervention approaches recommended for the remediation of speech impairment use a parent-as-therapist aide approach to family involvement. In this approach, parents are involved primarily in the provision of the intervention, with little involvement in intervention planning. From their descriptions in the literature, approaches that could be considered to use a parent-as-therapist aide model include the cycles approach (Hodson & Paden, 1991; Hodson, 2006), the psycholinguistic approach (Stackhouse, Pascoe, & Gardner, 2006), and the constraint-based nonlinear approach (Bernhardt, Stemberger, & Major, 2006). These intervention approaches appear predominantly to involve parents in the provision of home activities and make no mention of parental involvement in decision-making. Again, it is possible that clinicians may incorporate greater family involvement in these approaches when they use them in their clinical practice.

Family-Centered Approaches

In a family-centered approach to speech intervention the SLP would follow the parents' lead in all aspects of the assessment and intervention. Although they would provide their expert knowledge to guide the family's choices they would accept the families' decisions even if they did not professionally agree with them. Families would be encouraged to be involved in intervention planning and provision and intervention would focus on the family as well as the child. No reports of intervention approaches for speech impairment could be located that could be called truly family-centered. Although the PACT approach (Bowen & Cupples, 1998) does involve families significantly in the intervention it still appears that in this approach the professional does not completely follow the families' lead.

Family-Friendly Approaches

In family-friendly approaches to speech intervention family involvement in intervention planning and provision is encouraged and supported. However, the SLP still retains the role of the final decision-maker in the intervention. Several approaches to speech intervention such as PROMPT (PROMPTS for Restructuring Oral Motor Targets) (Hayden, 2006), PACT (Parents and Children Together) (Bowen & Cupples, 2006) and core vocabulary (Dodd, Holm, Crosbie, & McIntosh, 2006) could be considered to be family friendly. For example in the PROMPT approach to intervention, family members help choose priorities for intervention and are involved in the assessment and intervention activities. However, the SLP still leads the intervention process, selecting final intervention targets and determining when parents begin to conduct specific activities with the child. So, although the PROMPT approach involves families, it still allows the SLP to use their expertise to guide the intervention process.

Evidence Base of Effectiveness of Family Involvement in Speech Intervention

As noted by Bowen and Cupples (2006), although a number of current approaches to speech intervention incorporate family involvement, the relative impact of that involvement on the effectiveness of those intervention approaches is not known. We now consider the limited literature on the effects of family involvement on intervention for speech impairment. A number of studies have been conducted to investigate the effectiveness of various forms of family involvement in intervention for speech impairment. The majority of these studies were conducted prior to 1991 with the most recent study conducted in 1998 (Bowen & Cupples). It is important to note that the family members involved in the studies have all been parents. No studies have explored the involvement of other family members such as grandparents or siblings. The studies have investigated the impact of parental involvement in speech intervention using predominantly traditional or minimal pair intervention approaches. There is a dearth of evidence regarding the impact of parental involvement on more contemporary intervention approaches. Table 7-2 on page 200 outlines the details of the studies and identifies the forms of parental involvement evaluated in each study.

The studies focused on one or more of the following questions:

1. Are intervention programs incorporating parental involvement effective?
2. Is parent-administered speech intervention as effective as SLP-administered intervention?
3. Does parental involvement make speech intervention provided by a SLP more effective?

We now consider how the studies answered the above questions.

Table 7–1. Parental Involvement in Speech Intervention Studies (in Alphabetical Order)

Approach	Study	Parental Involvement
Minimal pairs	Blanche, Parsons, & Humphreys (1981)	No
Minimal pairs	Broen & Westman (1990)	Home program with training Involvement in goal-setting
Naturalistic speech intelligibility training	Conture, Louko, & Edwards (1989)	Parent education (group) Homework Attendance at intervention sessions Participation in intervention sessions
Minimal pairs	Elbert, Powell, & Swartzlander (1991)	No
Traditional Minimal pairs	Forrest & Elbert (2001)	No
Maximal pairs	Gierut (1989)	No
Maximal pairs	Gierut (1990)	Homework
Maximal pairs	Gierut (1991)	Homework
Maximal pairs	Gierut (1992)	Homework
Maximal pairs	Gierut (1999)	No
Maximal pairs	Gierut & Champion (2000)	No
Maximal pairs	Gierut & Champion (2001)	No
Maximal pairs	Gierut, Morrisette, Hughes, & Rowland (1996)	No
Whole language Minimal pairs	Hoffman, Norris, & Monjure (1990)	No
Traditional Minimal pairs Imagery	Klein (1996)	Attendance at intervention sessions Participation in intervention sessions Homework

continues

Table 7–1. *continued*

Approach	Study	Parental Involvement
Cycles approach	Montgomery & Bonderman (1989)	Homework
Minimal pairs	Powell & Elbert (1984)	No
Traditional therapy Minimal pairs	Powell, Elbert, Miccio, Strike-Roussos, & Brasseur (1998)	No
Minimal pairs	Saben & Ingham (1991)	No
Traditional therapy	Shriberg & Kwiatkowski (1990)	No
Traditional therapy Imagery	Stone & Stoel-Gammon (1990)	No
Minimal pairs Cycles approach Whole language	Tyler & Sandoval (1994)	Attendance at intervention sessions Participation in intervention sessions Homework
Cycles approach Whole language	Tyler & Watterson (1991)	No
Multiple oppositions	Williams (2000)	No
Traditional therapy	Wolfe, Blocker, & Prater (1988)	No

Are Speech Intervention Programs Incorporating Parental Involvement Effective?

The effectiveness of intervention programs involving a significant amount of parental involvement has been investigated in a number of studies (Bowen & Cupples, 1998; Broen & Westman, 1990; Costello & Bosler, 1976; Dodd & Barker, 1990; Shelton et al., 1972, 1975; Wing & Heimgartner, 1973). However, few of the studies have included a control group in the study design (Bowen & Cupples, 1998; Broen & Westman, 1990). Although the children in the remaining studies demonstrated improvement in their speech-sound production, the lack of a control group makes it difficult to determine whether the observed sound change was as a result of the home program or simply of maturation.

The two studies that did include a control group involved different forms of parental participation. Broen and Westman (1990) compared a group of children who received a home program to a group who received no intervention for their speech impairment. The parents of the 12 children in the experimental group attended weekly group sessions with the SLP. Individualized home activity kits were given to the parents each week to use at home with their children. The eight children in the control group received no intervention. The experimental group made significantly more progress than the control group. Thus, the study suggested that speech intervention given by parents was more effective than no intervention. However, the SLP was still involved with the intervention to a large extent (weekly sessions with parents), so it is unclear whether home programs given by parents with less intensive training would be more effective than no intervention at all.

Bowen and Cupples (1998) investigated the effectiveness of an intervention approach entitled Parents and Children Together (PACT), in which parents were encouraged to participate in intervention sessions, forming a triad with the SLP, parent, and child. The parents were also asked to conduct home activities with their child. The results of the study indicated that the PACT approach to speech intervention was more effective than no intervention at all (Bowen & Cupples, 1998). However, it is not known whether the speech intervention would have been just as effective without parental participation.

The results of these studies appear to indicate that speech intervention involving a significant amount of parental involvement can be effective. However, as only two of the reviewed studies contained control groups (Bowen & Cupples, 1998; Broen & Westman, 1990) the evidence base for the effectiveness of intervention involving a significant amount of parental involvement is not extensive.

Is Parent-Administered Speech Intervention as Effective as SLP-Administered Intervention?

A few studies have compared parental provision of home programs to that given by a SLP. Tufts and Holliday (1959) investigated the effectiveness of a home program administered by parents with a group of 30 children aged 4 to 6 years. The children presented with a moderate speech impairment of unknown origin. The participants were separated into three groups. Group A received no intervention, Group B received weekly group intervention with a SLP, and the parents of the children in Group C received weekly group training to treat their child's speech impairment while their children received no direct intervention from the SLP. A traditional therapy approach was used for both the SLP and parent-administered intervention conditions. After an intervention period of 7 months the children were reassessed. Surprisingly, the children who had not received intervention showed no change in their speech sound production over the period of the study. In contrast, the children in Groups B and C improved in speech sound production to a similar extent, thus suggesting that intervention provided by the parents was as effective as the group intervention with the SLP. It should be noted, however, that the intervention provided by the SLP was in a group of 10 children. It is not known whether the large size of this group affected the intervention outcomes. Individual intervention by the SLP may have been more effective than intervention provided by the parents.

In the second study, Eiserman, McCoun, and Escobar (1990) investigated whether speech intervention conducted by parents was as effective as intervention given by a SLP for 40, 3- to 5- year-old children with a moderate speech impairment. The participants were stratified for age and speech ability and then randomly assigned to one of two groups. The 20 children in the first group received weekly small group intervention with the SLP. The parents of the 20 children in the second group were visited fortnightly at their home by the SLP to receive training to conduct a home program. The training sessions were 40 minutes in duration and involved the SLP informally evaluating the child to determine the activities for the next fortnight. The SLP also demonstrated the home program activities and gave the parent an opportunity to practice the procedures with the child. The parents in this group were asked to work daily with their children for 20 to 30 minutes.

The results indicated that the children in the home training group made similar gains to the children who received intervention primarily from the SLP. This study indicated that a home program for speech intervention was just as effective as speech intervention provided primarily by a SLP. However, although the home program was primarily delivered by the parents, speech-language pathology input and support occurred during fortnightly sessions. A home program given with less intensive support might be less effective than regular intervention sessions with the SLP.

These two studies indicated that speech intervention provided primarily by parents can be just as effective as speech intervention provided primarily by a SLP. However, as the intervention given by the SLP in both studies was in a group format, it is uncertain whether individual intervention with the SLP may have led to better outcomes. Additionally, although the parents primarily administered the home programs, SLP input and support was still high (weekly or fortnightly sessions). A home program given with less intensive support might be less effective than regular intervention sessions with the SLP.

Does Parental Involvement Make Speech Intervention Provided by a SLP More Effective?

There are numerous ways in which parents can be involved in intervention for speech impairment. Some of these forms of involvement include provision of home activities, attendance at intervention sessions, participation in the sessions, and participation in intervention planning. To advise families of the most effective ways in which they can be involved in their child's intervention knowledge about the efficacy of different forms of parent and family involvement is useful. The efficacy of specific types of parent involvement has been investigated in a limited number of the studies listed in Table 7-2. We now consider the findings of these studies in relation to the form of parental involvement they investigated.

Homework Activities

Sommers (1962), Sommers et al. (1964), and Ruscello, Cartwright, Haines, and Shuster (1993) investigated whether the provision of homework activities by parents makes speech intervention given by a SLP more effective. Sommers (1962) investigated the effect of training parents to conduct speech homework activities with their children who had received either group or individual intervention. Eighty school-aged children with a speech impairment of unknown origin were given an intensive block of traditional speech intervention.

Table 7–2. Studies Investigating Parental Involvement in Speech Intervention (from Least to Most Involvement)

Form of Parental Involvement	Studies	Sample Size	Severity of Speech Impairment	Homogeneity of Groups	Length of Parental Intervention	Summary of Outcomes
Provision of homework activities (no training)	None have investigated outcomes	—	—	—	—	Unsure if effective
Provision of homework activities (training and education)	Sommers, 1962	80 children	Not specified	For age	4 × 50-minute training sessions a week for 4 weeks Homework activities	Children of parents trained to give homework activities made more progress than children of parents who were not trained
	Sommers et al., 1964	80 children	Not specified	For age, intelligence, and socioeconomic level	4 × 50-minute training sessions a week for 4 weeks Homework activities	Children of parents trained to give homework activities made more progress than children of parents who were not trained
	Ruscello, Cartwright, Hanes, & Shuster, 1993	12 children	Below 15th percentile on standardized test	For severity of speech impairment	Used computer program with child 1 × 8 weeks	Children in both groups made similar gains in speech-sound production

Form of Parental Involvement	Studies	Sample Size	Severity of Speech Impairment	Homogeneity of Groups	Length of Parental Intervention	Summary of Outcomes
Attendance at speech intervention sessions	Fudala, England, & Ganoung, 1972	92 children	Not specified	For severity of speech impairment	Attendance at 16 speech intervention sessions Homework activities	Better outcomes when parents attended sessions
Participation in speech intervention sessions	Fudala, England, & Ganoung, 1972	92 children	Not specified	For severity of speech impairment	Attendance and occasional participation in 16 intervention sessions Homework activities	No better outcomes when parents participated in sessions
	Bowen & Cupples, 1998	22 children	Ranged from mild to severe, mostly moderate	For age and severity of impairment	Varied—parental attendance and participation at 6–27 sessions Homework with parent from 6–24 times per week	Control group received no intervention—unsure if parental participation in sessions affected intervention outcomes
Home program (without training)	None have investigated outcomes	—	—	—	—	Unsure if effective

continues

Table 7–2. *continued*

Form of Parental Involvement	Studies	Sample Size	Severity of Speech Impairment	Homogeneity of Groups	Length of Parental Intervention	Summary of Outcomes
Home program (with training)	Tufts & Holliday, 1959	30 children	Moderate speech impairment	For intelligence, age and severity of speech impairment	Parental attendance at weekly group training sessions for 7 months	Children trained by parents made same gains as children who received group intervention with SLP
	Shelton, Johnson, & Arndt, 1972	8 children	Mild	No control group	1 × group session with SLP then 4 × 10-minute weekly meetings Home program	As no control group unsure if effective
	Wing & Heimgartner, 1973	6 children	Mild	No control group	1 × individual parent training session Weekly phone conference with SLP Home program— 10 minutes each day for 5–10 weeks	As no control group unsure if effective

Form of Parental Involvement	Studies	Sample Size	Severity of Speech Impairment	Homogeneity of Groups	Length of Parental Intervention	Summary of Outcomes
Home program (with training) *continued*	Shelton, Johnson, Willis, & Arndt, 1975	10 children	One standard deviation or more below mean	No control group	1 × individual parent training session Home program—5 days per week for 5 weeks.	As no control group unsure if effective
	Costello & Bosler, 1976	3 children	Not specified	No control group	2 × 1½–2 hour group sessions with therapist followed by 1 × 1 hr individual session with therapist Home program	As no control group unsure if effective
	Broen & Westman, 1990	20 children	Moderate-severe	No, children in control group had milder speech impairment	17 × 1½ hour parent classes Homework an average of 6 times a week	More effective than no intervention Just as effective as intervention given by SLP Extensive training and support necessary to obtain outcomes

continues

Table 7–2. *continued*

Form of Parental Involvement	Studies	Sample Size	Severity of Speech Impairment	Homogeneity of Groups	Length of Parental Intervention	Summary of Outcomes
Home program (with training) *continued*	Dodd & Barker, 1990	5 children	Not specified	No control group	11 × 120-minute weekly group sessions Home program	As no control group unsure if effective
	Eiserman, McCoun, & Escobar, 1990	40 children	Moderate	For severity of speech impairment, education of parents and age of child	40 fortnightly home visits from SLP for 7 months Homework activities with child 4 times weekly	Parent-administered intervention as effective as group SLP-administered intervention
Involvement in intervention planning	Broen & Westman, 1990	20 children	Moderate-severe	No, children in control group had milder speech impairment	17 × 1½-hour parent classes Homework an average of 6 times a week	Parent-administered intervention more effective than no intervention—unsure what impact parental involvement in intervention planning had on outcomes

SLP = speech-language pathologist.

Half of the children (40) received small group therapy (three to five children in a group) for 50 minutes and the other half (40) received individual speech therapy sessions of 30 minutes in duration. The intervention was intensive and took place 4 days a week, for a period of 4 weeks. Half of the parents of the children in each group (20 parents of the children from the group training condition and 20 parents of the children from the individual intervention training condition) were trained in group sessions for 45 minutes per day, 4 days per week for the duration of the study. Therefore, in both child training conditions (group or individual intervention) half of the parents of the children in the group received training to work with their child and half received no training.

The parent training sessions consisted of lectures covering speech development and error remediation, discussion, and observation of the children's speech intervention sessions. Both the trained and untrained parents were given homework activities to complete with their child. It was found that the children of the parents who were trained to do homework activities with their child made significantly more improvement in their speech sound production than the children of the parents who were not trained. This effect was present regardless of whether individual or group speech intervention was given by the SLP. This study indicated therefore that the provision of homework activities by trained parents can improve outcomes of speech intervention given by a SLP, even when that intervention is provided in an intensive block.

A similar study conducted by Sommers et al. (1964) produced comparable results: children whose parents were trained achieved greater speech change than those whose parents were not trained. In both of these studies, the frequency with which homework activities were conducted at home was not measured. The trained parents therefore may simply have given the homework activities more frequently than the untrained parents, so that the frequency of the homework might have been the cause of the difference in outcomes, rather than the parental training.

The third study investigated the effectiveness of parental involvement in computer-based speech intervention. Ruscello et al. (1993) investigated the effect of parents providing a weekly speech session to their child via a computer program. This could be considered a form of homework although the activity occurred within the speech-language pathology clinic. Twelve preschool-aged children (4–5 years of age) who scored below the 15th percentile on a test of speech sound production were provided with minimal pair speech intervention given via a computer program. All the children had normal hearing, receptive language, and structure and function of the speech mechanism. The children were split into two groups. Children in Group A received computer-based speech intervention with the SLP twice a week for 8 weeks (the sessions were 1 hour in length). In this group, the parents did not work with their children at home. The children in Group B received a combination of SLP and parent-administered intervention. Speech intervention sessions with the SLP were held for 1 hour, once a week for the 8 weeks of the study. In a second 1-hour period per week, the children's parents traveled to the clinic to give the computer-based intervention to their child. An SLP was available to answer questions but the training was led by parents. The parents were trained in the use of the computer program prior to working with their children. This training typically took approximately 3 hours.

At the post-test the children in each group had made similar gains in speech-sound production. No differences were found between the improvement made by the children whose parents were trained to work with them once per week and that made by the children who received intervention from the SLP only. This study may indicate that the training of parents to work with their child leads to outcomes similar to those obtained if the SLP only works with the child. However, as the parents were working with their children only once per week, it is difficult to generalize this finding to the use of daily homework activities.

The results of these three studies appear to indicate that parental involvement in the form of conducting home activities with their child while the child receives intervention from a SLP makes that intervention more effective, even when the child is receiving intensive speech intervention. However, the most significant effects on outcomes seem to have occurred when parents were provided with intensive training to give the homework. No studies have specifically investigated the effects of homework provision when parental training is not provided. Considering that homework provision is one of the most common ways that SLP clinicians involve parents in speech intervention (Watts Pappas et al., 2008) it is unfortunate that it is not known whether the provision of homework activities to untrained parents would improve speech intervention outcomes.

Parental Attendance at Intervention Sessions

There has been limited attention to the effects of parental attendance at speech intervention sessions. Fudala, England, and Ganoung (1972) investigated the effects of parental observation of their child's speech intervention sessions with a group of 92 school-aged children (ranging from first to fifth grades). The children, all of whom had a speech impairment of unknown origin, received traditional articulation group therapy sessions with the SLP for 16 weeks. Sessions were held for 1 hour, weekly. All the children's parents were given the same speech activities to conduct with their child at home; however, some parents attended sessions and some did not.

The children were separated into three groups. Parents of the 46 children in Group I did not attend any therapy sessions. The parents of the 23 children in Group IIA were requested to attend their child's speech therapy sessions once a month. Parents of the 23 children in Group IIB were asked to attend the sessions weekly. The parents in Group IIB also participated in the sessions to some extent, acting as the clinician in some of the group sessions toward the end of the study.

The same therapy and homework activities were given to all of the children. The results showed that the children in Groups IIA and IIB made more than double the improvement in speech sound production than those in Group I. However, the improvement made in Groups IIA and IIB was similar. These findings indicate that parental attendance at sessions improved the effectiveness of speech intervention. However, only monthly parental attendance at speech intervention sessions was required for this increase in outcomes to occur. Additionally, it should be noted that the parents who attended the sessions were also asked to conduct homework activities with their children. The observation may therefore have acted as a training tool for these homework tasks. Parental attendance at sessions without the use of homework activities might not have increased the outcomes of intervention.

Parental Participation in Intervention Sessions

In the study conducted by Fudala et al. (1972), as previously described, the parents in Group IIB (who attended their child's speech-language pathology sessions weekly) also participated in some of the sessions, acting as the clinician at times during the intervention. There was no difference in the improvement in speech sound production made by the children whose parents participated in the intervention and those who observed only. Therefore, the results of this study appear to indicate that the active participation of parents in intervention sessions may not make speech intervention any more effective. However, this parental participation occurred only toward the end of the period of the study and it was not noted how many times the parents participated in the intervention sessions. More frequent parental participation in intervention sessions might have led to a difference in outcomes.

Parental Participation in Intervention Planning

In a study conducted by Broen and Westman (1990), parents were given choices regarding the sounds chosen for treatment and the intervention activities used with their children. As the design of this study involved a comparison with a group of children who received no intervention, it is not possible to determine the impact of this aspect of parental participation on the effectiveness of intervention for speech impairment.

In summary, parental involvement in the form of attendance at speech-language pathology sessions and the provision of homework activities (with parental training to conduct them) have been shown to make intervention for speech impairment more effective. Parental participation in sessions, however, may not improve speech intervention outcomes. No study has specifically investigated whether parental involvement in the form of homework activities without training or parental involvement in intervention planning makes speech intervention any more effective. It is interesting to consider how these findings relate to how SLPs involve families in intervention in their clinical practice, which we will now discuss.

Clinical Practice: SLPs' Involvement of Families in Speech Intervention

The extent and nature of family involvement in *clinical* practice for speech impairment has not been widely researched. A small number of studies conducted in various English-speaking countries have provided some limited information regarding the extent to which SLPs involve parents in speech intervention. A survey conducted by McLeod and Baker (2004) of Australian SLPs' intervention practices indicated that 88% of respondents reported they involved parents in speech intervention. What was not specified was the exact type of involvement the parents had in the intervention and whether family-friendly practices, such as parental involvement in intervention planning, were used. A similar survey of 98 SLPs from the United Kingdom reported that 76.5% of respondents used parental involvement as a therapy strategy (Joffe & Pring, 2008). Again, the extent and nature of that involvement was not specified. Considering assessment practices, a survey conducted in the United States by Skahan, Watson, and Lof (2007) found that only 35% of SLPs reported that parents typically accompanied their child to assessment sessions for speech impairment.

The authors of this chapter conducted an extensive survey of the practices of 277 Australian SLPs regarding their involvement of parents in intervention for speech impairment (Watts Pappas et al., 2008). The survey found that involvement of parents in speech intervention was common and took place in a variety of ways. The majority of SLPs indicated that parents always or usually attended assessment (84%) and intervention (80%) sessions for their child with speech impairment. As part of the assessment, 91% of respondents always or usually acquired background information about the child and the child's difficulties from the parents and 82% reported that they always or usually discussed the findings of the assessment with parents. However, although parents were usually present at intervention sessions only 35% of the SLPs indicated they always or usually asked parents to participate in the sessions.

The way in which the SLPs most commonly involved parents was by asking them to provide home activities to their child (Watts Pappas et al., 2008). 95% of respondents indicated they always or usually gave home activities to parents and 59% usually or always gave parents home programs to conduct with their child prior to regular intervention. The area in which parents were least likely to be involved was in intervention planning. Although 67% of the SLPs reported that they usually or always involved parents in goal-setting, only 38% of the respondents always or usually allowed parents to make the *final* decisions about intervention goals.

The SLPs indicated that they used some family-friendly/family-centered practices in their work with families in intervention for speech impairment. These included considering parents' time and priorities when providing homework (94%), supporting parents to help identify home activities in which goals could be targeted (79%), asking parents about the impact of the child's speech impairment on the family (77%), giving parents an opportunity to discuss the child's strengths as well as weaknesses (76%), incorporating home activities into the daily routine (73%), and asking parents if they agreed with the assessment findings (68%). Other family-friendly or family-centered practices were used less frequently; only 56% of the SLPs always or usually gave parents the option of when to begin intervention for their child and 53% allowed parents to suggest changes in goals or activities. The family-centered practices least used centered around family decision-making. Only 44% of SLPs always or usually gave parents the option of determining the extent of their involvement in the intervention, as indicated previously, only 38% allowed parents to make final decisions regarding the goals for intervention and 17% gave parents an option regarding the service delivery format provided to their child.

In the Watts Pappas et al. (2008) survey the participants' workplace was found to be an influencing factor in the way they involved parents in speech intervention with SLPs who worked in an educational setting much less likely to have parents present at intervention sessions. The SLPs' own parental status did not influence their responses to the selected questions; however, SLPs who were trained in either the Hanen ITTTT (It Takes Two To Talk®) (Girolametto, Verbey, & Tannock, 1994) or the Lidcombe Program (Onslow, Packman, & Harrison, 2003) were significantly more likely to involve parents in the intervention sessions.

It appears that the majority of SLPs across several (English-speaking) countries involve parents in intervention for speech impairment. This involvement appears to occur mostly in the form of attendance at intervention and assessment sessions and the provision of home activities. Although some family-centered and family-friendly practices are used, the majority of SLPs do not appear to use family-centered practices in decision making about speech intervention, with parents rarely allowed to make the final decisions about their child's intervention.

SLPs' Perceptions of Parental Involvement in Speech Intervention

Although SLPs may involve families in certain ways in speech intervention their beliefs about how families *should* be involved may be different to their actual practice. A few studies have investigated

SLPs' perceptions of working with families in intervention for *speech* impairment (Watts Pappas et al., 2008; Watts Pappas, McAllister, & McLeod, 2009a). (SLPs' views on parental involvement in early intervention in general are reviewed in Chapter 2). Two hundred and seventy-seven SLPs participated in the previously described survey investigating SLPs' practices and beliefs regarding parental involvement in intervention for speech impairment (Watts Pappas et al., 2008) and 6 SLPs participated in a focus group investigating their experiences, feelings, and beliefs regarding working with families in speech intervention (Watts Pappas et al., 2009a). The SLPs in these two groups shared many similar beliefs regarding working with families. Both groups believed that parental involvement in speech intervention was important and greatly impacted on the intervention's effectiveness. As one of the SLPs in the focus group stated:

> My point of view is [that] the therapy is such a very small part of the child's life, that if they're [the parents] not able to follow up by doing some home practice . . . then there is no point in coming (Watts Pappas, 2007, pp. 280–281).

However, although the SLPs felt that parental involvement was important they described experiencing barriers to working with parents and families in practice (Watts Pappas et al., 2008; 2009a). Many SLPs identified barriers in their workplace such as a lack of time and support from managers that prevented them from working with families as much as they felt was ideal. Working in an educational setting was identified as being particularly problematic in involving families (Watts Pappas et al., 2008). Another identified barrier was the SLPs' skills and confidence in working with parents, particularly in intervention for speech impairment (Watts Pappas et al., 2008, 2009a). Speech intervention approaches were perceived as challenging for parents to follow through with at home and difficult to adapt to the home environment (Watts Pappas et al., 2009a). University training was also perceived to be inadequate to fully prepare SLPs for their interaction with families in the workplace (Watts Pappas et al., 2009a).

Interestingly, the factor that the SLPs most often reported to impact on their work with families was the parents themselves (Watts Pappas et al., 2008, 2009a). The two groups of SLPs identified various parent factors that impacted on how they were able to involve families in the intervention. These included the parent's skills in working with their child and their available time for things such as attendance at sessions and providing homework. Some SLPs also felt that parents' beliefs and expectations about their participation could limit their willingness to be involved. As one of the respondents to the survey stated "Some families are not as involved as I'd like, hampered by their perception that therapy, like education is 'done to' their child by an 'expert.'"

In the Watts Pappas et al. studies (2008, 2009a) many of the SLPs expressed frustration when parents did not wish to be involved in the intervention as much as the SLPs would have preferred. In fact, throughout the responses to the focus group and survey the SLPs demonstrated a general negativity toward parents who did not wish to be involved in their child's intervention. The SLPs' belief in the importance of parental involvement to intervention outcomes and their wish to give effective intervention to the child was a possible reason for their frustration with parents who reject involvement.

Although the SLPs felt parental involvement in speech intervention was important they assigned varying levels of importance to different forms of parent and family involvement. For example, although the SLP participants in the focus group and survey did not necessarily expect parents to be involved in all aspects of the intervention, they firmly believed that parents should do home activities with their child (Watts Pappas et al., 2008, 2009a). Seventy-five percent of respondents to the survey agreed or strongly agreed that parents should be able to find time to do home activities (Watts Pappas et al., 2008). Parental attendance and participation in the intervention sessions was also perceived as important by some SLPs. In comparison, parent and family involvement in intervention planning was given a lower priority (Watts Pappas et al., 2008). Although the SLPs generally believed that families should be given the opportunity to be involved in the intervention planning for their child, they saw the SLP as holding the role of the primary decision-maker. Parents were perceived to both need and want guidance from the SLP. This belief was encapsulated by a theme from the analysis of the focus group interview entitled "SLP should take the lead" (Watts Pappas, McAllister, & McLeod, 2009a). Additionally, the SLPs saw themselves as the specialists in speech and language. Although they recognized the parents' knowledge and expertise about their child, they perceived the professionals' skills as more important in the therapeutic situation. As the specialists, the SLPs felt it was their responsibility to take the lead in intervention planning and provision.

Families' Perspectives of Involvement in Speech Intervention

Considering the SLPs' strong views about the importance of family involvement in speech intervention it is interesting to consider whether families also hold this view. We have limited reports of families' perspectives of their involvement in intervention for speech impairment (Broen & Westman, 1990; Eiserman et al., 1990; Fudala et al., 1972; Watts Pappas et al., 2009b). The previously described studies of Broen and Westman (1990), Eiserman and colleagues (1990) and Fudala and colleagues (1972) administered brief surveys to parents as part of their investigation of the impact of parental involvement in speech intervention. The results of these surveys indicated that overall, parents were satisfied with the service their child had received. In addition, the majority of parents in the surveys conducted by Broen and Westman (1990) and Eiserman et al. (1990) indicated that they would prefer a service delivery model that incorporated parental involvement to a model which consisted of speech intervention given primarily by a SLP. Parents in the study conducted by Fudala et al. (1972) indicated that although they would be happy to continue to be involved in their child's intervention, they would prefer to do so at a decreased level— attendance at sessions once a month rather than weekly.

One study has been conducted that has investigated parental involvement in speech intervention using the more in-depth method of interviewing (Watts Pappas et al., 2009b). In this study, interviews were conducted with 7 parents (6 mothers and 1 father) of 6 children receiving a four- to six-session block of intervention for their child with a speech impairment. The parents were interviewed three times —twice during the intervention and once after their child's intervention block had been completed. The interviews explored the parents' feelings about their involvement in the intervention and their relationship with their SLP. One of the major themes that arose from the analysis of the interviews was the parents' desire to do the right thing by their child. The parents interpreted doing the right thing by their child as accessing timely, effective intervention for their children, using the SLPs' expertise, being involved in the intervention in whatever way was required, and ensuring intervention was a positive experience for their child. The parents in this study perceived their child's speech difficulty as short-term and remediable and valued impairment-focused intervention that was as efficient as possible. They looked to their SLP to provide expert guidance regarding the intervention goals and activities and saw the intervention sessions as the SLPs' time to work with their child. Although most of the parents expected to be involved only be doing home activities they were open to being involved in the intervention in whatever way their SLP asked. The parents' main priority was their child's well-being and if the intervention was a negative experience for their child they took steps to rectify this, including discontinuing the intervention. Although they appreciated being asked for their opinion and treated with respect, the parents looked to the SLP for the lead in the intervention.

Other factors that impacted the parents' experience of involvement in their child's speech intervention in the Watts Pappas et al. (2009b) study included service delivery factors (such as wait-times and ease of accessing a referral) and SLP factors. Parents valued services that had reduced wait-times, were close to their home, had easy parking, and child-friendly clinic rooms. They also valued SLPs who were approachable and friendly, respectful of their opinions and beliefs, who communicated effectively, established a good rapport with their child, and were technically competent.

Although parents appear to be generally positive about their involvement in speech intervention, this perception may differ from parent to parent. Parents' expectations about the extent of their involvement may play a significant role in their perceptions of and willingness to be involved in their child's intervention. The perceived remediable nature of speech impairment may also impact on how parents view their involvement. However, the limited number of studies which have investigated parents' and families' views provide us with an incomplete picture of families' perceptions of involvement in speech intervention. Further study is required to determine the range of parents' feelings about involvement and whether these feelings change according to the type and severity of the child's difficulty.

Nexus Between Research, Clinical Practice, and Families' Views on Family Involvement in Speech Intervention

SLPs believe in the importance of parental involvement in speech intervention and attempt to engage families in the intervention process. However, many experimental studies of contemporary intervention approaches for speech impairment make limited mention of parental involvement in their descriptions of the intervention technique. Due to the limited information available regarding how to involve families in common speech intervention approaches and a perceived paucity of training at the university level, SLPs may feel a lack of confidence and expertise in working with families in intervention for speech impairment. SLPs are more likely to use forms of parental and family involvement that have been shown to have the greatest impact on the outcomes of intervention, such as parental attendance at intervention sessions and parental provision of homework activities. However, the evidence-base for the benefits of family involvement in intervention for speech impairment is dated and may not be representative of regular clinical practice (for example, the provision of intensive training to families regarding how to provide home activities may not occur in routine clinical practice). Due to this gap in the literature, SLPs have no clear evidence of what the effects of parent and family involvement in intervention for speech impairment might be.

Families appear to be keen to be involved in their child's speech intervention provision. However, like SLPs, it seems that many parents believe the professional should take the lead role in intervention planning. Although parents and SLPs both consider family involvement in speech impairment to be important they may have different perceptions and expectations of the form of that involvement. For example, in the Watts Pappas et al. (2009b) study, although parents were happy to be involved in the intervention in whatever way was required, they had strong expectations that the SLP would work with their child in the intervention sessions. SLPs may need to consider individual family's expectations and beliefs about involvement when attempting to engage them in the intervention. To work effectively with families in clinical practice, SLPs need to consider the experimental evidence of the effectiveness of family involvement in speech intervention, the family's beliefs and expectations, as well as address barriers to working with families in their workplace.

Case Study of Family Involvement in Speech Intervention

Introduction

This case study illustrates the application of family-friendly practice to a child with speech impairment. The case is based on the first author's clinical practice. However, details have been changed to ensure anonymity.

Joshua was seen for a block of six sessions for speech intervention at his local community health center. Because community health centers are government funded in Australia, this limited the amount of intervention that could be provided. At the time of the intervention, children who were not attending a full-time educational program were eligible for treatment at the service. Children were provided with six session blocks of intervention separated by 12-week breaks. Waiting times for the service were long: 12 to 18 months from the time of referral.

Joshua was referred to the community health center by his parents due to concerns regarding his speech-sound production. He was 4 years, 5 months of age at the time of the referral and after remaining on the waiting list for approximately 13 months was offered an initial assessment appointment at the age of 5 years, 6 months. Joshua was offered a six-session block of intervention. As Joshua began attending school after this block of intervention was completed, he was not eligible for any further intervention from the service.

Assessment

Appointment Scheduling

Joshua's parents were called to arrange a time for the assessment appointment. Calling rather than mailing out an appointment ensured that the appointment time was convenient for the family. On the telephone, the SLP spoke to Joshua's mother, Jane, who was invited to bring along support people to the assessment if she wished. One of the findings of research conducted with families is that they often do not know what to expect when attending an SLP assessment session (Watts Pappas et al., 2009b). To put Jane at ease, the SLP discussed with her what would happen at the assessment session and gained information about her main concerns regarding Joshua's speech and language skills. Some parents report that they are uncomfortable talking about their child's difficulties in front of their child (Watts Pappas et al., 2009b). Considering this, Jane was given the option of having a telephone meeting with the SLP before the assessment to take the case history information. Jane accepted this offer as she reported that Joshua was very sensitive about his speech difficulty. Two appointments therefore were arranged—a case history appointment by telephone and an appointment for Joshua to be assessed in the clinic.

Assessment Activities

During the telephone appointment, a case history was taken from Joshua's mother, Jane, covering background medical and developmental information, family history, and the impact of Joshua's difficulties on his family and his ability to participate in the activities of his daily life. During the clinic assessment session, Joshua's speech-sound production in single words was assessed using a standardized test of articulation and phonology. The assessment tested the production of all English consonants in initial, medial, and final positions of words. Production of consonant clusters and multisyllabic words was also assessed. Joshua's expressive and receptive language was assessed using a standardized test of language production. An oromotor assessment, an assessment of stimulability, and an assessment of Joshua's speech-sound production and expressive language in conversation were also conducted.

Family Involvement in Assessment

During a telephone conversation, Joshua's mother, Jane, was asked about her concerns regarding Joshua's speech and language skills and given the opportunity to discuss how they impacted on the family and his daily activities. Jane also provided information about Joshua's background medical and developmental history, Joshua's feelings about his speech difficulties, and his favorite toys/activities. Her expectations about involvement in the intervention were then discussed. Previous research has indicated that SLP and family expectations and beliefs about intervention involvement can vary (Watts Pappas et al., 2009b). Therefore, obtaining information about parents' expectations about involvement is considered an important element of the assessment. During the assessment session conducted in the clinic, Jane was invited to sit at the table with Joshua and the SLP. She provided encouragement to Joshua during the assessment and indicated whether Joshua's performance in the assessment was typical. Jane also provided interpretation of some of Joshua's conversational speech during a play activity. She particularly helped motivate Joshua during the oromotor assessment in which he was initially reluctant to participate.

Assessment Results

Joshua was an only child who achieved his major motor and speech developmental milestones at the appropriate ages. He had no history of middle ear infections or serious accidents or illnesses. His hearing had been tested and was within normal limits; no family history of speech and language difficulties was present. Joshua was attending a repeat year of preschool due to his parent's concerns regarding the intelligibility of his speech. Jane reported that Joshua's speech was very difficult for unfamiliar listeners to understand and that his speech was also occasionally misunderstood by his family. When this happened, it caused great frustration for both Joshua and his parents. Joshua was very aware and extremely sensitive about his speech difficulties. He sometimes found it difficult to make friends at his preschool, possibly due to his speech difficulties. He liked playing with animals (particularly zoo animals) and was also interested in dinosaurs. Jane had expected to be involved in Joshua's intervention by doing home activities with him. Her goal for the intervention was for his speech to become easier for others to understand.

Joshua's speech was characterized predominantly by his multiple phoneme collapse of most fricatives (all except "v" which was replaced with "b") and all affricates to "d." This collapse occurred in initial, medial, and final word positions. Joshua was not heard to produce any fricative or affricate sounds in his single word productions or conversational speech. Joshua reduced and usually simplified all consonant clusters. His strengths were that he was able to produce multisyllabic words without reduction (up to 5 syllables) and he was stimulable for the: "sh," "f," and "s" sounds in isolation. Oromotor assessment indicated a normal oral structure and movement of the lips, tongue, and jaw in nonspeech tasks. The results of the language assessment indicated normal expressive and receptive language skills. Due to his significantly reduced phonemic inventory and multiple phoneme collapses, Joshua's intelligibility in conversational speech was poor. Joshua was aware of his speech difficulties and often became frustrated when he was not understood. The difficulties were causing his parents much concern (they were the primary reason Joshua was repeating a year of preschool). They were particularly concerned about how Joshua's difficulties would impact his school performance in the following year.

Feedback

Jane was invited to attend a feedback session with the SLP to discuss the results of the assessment and plan the goals of the intervention.

Both Jane and her husband Paul attended this session. Jane was given the option of attending the feedback session without Joshua present, which she decided to do. In the feedback session the SLP discussed the results of the assessment and gave the parents a report outlining the findings. The SLP then went through the report with the parents and asked if they agreed with the findings. The SLP also discussed the plan for the intervention. Previous research has indicated that, although parents appreciated being asked for their opinion, they looked to the expert SLP to lead the intervention (Watts Pappas et al., 2009b). In this meeting, therefore, although the SLP involved the parents in choosing intervention targets, she recommended the intervention approach and provided the parents with a list of possible targets to choose from. Due to Joshua's multiple phoneme collapse the SLP suggested that the multiple oppositions approach to intervention (Williams, 2000) would be a good approach to remediate his speech impairment. The SLP outlined a group of sounds that could be chosen to be used with this approach. With consultation with Joshua's parents, the "s," "z," "sh," and "j" sounds were chosen to be targeted for intervention.

Intervention

Intervention Approach

The multiple opposition approach is a contrastive approach to speech intervention in which a sound the child uses to replace many error sounds is contrasted with the group of sounds it replaces. For example, if the child produced the "f," "s," "k," and "sh" sounds as "d," a set of multiple oppositions to use with this child would be *fee, see, she, key,* and *dee* (Willliams, 2000). The theory behind this approach is that the child's learning is directed across their phonological system rather than focused on a particular sound or rule. Joshua's target sounds of "s," "sh," and "j" were contrasted with his error replacement sound of "d" in sets of words such as *shoe, do, dew* and *sue,* and *ship, dip, jip,* and *sip.* The intervention involves asking the child to repeat each word of the set with the error replacement word after the examiner. Using one of the previous examples, Joshua was asked to repeat *shoe do* after the SLP, then *sue do,* and so on. As the intervention progressed, the "f" and "z" sounds were also added to the word sets. Some phonetic placement cues were needed to elicit Joshua's production of the words. As Joshua's production at the single word-level improved, scripted activities using the words at a sentence and conversational level were included, for example, songs involving the words or a play activity such as a tea party.

Family Involvement in Intervention Sessions

In the intervention sessions, Joshua's mother, Jane, was invited to sit at the table with her son and the SLP, which she was happy to do. Physically locating Jane closer to Joshua and the SLP made Joshua more comfortable and also allowed Jane to be more involved in the intervention activities. Once the SLP had introduced the intervention technique she also invited Jane to participate in the intervention activities, explaining that this would make it easier for her to work with Joshua at home; Joshua may be more accepting of his mother doing the activities with him at home and it would also be a chance for Jane to practice with the SLP to help her perfect her technique. In previous research it was found that parents generally expected that the SLP would work with their child in the intervention sessions and that the parents would observe: parents considered this an important part of the SLPs' role (Watts Pappas et al., 2009b). When asking parents to be involved in the interventions sessions, it is useful to be aware that they may have not expected this level of involvement and explain to them the importance of their participation.

Jane and the SLP took turns giving the multiple oppositions activities. Games were included in these activities to ensure Joshua's motivation (for example, a turn of a ball tower game after a group of responses). Joshua's mother was asked to practice the activities covered in the intervention sessions at home. Previous research has revealed that some parents feel they are not supported to give speech activities at home to their child (Watts Pappas et al., 2009b). In the interviews, parents spoke about being given limited information about how to conduct activities or games to keep their child's motivation. Care was taken, therefore, to ensure that Jane felt confident about how to do the activities with Joshua as well as provide her with materials and games to increase Joshua's motivation to do the work at home. For example, a home practice scrapbook was given to Jane. In this book, the SLP wrote instructions of how to do the activities with Joshua as well as included simple games such as bingo to play while doing the activities.

Joshua's mother was also involved in generating some of the more advanced activities which included the target words in conversational tasks, often bringing activities along to the sessions which incorporated the target opposition words. For example, Joshua and Jane would write stories together incorporating the target words. Joshua would then retell the stories. The partnership between the SLP and the parent ensured that the intervention activities were aligned with Joshua's interests and included activities which were easily replicated at home.

Intervention Outcomes

After a six-session intervention block and an 8-week break from intervention, Joshua was reassessed. Over the course of the block of intervention, Joshua had acquired all of the sounds which were targeted in the intervention: "f," "s," "z," "sh," and "j" in the initial position of words. No other changes to his phonemic inventory occurred during this period, possibly indicating that the intervention was the cause of the sound change. Unfortunately, after this block of intervention, Joshua was no longer eligible for further intervention at the community health center as he had started attending school. His mother was provided with some further activities to follow up with at home and he was referred to the SLP working at the school Joshua was attending. Jane indicated she enjoyed being involved in the intervention and was happy with the progress that Joshua had made. By providing a family-friendly approach to intervention for speech impairment, the SLP was able to provide an evidence-based, effective intervention approach while involving the family to individualize this approach to Joshua. The SLP led the intervention process but involved Joshua's parents in the intervention planning and provision, thereby possibly making the intervention more effective and ensuring it was acceptable to Joshua and his family.

Summary and Conclusion

SLPs' beliefs and practice regarding working with families in intervention for speech impairment has changed significantly over time. Although in the past parents and families have been excluded from the intervention process, the majority of SLPs now involve families in intervention for speech impairment. A family-friendly practice model in which families are given the opportunity to be involved in intervention planning, but in which SLPs retain the responsibility as primary decision-makers, appears to be the most desired model for both parents and SLPs in speech intervention.

Although the research regarding the effect of family involvement in speech intervention does not provide clear evidence that parental involvement makes speech intervention more effective, both SLPs and parents believe that family involvement in speech intervention is important. However, SLPs report they experience many barriers to working with families in speech intervention including workplace barriers, family barriers (such as parents' skills, time, and inclination to be involved), and a lack of information regarding how to incorporate families into common intervention approaches for speech impairment. Studies of families' perspectives of their involvement in speech intervention have shown that they value services that are accessible, provided by SLPs who are competent, friendly, respectful of the parent's knowledge, and who relate well to their child. They also value being adequately supported to be involved in their child's intervention provision. If SLPs wish to engage parents and families in intervention for speech impairment they should consider parents' perspectives of their involvement and use these insights to more successfully form parent/professional partnerships.

References

Bauman-Waengler, J. (2004). *Articulatory and phonological impairments: A clinical focus* (2nd ed.). Boston: Pearson Education.

Bernhardt, B. H., Stemberger, J., & Major, E. (2006). General and nonlinear intervention perspectives for a child with a resistant phonological impairment. *Advances in Speech-Language Pathology, 8*(3), 190–206.

Bernthal, J. E., & Bankson, N. W. (Eds.). (2004). *Articulation and phonological disorders* (5th ed.). Boston: Pearson Education.

Bird, J., Bishop, D. V. M., & Freeman, N. H. (1995). Phonological awareness and literacy development in children with expressive phonological impairments. *Journal of Speech and Hearing Research, 38*, 446–462.

Blanche, S. E., Parsons, C. L., & Humphreys, J. M. (1981). A minimal-word-pair model for teaching the linguistic significant difference of distinctive feature properties. *Journal of Speech and Hearing Disorders, 20*, 291–296.

Bowen, C. & Cupples, L. (1998). A tested phonological therapy in practice. *Child Language Teaching and Therapy, 14*(1), 29–50.

Broen, P. A., & Westman, M. J. (1990). Project parent: A preschool speech program implemented through parents. *Journal of Speech and Hearing Disorders, 55*, 495–502.

Conture, E. G., Louko, L. J., & Edwards, M. L. (1989). Simultaneously treating stuttering and disordered phonology in children: Experimental treatment, preliminary findings. *American Journal of Speech-Language Pathology, September,* 72–81.

Costello, J., & Bosler, S, (1976). Generalization and articulation instruction. *Journal of Speech and Hearing Disorders, 41*, 359–373.

Dodd, B. (1995) *Differential diagnosis and treatment of children with speech disorder.* London: Whurr.

Dodd, B., & Barker, R. (1990). The efficacy of utilizing parents and teachers as agents of therapy for children with phonological disorders. *Australian Journal of Human Communication Disorders, 18*(1), 29–45.

Dodd, B., Holm, A., Crosbie, S., & McIntosh, B. (2006). A core vocabulary approach for management of inconsistent speech disorder. *Advances in Speech-Language Pathology, 8*(3), 220–230.

Eiserman, W. D., McCoun, M., & Escobar, C. (1990). A cost-effectiveness analysis of two alternative program models for serving speech-disordered preschoolers. *Journal of Early Intervention 14*(4), 297–317.

Elbert, M., Powell, T. W., & Swartzlander, P. (1991). Toward a technology of generalization: How many exemplars are sufficient? *Journal of Speech and Hearing Research, 34,* 81–87.

Felsenfeld, S., Broen, P. A., & McGue, M. (1992). A 28-year follow-up of adults with a history of moderate phonological disorder: Linguistic and personality results. *Journal of Speech and Hearing Research, 35*(5), 1114–1125.

Felsenfeld, S., Broen, P. A., & McGue, M. (1994). A 28-year follow up of adults with a history of moderate phonological disorder: Educational and occupational results. *Journal of Speech and Hearing Research, 37*, 1341–1353.

Forrest, K., & Elbert, M. (2001). Treatment for phonologically disordered children with variable substitution patterns. *Clinical Linguistics and Phonetics, 15*(1), 41–45.

Fudala, J. B., England, G., & Ganoung, L. (1972). Utilization of parents in a speech correction program. *Exceptional Children, 1,* 407–412.

Gierut, J. A. (1989). Maximal opposition approach to phonological treatment. *Journal of Speech and Hearing Disorders, 54,* 9–19.

Gierut, J. A. (1990). Differential learning of phonological oppositions. *Journal of Speech and Hearing Research, 33*, 540–549.

Gierut, J. A. (1991). Homonymy in phonological change. *Clinical Linguistics and Phonetics, 5*(2), 119–137.

Gierut, J. A. (1992). The conditions and course of clinically induced phonological change. *Journal of Speech and Hearing Research, 35*, 1049–1063.

Gierut, J. A. (1999). Syllable onsets: Clusters and adjuncts in acquisition. *Journal of Speech, Language, and Hearing Research, 42*, 708–726.

Gierut, J. A., & Champion, A. H. (2000). Ingressive substitutions: Typical or atypical phonological pattern? *Clinical Linguistics and Phonetics, 14*(8), 603–617.

Gierut, J. A., & Champion, A. H. (2001). Syllable onsets II: Three-element clusters in phonological treatment. *Journal of Speech, Language, and Hearing Research, 44*(4), 886–905.

Gierut, J. A., Morrisette, M. L., Hughes, M. T., & Rowland, S. (1996). Phonological treatment efficacy and developmental norms. *Language, Speech, and Hearing Services in Schools, 27*, 215–230.

Girolametto, L. E., Verbey, M., & Tannock, R. (1994). Improving joint engagement in parent-child interaction: An intervention study. *Journal of Early Intervention, 18*(2), 155–167.

Hayden, D. (2006). The PROMPT model: Use and application for children with mixed phonological-motor impairment. *Advances in Speech-Language Pathology, 8*(3), 265–281.

Hodson, B. W. (2006). Identifying phonological patterns and projecting remediation cycles: Expediting intelligibility gains of a 7-year-old Australian child. *Advances in Speech-Language Pathology, 8*(3), 257–264.

Hodson, B. W., & Paden, E. P. (1991). *Targeting intelligible speech: A phonological approach to remediation* (2nd ed.). Austin, TX: Pro-Ed.

Hoffman, P. R., Norris, J. A., & Monjure, J. (1990). Comparison of process targeting and whole language treatments for phonologically delayed preschool children. *Language, Speech, and Hearing Services in Schools, 21*, 102–109.

Joffe, V., & Pring, T. (2008). Children with phonological problems: A survey of clinical practice. *International Journal of Language and Communication Disorders, 43*(2), 154–164.

Klein, E. S. (1996). Phonological/traditional approaches to articulation therapy: A retrospective group comparison. *Language, Speech, and Hearing Services in Schools, 27*, 314–323.

Law, J., Boyle, J., Harris, F., Harkness, A., & Nye, C. (2000). The relationship between the natural history and prevalence of primary speech and language delays: Findings from a systematic review of the literature. *International Journal of Language and Communication Disorders, 35*(2), 165–188.

McKinnon, D. H., McLeod, S., & Reilly, S. (2007). The prevalence of stuttering, voice and speech-sound disorders in primary school students in Australia. *Language, Speech, and Hearing Services in Schools, 38*(1), 5–15.

McLeod, S., & Baker, E. (2004). Current clinical practice for children with speech impairment. In B. E. Murdoch, J. Goozee, B. M. Whelan, & K. Docking

(Eds.), *Proceedings of the 26th World Congress of the International Association of Logopedics and Phoniatrics*. Brisbane: University of Queensland.

McPherson, E., Morris, M., & Ferguson, A. (1987, March). What do parents think of home programs? *Australian Communication Quarterly*, pp. 16–20.

Moll, K. L., & Darley, F. L. (1960). Attitudes of mothers of articulatory-impaired and speech-retarded children. *Journal of Speech and Hearing Disorders, 25*, 377–384.

Montgomery, J. K., & Bonderman, I. R. (1989). Serving preschool children with severe phonological disorders. *Language, Speech, and Hearing Services in Schools, 20*, 76–84.

Onslow, M., Packman, A., & Harrison, E. (2003). *The Lidcombe Program of Early Stuttering Intervention: A clinician's guide*. Austin, TX: Pro-Ed.

Pascoe, M., Stackhouse, J., & Wells, B. (2006). *Persisting speech difficulties in children: Children's speech and literacy difficulties 3*. Padstow, Cornwall: Whurr.

Powell, T. W., & Elbert, M. (1984). Generalization following the remediation of early- and later-developing consonant clusters. *Journal of Speech and Hearing Disorders, 49*, 211–218.

Powell, T. W., Elbert, M., Miccio, A. W., Strike-Roussos, C., & Brasseur, J. (1998). Facilitating [s] production in young children: An experimental evaluation of motoric and conceptual treatment approaches. *Clinical Linguistics and Phonetics, 12*, 127–146.

Ruscello, D. M., Cartwright, L. R., Haines, K. B., & Shuster, L. I. (1993). The use of different service delivery models for children with phonological disorders. *Journal of Communication Disorders, 26*, 193–203.

Saben, C. B., & Ingham, J. C. (1991). The effects of minimal pairs treatment on the speech-sound production of two children with phonologic disorders. *Journal of Speech and Hearing Research, 34*, 1023–1040.

Shelton, R. Johnson, A., & Arndt, W. B. (1972). Monitoring and reinforcement by parents as a means of automating articulatory responses. *Perceptual and Motor Skills, 35*, 759–767.

Shelton, R., Johnson, A., Willis, V., & Arndt, W. (1975). Monitoring and reinforcement by parents as a means of automating articulatory responses: II. Study of preschool children. *Perceptual and Motor Skills, 40*, 599–610.

Shriberg, L. D., Gruber, F. A., & Kwiatkowski, J. (1994). Developmental phonological disorders III: Long-term speech-sound normalization. *Journal of Speech and Hearing Research, 37*, 1151–1177.

Shriberg, L. D., & Kwiatkowski, J. (1990). Self-monitoring and generalization in preschool speech-delayed children. *Language, Speech, and Hearing Services in Schools, 21*, 157–170.

Simon, C. S. (1998). When big kids don't learn: Contextual modifications and intervention strategies for age 8–18 at-risk students. *Clinical Linguistics and Phonetics, 12*(3), 249–280.

Skahan, S. M., Watson, M., & Lof, G. L. (2007). Speech-language pathologists' assessment practices for children with suspected speech sound disorders: Results of a national survey. *American Journal of Speech-Language Pathology, 16*, 246–249.

Solomon, A. L. (1961). Personality and behavior patterns of children with functional defects of articulation. *Child Development, 23*, 731–737.

Sommers, R. K. (1962). Factors in effectiveness of mothers trained to aid in speech correction. *Journal of Speech and Hearing Disorders, 27*, 178–186.

Sommers, R. K., Furlong, A. K., Rhodes, F. E., Fichter, G. R., Bowser, D. C., Copetas, F. G., et al. (1964). Effects of maternal attitudes upon improvement in articulation when mothers are trained to assist in speech correction. *Journal of Speech and Hearing Disorders, 29*(2), 126–132.

Stone, J. R., & Stoel-Gammon, C. (1990). One class at a time: A case study of phonological learning. *Child Language Teaching and Therapy, 6*, 173–191.

Tufts, L. C., & Holliday, A. R. (1959). Effectiveness of trained parents as speech therapists. *Journal of Speech and Hearing Disorders, 24*, 395–401.

Tyler, A. A., & Watterson, K. H. (1991). Effects of phonological versus language intervention in preschoolers with both phonological and language impairment. *Child Language Teaching and Therapy, 7*, 141–160.

Watts Pappas, N. (2007). *Parental involvement in intervention for speech impairment.* Unpublished doctoral dissertation, Charles Sturt University, Bathurst, Australia.

Watts Pappas, N., McAllister, L., & McLeod, S. (2009a). *Working with families in paediatric speech intervention: Speech language pathologists' beliefs and practices* (manuscript in preparation).

Watts Pappas, N., McAllister, L., & McLeod, S. (2009b). *Family involvement in paediatric speech intervention: What do parents think?* (manuscript in preparation).

Watts Pappas N., McLeod, S., McAllister, L., McKinnon, D. H. (2008). Parental involvement in speech intervention: A national survey. *Clinical Linguistics and Phonetics, 22*(4), 335–344.

Watts Pappas, N., McLeod, S., McAllister, L., & Simpson, T. (2005). Partnerships with parents in speech intervention: A review. In L. Brown & C. Heine (Eds.), *Speech Pathology Australia National Conference* (pp. 62–73). Melbourne: Speech Pathology Australia.

Williams, A. L. (2000). Multiple oppositions: Case studies of variables in phonological intervention. *American Journal of Speech-Language Pathology, 9*, 289–299.

Wing, D. M., & Heimgartner, L. M. (1973). Articulation carryover procedure implemented by parents. *Language, Speech, and Hearing Services in Schools, 4*, 182–195.

Wolfe, V. I., Blocker, S. D., & Prater, N. J. (1988). Articulatory generalization in two word-medial ambisyllabic contexts. *Language, Speech, and Hearing Services in Schools, 19,* 251–258.

Wood, K. S. (1946). Parental maladjustment and functional articulatory defects in children. *Journal of Speech Disorders, 11,* 255–275.

Chapter 8

Working with Families of Children Who Use AAC

Julie Marshall and Juliet Goldbart

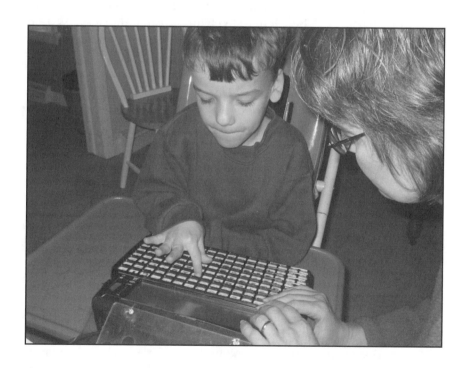

Recent Contextual Factors Impacting on AAC and Families/Parents

Augmentative and alternative communication (AAC) supplements (augmentative) or replaces (alternative) spoken language for children and adults. AAC can be divided into aided and nonaided types. It can be used with children and adults of all ages and with children who have a wide range of different types of speech, language, and communication difficulties, including those with cerebral palsy, craniofacial anomalies, specific language impairment, hearing impairment, learning difficulties, autistic spectrum disorders, and acquired brain injury. AAC systems encompass high-tech communication aids, (e.g., Voice Output Communication Aids [VOCAs]/ Speech Generating Devices [SGDs]), which are often based on portable computers, light-tech aids such as e-tran (Eye Transfer) frames, no-tech aids such as symbol books or charts and the Picture Exchange Communication System (PECS), and unaided systems, such as formal signing languages or systems (e.g., British or American Sign Language and Makaton), gesture, and eye pointing.

The development of the field of AAC with children has been influenced by many factors, some of which are specific to AAC (or children using AAC), some specific to children with speech, language, and communication difficulties and some are more general. Some of these factors influence and are influenced by family involvement issues.

In many countries, the past 30 to 40 years have seen transitions within education; including, in some countries the first legal right to education for all children, whatever the nature and extent of their abilities or disabilities. In those countries where educational provision is available for children with disabilities, there have been changes in the designation and location of this provision, from specialist segregated schooling to a diverse range that includes full inclusion with appropriate support, partial inclusion (i.e., split placement), unit-based provision within mainstream schools, special and mainstream schools that share a campus, and separate special schools.

Across speech-language pathology, particularly in minority world[1] countries, there has been an increasing recognition of the importance

---

[1]We have chosen to use the terms majority/minority world countries or countries with a low/high Human Development Index (The HDI is a scale developed in 1990 and based on measures of longevity, education and per capita Gross Domestic Product.)

of the context of the child's situation to communication development and (re)habilitation. Context includes such factors as communication partners, the family and the wider society, family constellations, the presence or absence of objects such as toys, books, television, DVDs, and so forth, housing, the socioeconomic situation, and educational/ social facilities. Speech-language pathology intervention should not ignore these influences.

A gradual move from the medical (or individual) model of health and disability (e.g., Barnes & Swain, 2003) toward a more social model, has further influenced understanding of the role of the family and context in disability. One significant outcome of this move has been the publication of the International Classification of Functioning, Disability and Health (ICF) (WHO, 2001), with its inclusion of contextual factors and a growing recognition of their importance in measuring SLP (including AAC) outcomes.

There is growing recognition within the AAC field, as well as in wider health, education, and social care provision, of the impact of culture on the provision and uptake of services. If culture is defined as including factors such as socioeconomic status, educational status, gender, sexuality, (dis)ability status, age, and not just language/s spoken, religion, and ethnic group, then diversity within almost any setting is likely. This recognition of increasing diversity and the relevance of culture, may impact on AAC provision in many ways.

Increasing global mobility has meant that, even in those countries where monolingualism has been in the majority, there has been an increase in diversity of languages spoken, with a corresponding impact on the provision of SLP and, in turn, AAC. Importantly, in many countries, SLPs tend to come from the cultural and linguistic "dominant"[2] or "mainstream" group in society. This may have implications for working with families who may not share the views, expectations, and practices of the dominant culture.

This term is used by the United Nations Development Program in its annual Human Development Report. A HDI of below 0.5 indicates low development and a HDI of more than 0.8 indicates high development. Thus, the United Kingdom would be labeled a minority world country.

[2]Here we use "dominant" in a similar way to Knowles and Peng (2005): "a *dominant* group need not be a numerical majority (although it often will be). Rather, a group is dominant if it possesses a disproportionate share of societal resources, privileges, and power" (p. 223). In the United Kingdom the dominant group could be described as being white, monolingual, post-16 educated and middle-class, although it is acknowledged that such definitions are disputed.

In one respect, these issues are uniquely important in the field of AAC, in that professionals (often, but not exclusively, SLPs) typically select the vocabulary available to the children, and sometimes even morphologic and syntactic forms. This means that it is imperative to understand the child's context and this should include the close involvement of families. Thus, a number of influences have come to bear on AAC provision with and for children and their families. We now examine the published literature about children and families with this client group.

The Evidence Base Regarding the Effectiveness of Family Involvement Where a Child Uses AAC

It is now recognized that many children of different ages and with different types of speech, language and communication difficulties may require AAC for either short- or long-term use, for communicating with some or all communication partners and for communicating about some or all topics. A child's difficulty with speech, language, and communication may be recognized or suspected by many, including the child's family, educators or SLP, or the child him or herself. Furthermore, the suggestion that AAC may be helpful may be made by one or more of the groups above and, correspondingly, may or may not be welcomed by others. Differences in factors, such as:

- how well a communication partner understands a child and his or her needs
- whether communication between a given communication partner and a child is mainly based on yes/no questions, familiar topics, or context,
- whether the priority is the child's *current* communication levels (semantically, grammatically or pragmatically), communication partners, communication contexts, and/or *future* communication levels, partners, and so on,

may all influence how the introduction of AAC is viewed, the type of system that is preferred, and the goals of the system.

Additionally, the child's and family's values and attitudes toward AAC, professional skills, knowledge, finances, and support that are available, as well as the skills and needs of the child him- or herself, may all influence whether and how AAC is introduced. It is also now clear that simply introducing an AAC system is insufficient and that implementation is time-consuming and complex. Family involvement in that process is increasingly recognized to be important.

Issues relating to family involvement in communication intervention for children learning to communicate through augmented means include many of those relevant to families of children with other severe and pervasive communication impairments. There are, however, some specific issues which relate specifically to AAC and these are described.

A number of authors have suggested that parental involvement in AAC is important (e.g., Angelo, Jones, & Kokoska, 1995; Cress, 2004; Lund & Light, 2007). Lund and Light's (2007) findings explicitly contrast "Low expectations of family members" (p. 326), which act as a barrier to long-term success with AAC, with the positive impact of "Strong parental advocacy" and "Family involvement in intervention" (p. 326). Jones et al. (1998), in a study of middle-class North American families, suggested that parents relied on professionals for support. Furthermore, Angelo (2000) reported both positive and negative experiences of families regarding acquiring an AAC device. Starbie et al. (2005) reported on a family-centered approach to AAC intervention that had positive results with one family. However, in common with the first study reported above, this was a well-educated North American family and it is important to be aware that different types of families may want different services.

Not all studies report that parental involvement is positive and there is a significant step between believing that family involvement is important and involving families appropriately and successfully. For example, McCord and Soto (2004) reported that the Mexican-American parents that they interviewed about AAC, felt distanced from decision-making, that the AAC provided did not always contain relevant vocabulary for family interaction, and high–tech AAC was not always used at home. Allaire, Gressard, Blackman, and Hostler's (1991) study of North American families found that parents and professionals did not always agree about the children's communication modes. In our own research with families in England (Goldbart & Marshall, 2004; Marshall & Goldbart, 2008), we found that parents felt that AAC implementation placed many demands on them, in that high-tech AAC was costly and slow to acquire and that, for many families, much of the initial work around AAC had been initiated by themselves.

Granlund, Bjork-Akesson, and Alant (2005) suggest that families take on a number of roles during AAC intervention:

- that of decision-maker;
- as communication environment;
- as consumers;
- as trainers
- as a family in crisis.

The extent to which each of these will be relevant to a particular family may vary both over time and according to characteristics of the child, the family, and their environment. So, SLPs need to be flexible, recognizing which of these roles is/are operating and providing support accordingly.

It has already been mentioned in the previous section that cultural factors may be influential in the successful acquisition and use of AAC. Huer (1997) has suggested that linguistic and cultural factors are important and it has been suggested that adaptations to service provision and dialogue with families are needed to facilitate AAC use where families are either not part of the mainstream society or have a culture very different from the professionals with whom they are dealing (Huer, Parette, & Saenz, 2001; Huer & Saenz, 2001).

Several authors have provided guidance for working with families from a range of backgrounds. For example, Parette, Huer, and Wyatt (2002), writing about African-American families, remind us that caregivers may be drawn from extended family networks and from the wider community, so consideration must be given to this wider range of communication partners. Alant (1996) has described a school-based approach for AAC intervention in South Africa that includes both staff and families. She, too, considers that it is important to know about the family structure and context, as well as the AAC device, in order to maximize successful implementation. Parette, Brotherson, and Huer (2000) reported that North American families from a number of different ethnic backgrounds, wanted professionals to understand them, their ethnicity, and values better with better dialogue. They also wanted information in home languages.

Cultural factors in social interaction may also be important. For example, McCord and Soto's (2004) participants found AAC devices a barrier to intimacy. Vocabulary may be different, not only between the home and school setting (as is the case for many families) but may also be very different from professionals' expectations of home settings. Families in McCord and Soto's (2004) study prioritized rate of communication over complexity and there are suggestions in our own research that this view may be shared by our white participants in the United Kingdom. Attitudes towards technology may vary. Huer (2000) examined differences in perceptions of graphic symbols in participants from four different ethnic backgrounds: African-American, Chinese, European-American, and Mexican. Although rank order in terms of translucency of three commonly used symbol systems in the United States: PCS, DynaSyms, and Blissymbols, was the same for the four groups, there was some suggestion that the African American group perceived the symbols a little differently. More research is needed on this topic but Huer recommends that SLPs discuss symbol selection with their clients and their families.

It has been suggested by Parette, Huer, and Brotherson (2001) that, at least for professionals in North America, cultural issues are not foregrounded. This finding is echoed in Lund and Light's (2007) interviews with long-term users of AAC and their families, and is reflected in our own experiences with SLPs in the United Kingdom and suggests that there remains much for us to learn about the complexities of successful work with families from a wide range of cultures.

In the United Kingdom, we carried out a study talking to parents of children who used AAC to understand their perspectives (Goldbart & Marshall, 2004; Marshall & Goldbart, 2008). We found that parents differed in their views and their responses to their child's communication difficulties but there were common themes. Many parents had put in huge amounts of effort to develop communication systems with their children and recognized the impact of restricted communication. Unsurprisingly, they expressed strong emotions about having children with communication difficulties and talked a lot about the kind of demands that were placed on them and, for some parents, the need to be "pushy" (a label that has rather negative connotations in British English) and to fight constantly to get what they perceived their child needed. They did not always feel that their expert knowledge of their child was recognized. These interviews provided a great deal of rich information about parents. The data were based only on the words of 11 families in one part of one country and so we cannot claim that they are representative of all parents. However, what they do seem to demonstrate is the value of prioritizing spending time talking to and listening to parents, in order to fully understand their perspectives.

Although we did not set out to make this an explicitly cross-cultural study, this, and other research with parents in which we have been involved (e.g., Marshall, Goldbart, & Phillips, 2007), indicate that, in some respects, parents and professionals can be regarded as belonging to two separate subcultures (or communities of practice) and that professionals need to find ways to bridge these potential gaps.

One important but often neglected issue concerns the demands on parents' time of working with their child or collaborating with professionals. One aspect of this is family constellation; who makes up the family group? Lone parent families are common in many countries, with consequent additional pressures on the sole carer. In many minority world settings it is now common for both parents in a two-parent family to be working outside the home, again reducing time for additional commitments. Goldbart and Mukherjee (1999) studying parents of children with cerebral palsy (CP) in West Bengal, India, found three different types of family structure:

- *nuclear*, with two parents and one or more children,
- *extended*, where the nuclear family was augmented by an unmarried relative of one of the parents, and
- *joint*, where three or more generations lived together; typically one or more grandparents and one or more of their sons with their wives and children:

It is sometimes suggested that extended or joint families provide additional support for families with a child with a disability as there are more adults available to share domestic responsibilities. In this West Bengal study Goldbart and Mukherjee found that women, usually the mothers of the children with CP, carried the overwhelming responsibility for domestic work and child care. Female relatives did play a greater role in joint and extended families than in nuclear families; however, this was balanced by the fact that in joint and extended families there are likely to be more people to cook, clean, and care for. Families in our U.K. study also reported heavy demands on their time, saying, for example: "It is very frustrating because I can see there is a huge potential but there just aren't enough hours in the day to be able to do it" and "If I had more time I would do more but time is a problem" (Goldbart & Marshall, 2004, p. 203).

Thus, we can see that there is research that supports the need for working with families in AAC intervention and that some of this research has focused specifically on the impact of cultural diversity on service provision. In the following section we take this research and the four models of delivering SLP already identified earlier in this book, and apply it to AAC intervention with children and briefly suggest implications for improved clinical practice.

Implications of Research for Models of Service Delivery

Typically, although not exclusively, children who become candidates for AAC have significant and complex communication needs that are apparent when they are quite young. Consequently, they and their families should be receiving guidance on early communication from SLPs or other professionals well before school entry. Later, children learning language and communication by augmented means will need SLP to support both their educational progress and their social development. The former would most appropriately be delivered within the school setting. The latter has implications for the child in the school setting, in the home setting, and in middle and later childhood, at least, in the wider social sphere.

We can now consider the advantages and disadvantage of the four models of delivering SLP in relation to children learning language through AAC. We draw on examples from our own research and other research on families.

Therapist-Centered Approaches

The advantages of therapist-centered approaches would include the benefit of the direct application of the SLP's expertise and immediate responsiveness to the child's progress or any difficulties he or she is experiencing. The SLP can identify priorities according to his or her clinical, theoretical, and research-driven experience and knowledge. If parents are not able to engage with therapy for whatever reason, then intervention can still continue and parents do not feel guilty. Our interviews with parents (Goldbart & Marshall, 2004; Marshall & Goldbart, 2008) supported these points, with parents expressing guilt that they were unable to provide as much input as their child needed. They also wanted to make the most of SLPs' expertise. This was particularly important when the parents were aware that the therapist to whom their child was referred actually had particular competence in the area of AAC. There are, however, considerable disadvantages with this approach, as the people around the child do not develop competence either in interaction with the child or in operational aspects of the AAC equipment. This may restrict the child's competence in communicating with nonexperts and those outside the therapy setting, in particular, child-child interaction. Developing communicative competence (using AAC) is largely limited to the therapy context; hence generalization is likely to be more difficult. Communication priorities may not be those of the family or the child and the vocabulary selected by SLPs may not be relevant to the child's interactions with family and friends (McCord & Soto, 2004).

Parent-as-Aide Approaches

In the parent-as-aide approach the parent develops some level of competence in both interaction with child and operational aspects of AAC use, according to the SLP's priorities. Consequently, the child gains a competent communication partner in the home and greater opportunity for home practice. Through collaboration, the parent develops a closer relationship with the therapist and may have some input into identifying priorities, selection of appropriate vocabulary, and manageable modes of communication at home. It is clear from our research (Goldbart & Marshall, 2004) that the great majority of parents want to work in partnership with SLPs and do not consider themselves to be experts in AAC intervention. One parent said explicitly "We're not speech and language therapists . . . , we've never done this before, we rely on people like them" (Goldbart & Marshall, 2004, p. 204).

In the parent-as-aide approach, however, valuable therapy time is taken up with training the parent. Parents may struggle to implement activities or programs at home, especially with limited insight into what they are doing and why. Lack of understanding of activities may affect parents' motivation to do homework and SLP's priorities still may not have a close match with the parents' or child's. The parents have limited knowledge to pass on to others working with the child; for example, teachers and other therapists. This approach puts an additional burden on parents who may already be overstretched and stressed by the additional responsibilities involved in raising a child with a disability. The parents in McCord and Soto's (2004) study felt distanced from decision-making regarding their child's AAC as did some of the parents in our own research (Goldbart & Marshall, 2004; Marshall & Goldbart, 2008). This may be particularly problematic if the parents and SLPs do not share a common culture.

Family-Centered Approaches

Parents involved in family-centered approaches will be better placed to advocate for their children in other settings and to pass on skills to friends and other family members. Priorities will reflect those of the family and therefore be more readily integrated into the family routine. Both of these should extend the opportunities the child has to communicate with those outside SLP and parents. Vocabulary selected will be influenced by parents' understanding of the home situation. Parents should develop a greater understanding of the long-term aims of communication intervention and Dunst et al. (2001) stressed the importance, and advantages of incorporating therapy objectives into family routines.

Families, however, may be reluctant or feel insufficiently knowledgeable to be full partners in decision-making (Goldbart & Marshall, 2004). In this way of working more time is taken in discussion with, and in training parents, leaving less time for hands-on work with the child. This may be particularly acute when parents do not share the SLPs' assumptions about aspects such as parenting practices, the role of play, adult-child communication, and parents' role in language learning. Parents' priorities may conflict with those of the SLPs. There may also be conflicts between social and family priorities in AAC and education. At times parents may be too overwhelmed with other issues to take such a lead role in communication but might welcome it at other times. This approach implies a heavy responsibility for parents in carrying out work and also advocating about intervention to professionals and other family members.

Family-Friendly Approaches

Family-friendly approaches would seem to have considerable advantages as families are as engaged in decision-making and intervention as they want to be at any given time. Their priorities for communication and the child's other needs are respected and selected priorities emerge through negotiation.

Despite this, even this level of participation may be an unmanageable burden for some families at some points. Children's communication may receive relatively low priority if there are other pressing needs within the family, whether related to the child or to other family issues. SLPs need to invest time and effort in building strong relationships with families, and in discussing the nature of communication and its importance in education and daily life, so that agreement can be reached on appropriate levels of priority to allocate to communication. Our research suggests that most parents have given a lot of thought to the importance of communication in their child's life (Marshall & Goldbart, 2008).

Considering all these approaches, we also need to bear in mind Granlund et al.'s (2001, 2005) finding that the roles parents take on will vary over time and among families. Where SLPs develop good working relationships with families, they will be better placed to discuss with parents which roles are appropriate at any given time.

Implications/Suggestions for Good Practice

Best practice in AAC in terms of family involvement has many features in common with good practice with families in other areas of SLP. However, because of the nature of AAC and the frequently complex needs of the children, there are some specific considerations. In this final section we focus on suggestions that relate to intervention where a child needs or uses AAC.

Even if there is limited time to offer to each individual child, we advocate prioritizing working with the family, listening to them, and understanding their perspectives. Without this, any advice given to families may be wasted. Genuine collaboration requires an understand of parental perspectives, including their view of their children's communication (e.g., Allaire, Gressard, Blackman, & Hostler, 1991). This will allow understanding of family views about AAC and technology and of the vocabulary and communication needs of the child in the home situation.

Not all parents are the same. Jones, Angelo, and Kokoska (1998) found that middle-class parents of children using AAC in their study, relied on professional support, although it is, as yet, unclear if parents from different social, economic, and cultural backgrounds behave in the same ways. This has particular implications when we are suggesting, for example, in AAC work that parents practice with their child, program a communication aid, and use it in the home. Furthermore, whether or not parents will tell SLPs what they think of their suggestions may depend on their own culture and their expectations of interactions with professionals.

Can parent involvement be reframed away from the negative connotations associated with "pushy" parents? Our research, and a wider United Kingdom consultation for the Every Disabled Child Matters Campaign (ECDM, 2007), suggest that parents do not acquire the services or resources that they perceive their child needs unless they are assertive and put in a large amount of effort. This will depend on the resources and service delivery models in the area where parents live and has implications for the way in which professionals accept the different styles that parents use to express their needs and desires for their child.

Given the pressing need to build up the evidence base in SLP in general and AAC in particular, it is valuable for SLPs to document what they do. The framework for describing participants and environments in AAC research, designed by Pennington, Marshall, and Goldbart (Marshall, Pennington, & Goldbart, 2005; Pennington, Marshall, & Goldbart, 2007) may be useful in helping to describe clinicians' practice, so that others can see if it is applicable to their situation. It will also help in the accumulation of case study data. This is particularly important in the AAC field which is small and with very heterogeneous clients.

Finally, there is a need to understand more about how cultural factors might impact on parents and SLPs working together with children who need or use AAC. For example, what is the impact of:

- Family beliefs about the causes of the child's disability?
- Family ideas about how language is acquired and priorities for AAC intervention?
- Family's attitudes toward whether intervention is appropriate, allowed, or necessary?

■ Who in the family has time and opportunity to work with their child?

■ Parents' feelings about engagement in services (e.g., McCord & Soto, 2004)? Is it that parents are not included by professionals or that engagement does not fit their culture?

Summary

In summary, the field of AAC is young, with a limited research base and the work is often with children who are heterogeneous and who frequently have complex needs. Studies of family involvement with this client group are more recent still, as is the added consideration of cultural factors. We can see that much of the advice/good practice regarding working with families elsewhere in this book is applicable to this client group, but there are some considerations that are particularly relevant to children who use AAC and their families. We are not able to provide all of the answers in this chapter but hope that the questions and issues that we have raised are sufficient to stimulate changes in practice and continued research.

References

Alant, E. (1996). Augmentative and alternative communication in developing countries: Challenge of the future. *Augmentative and Alternative Communication, 12*, 1–12.

Allaire, J., Gressard, R., Blackman, J., & Hostler, S. (1991). Children with severe speech impairments: Caregiver survey of AAC use. *Augmentative and Alternative Communication 7*, 248–255.

Angelo, D. (2000). Impact of AAC devices on families. *Augmentative and Alternative Communication, 16*, 37–41.

Angelo, D., Jones, S., & Kokoska, S. (1995). A family perspective on AAC: Families of young children. *Augmentative and Alternative Communication, 11*, 193–201.

Barnes, C., & Swain, J. (Eds.). (2003). *Disabling barriers, enabling environments* (2nd ed.). Buckingham: Open University Press.

Cress, C. (2004). Augmentative and alternative communication and language understanding and responding to parents' perspectives. *Topics in Language Disorders, 24*, 51–61.

Dunst, C., Bruder, M., Trivette, C., Hamby, D., Raab, M., & McLean, M. (2001). Characteristics and consequences of everyday natural learning opportunities. *Topics in Early Childhood Special Education, 21*, 68-92.

Every Disabled Child Matters. (2007). *'If I could change one thing . . . ':* Parents' views. Retrieved 1/30/2008 from http://www.edcm.org.uk/Page.asp?originx _7962hg_2442312584137k31h_20079204746d

Goldbart, J., & Marshall, J. (2004). Pushes and pulls on the parents of children using AAC. *Augmentative and Alternative Communication, 20*(4), 194-208.

Goldbart, J., & Mukherjee, S. (1999). The appropriateness of Western models of parent involvement in Calcutta, India. Part 2: Implications of family roles and responsibilities. *Child: Care, Health and Development, 25*(5), 348-358.

Granlund, M., Bjork-Akesson, E., & Alant, E. (2005). Family-centred early childhood intervention: New perspectives. In E. Alant & L. Lloyd (Eds.), *Augmentative and alternative communication and severe disabilities: Beyond poverty* (pp. 221-242). London: Whurr.

Granlund, M., Bjork-Akesson, E., Olsson, C., & Rydeman, B. (2001). Working with families to introduce augmentative and alternative communication systems. In H. Cockerill & L. Carroll-Few (Eds.), *Communicating without speech: Practical augmentative and alternative communication* (pp. 88-102). New York: Cambridge University Press.

Huer, M. (1997). Culturally inclusive assessments for children using AAC. *Journal of Children's Communication Development, 19*, 23-34.

Huer, M. (2000). Examining perceptions of graphic symbols across cultures: Preliminary study of the impact of culture/ethnicity. *Augmentative and Alternative Communication, 16*(3), 180-185.

Huer, M., Parette, H., & Saenz, T. (2001). Conversations with Mexican Americans regarding children with disabilities and AAC. *Communication Disorders Quarterly, 224*, 197-206.

Huer, M., & Saenz, T. (2002). Thinking about conducting culturally sensitive research in augmentive and alternative communication. *Augmentative and Alternative Communication, 18*(4), 267-273.

Jones, S., Angelo, D., & Kokoska, S. (1998). Stressors and family supports: Families with children using augmentative and alternative communication technology. *Journal of Children's Communication Development, 20*, 37-40.

Knowles, E., & Peng, K. (2005). White selves: Conceptualising and measuring a dominant-group identity. *Journal of Personality and Social Psychology, 89*(2), 223-241.

Lund, S. K., & Light, J. (2007). Long-term outcomes for individuals who use augmentative and alternative communication: Part III—contributing factors. *Augmentative and Alternative Communication, 23*(4), 323-335.

Marshall, J., & Goldbart, J. (2008). "Communication is everything I think." Parenting a child who needs augmentative and alternative communication. (AAC). *International Journal of Language and Communication Disorders, 43*(1), 77–98.

Marshall, J., Goldbart, J., & Philips, J. (2007). Parents' and speech and language therapists' explanatory models of language development, language delay and intervention. *International Journal of Language and Communication Disorders, 42*(5), 533–555.

Marshall, J., Pennington, L., & Goldbart, J. (2005). Describing participants, partners and environments in AAC research. In S. von Tetzchner & M. de Jesus Goncalves (Eds.), *Theoretical and methodological issues in research on Augmentative and Alternative Communication* (pp. 63–72). Toronto, Canada: ISAAC.

McCord, M., & Soto, G. (2004). Perceptions of AAC: An ethnographic investigation of Mexican-American families. *Augmentative and Alternative Communication, 20*(4), 209–227.

Parette, H., Brotherson, M., & Huer, M. (2000). Giving families a voice in AAC decision-making. *Education and Training in Mental Retardation and Developmental Disabilities, 23*, 177–190.

Parette, P., Huer, M., & Brotherson, M. (2001). Related service personnel perceptions of team AAC decision-making across cultures. *Education and Training in Mental Retardation and Developmental Disabilities, 31*(1), 69–82.

Parette, H., Huer, M., & Wyatt, T. (2002). Young African American children with disabilities and Augmentative and Alternative Communication issues. *Early Childhood Education Journal, 29*(3), 201–207.

Pennington, L., Marshall, J., & Goldbart, J. (2007). Describing participants in AAC research and their communicative environments: Guidelines for research and practice. *Disability and Rehabilitation, 29*(7), 521–535.

Starbie, A., Hutchins, T., Favro, M., Prelock, P., & Bitner, B. (2005). Family centred intervention and satisfaction with AAC device training. *Communication Disorders Quarterly, 27*, 47–62.

World Health Organization. (2001). ICF: *International classification of functioning, disability and health*. Geneva: Author.

Chapter 9

Working with Families of Children with Dysphagia: An Interdisciplinary Approach

Bernice A. Mathisen

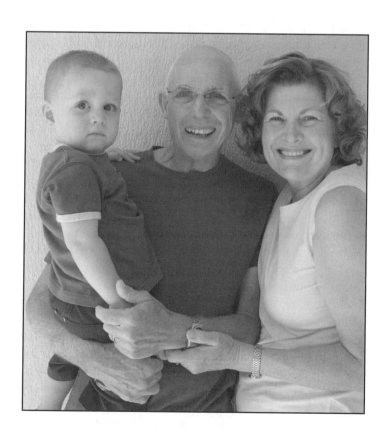

Introduction

Families can be defined as those individuals with a shared interest in the well-being of a child (Hanson, Jeppson, Johnson, & Thomas, 1997). Families have always been the focus in pediatric dysphagia, defined as an inherently heterogeneous population of children with feeding and swallowing problems from neonatal life to late adolescence (Arvedson & Brodsky, 2002).

Pediatric Dysphagia: A Definition

There is no universally accepted classification system of dysphagia, due to its inherent complexity and the frequent co-occurrence of associated disorders, which makes epidemiologic research particularly difficult (Mathisen, & Jakobs, 2004b). In 2007, Jakobs proposed a 10-point system (Table 9–1) based on the primary medical diagnosis(es), where diagnostic categories may also be associated with a major behavioral problem for example, food refusal.

This classification system could be used across disciplines and in association with the International Classification of Functioning, Disability and Health (ICF) (WHO, 2001) and the International Classification of Functioning, Disability and Health—Children and Youth Version (ICF-CY) (WHO, 2007) focusing on the well-being of the child in the environment of the family, rather than on impairment alone (Lefton-Greif & Arvedson, 2007). The ICF-CY is a timely and holistic biopsychosocial model (McLeod & Threats, 2008), emphasizing functionality but can also specify breakdown of body functions and structures such as oral-motor dysfunction for example, sucking (b5100), biting (b5101), chewing (b5102), or gastrointestinal dysfunction such as regurgitation and vomiting (b5106) (see Appendix 9A).

Few systematic data on the prevalence and incidence of dysphagia in children are available but parent reports of feeding problems in the general population are high. Lindberg, Bohlin, and Hagekull (1991) identified a 25% prevalence of early feeding problems up to 6 months in the general population and 10% ongoing problems after this age. Forsyth, Leventhal, and McCarthy (1985) reported a rate as high as 35% when mothers were interviewed. In infants and children with lifelong disability such as cerebral palsy, the incidence of dysphagia

Table 9–1. Major Pediatric Dysphagia Diagnostic Categories Based on Jakobs (2007)

1. Neurologic (e.g., cerebral palsy, autism spectrum disorder, traumatic brain injury)
2. Syndromic (e.g., Down syndrome)
3. Chromosomal
4. Metabolic
5. Anatomic and structural (e.g., clefts of the lip and palate)
6. Respiratory (e.g., tracheomalacia)
7. Cardiac (e.g., aplastic heart disease)
8. Gastrointestinal (e.g., gastroesophageal reflux disorder or GERD)
9. Functional (e.g., failure to thrive)
10. Psychopathologic (e.g., dysphagia associated with infant or carer diagnosis of mental health problem such as postnatal depression or anxiety disorder)

Based on Jakobs (2007).

has been reported as 85 to 90% and severe, causing parents much concern (Arvedson & Brodsky, 2002; Sullivan, Lambert, Rose, Ford-Adams, Griffiths, & Johnson, 1998) or 57% with sucking problems and 38% with swallowing problems in the first 12 months of life (Reilly, Skuse, & Poblete, 1996).

Historical Overview of Family Involvement in Pediatric Dysphagia

The involvement of speech-language pathology (SLP) in the management of children with pediatric dysphagia began 20 years ago to address challenging swallowing and communication problems of children with cerebral palsy. In Gisel and Patrick's seminal work of 1988, the interrelationship between dysphagia and protein calorie-malnutrition in cerebral palsy was first recognized. With this finding, came awareness that children with cerebral palsy were treatable, in terms of their impoverished nutritional status and that this was related to their poorly developed eating, drinking, and swallowing skills. As a result, the first interdisciplinary dialogue around feeding was begun between physicians, dieticians, and occupational therapists to be followed by many other health and education professionals (including SLPs) with a shared interest in this population.

Interdisciplinary collaboration between a speech-language pathologist and occupational therapist in the United States produced a parent-friendly textbook entitled *Pre-Feeding Skills: A Comprehensive Resource for Mealtime Development*, a seminal work which firmly avowed the need for SLPs to incorporate "feeding assessment and intervention" into their professional armoury (Morris & Klein, 1987). The text was designed to be a practical resource for health professionals and parents of children with pediatric dysphagia and was written in a user-friendly style, allowing for printing of clear information sheets on a wide variety of topics. Encouraged by extensive American legislative reform to ensure appropriate early intervention and educational opportunities for their children, parents went looking for professionals who could deliver "feeding" services. This created a huge impetus for the expansion of further research initiatives, postgraduate teaching opportunities, and interdisciplinary professional activity by speech-language pathologists and their professional partners in health and education, for example, medical specialists, occupational therapists, physiotherapists, dieticians, specialist dentists, nurses, and educationalists across the world.

In the 1980s, it was suggested by some that dysphagia was not the role of the SLP or that, if it was, it was a postgraduate specialty as in the United Kingdom, until recently. Fierce debate ensued around whose job it was to provide these services, the nature of the relationship between speech, language and swallowing (Mathisen, 2001) or speech and oral-motor therapy with proponents of both positions locking horns in the literature. Although there is some support for the hypothesis of integrative motor control and codevelopment of feeding and communication (Massey, Hird, & Simmer, 2004), there are major differences too and practitioners need to remember that *specificity* is a key feature to keep in mind when designing motor programs. For example, if speech is to be targeted, speech tasks need to be used by SLPs and if eating, drinking, and swallowing are to be targeted, those specific skills need to be incorporated into intervention plans. However, the consensus now is that the assessment and intervention of *both* communication and swallowing across the life span rests firmly in the scope of practice of speech-language pathology but should be shared with other disciplines for optimal outcomes for families (Threats, 2007). Therefore, a family-centered approach to the care of infants and children with pediatric dysphagia can only flourish where there are no smouldering "turf battles" between disciplines for power or prestige (Mathisen, 1999, 2003).

Since the 1980s, research in the area of dysphagia has continued at an exponential pace (Bell & Alper, 2007). The evidence base for dysphagia management in children is emerging rapidly (Reilly & Perry, 2001; Reilly & Ward, 2005) and there is increasing attention to the particular ethical and legal challenges associated in dysphagia intervention for infants and children (Arvedson & Lefton-Greif, 2007). Specific textbooks on pediatric dysphagia have appeared (Arvedson & Brodsky, 2002; Tuchman & Walter, 1994; Wolf & Glass, 1992) with a consistent emphasis on family involvement and the importance of interdisciplinary teamwork (Drinka & Clark, 2000). Standardized feeding assessments are available for research and clinical purposes with infants and children with dysphagia associated with varying etiologies (Als et al., 2003; Case-Smith, Cooper, & Scala, 1989; Gore & Wood, 2006; Kenny, Koheil, Greenberg, Reid, Milner, Moran, & Judd, 1989; Lefton-Greif & Sheppard, 2005; Palmer, Crawley, & Blanco, 1993; Reilly, Skuse, Mathisen, & Wolke, 1995; Reilly, Skuse, & Wolke, 2000; Sheppard, 2002a, 2002b; Skuse, Stevenson, Reilly, & Mathisen, 1995). As a measure of the increasing maturity of the field of pediatric dysphagia, a state of the art review was completed by a prestigious group of researchers and clinicians in the United States (see Pediatric Dysphagia: The 10th Anniversary Issue, Volume 28(3), 2007 in *Seminars in Speech and Language*). Throughout the body of research literature that supports clinical practice in pediatric dysphagia, a consistent and primary principle is the centrality of family involvement and an ever increasing emphasis on a truly holistic focus by SLPs and their professional partners, addressing the physical, social, emotional, and spiritual needs of the child in the context of their family system (Burgman, 2005; Mathisen & Mathers, 2006; Strong, 2008).

Evidence Base of Effectiveness of Family Involvement

The area of evidence-based intervention for pediatric dysphagia is in its infancy, with no randomized control trials completed. However, there is growing evidence to support SLP assessment and intervention of feeding and swallowing disorders in various clinical populations, such as preterm infants, in relation to transitioning from non-nutritive to nutritive sucking and with regard to various assessment and treatment options. Major gaps in the literature are filled by expert opinion and clinical experience at present but this will be replaced by more robust evidence in the short-term (Sheppard & Fletcher, 2007).

A thorough search of relevant databases (Medline/PubMed, Embase, Eric/ProQuest, Scopus, PsychINFO, Linguistics and Language Behavior Abstracts (LLBA), and the Cochrane Library of Systematic Reviews and Clinical Trials) revealed no completed randomized control trials (RCTs) in the published literature on the effectiveness of family involvement of children with dysphagia. The lack of completed RCTs makes it impossible to compare the relative benefit and/or potential for harm of the wide range of service delivery models that are currently in place for children with dysphagia. As stated previously, published case series and cohort studies suggest that family engagement is a central tenet of all models of service; however, the strength and nature of this engagement has yet to be reported in the literature. There is an urgent need to investigate the validity of this clinical assumption, but this is difficult, given the wide variability of the population of children with dysphagia (Mathisen & Jakobs, 2004) and serious ethical concerns remain in withholding care for medically-fragile children and their equally vulnerable parents (Arvedson & Lefton-Greif, 2007).

Importance of Family Involvement in Intervention for Pediatric Dysphagia

Feeding is a complex and dynamic system (Fischer & Pare-Blagoev, 2000; Goldfield, 2007). It is a sensitive indicator of the nature of the interrelationship between the child and the person doing the feeding and the result of negotiation through sensitive periods for acquiring feeding skills (Fischer & Silverman, 2007). Satter (cited in Morris & Klein, 2000) emphasized that this relationship is based firstly in *trust* and then in the cultural, social, emotional, and family dynamics operating at the time. Parents and children have different but complementary roles at every mealtime. The parent provides appropriate and nutritious food, drink, and feeding equipment and a sensitive and supportive environment and the child decides on what and how much to consume of what is offered. Thus, feeding affirms the child's rights to be responsible for his or her own intake in a respectful way and provides a naturalistic social setting for all communicative attempts (Mathisen, 2001).

Importantly, mealtimes provide a window into the psychoemotional health of the whole family, which may be comorbid to the dysphagia (Mathisen, 2002). There is evidence in the literature for a relationship with:

- parental (in particular, maternal) mental health factors and preterm birth (Nilsson, Lichtenstein, Cnattingius, Murray, & Hultman, 2002),
- infant under-nutrition at 6 months corrected age after controlling for birthweight (Rahman, Iqbal, Bunn, Lovel, & Harrington, 2004),
- low compliance with preventive and child-health promotion measures such as well-child visits in preschool years (Minkovitz, Strobino, Scharfstein, Hu, Miller, Mistry, & Swartz 2005),
- suboptimal breastfeeding (Galler, Harrison, Biggs, Ramsey, & Forde, 1999),
- repeated emergency hospital admissions (Bartlett, Kolodner, Butz, Eggleston, Malveaux, & Rand, 2001), and
- poor cognitive development (Murray & Copper, 2003).

Qualitative research has revealed new and deep insights into the extent of the impact of preterm birth on mothers with very low and extremely low birth weight infants in neonatal intensive care and how this affects the whole family (MacDonald, 2007). Mothers reported that they (and their partners) were "caught off guard" by the birth and severely traumatized. They experienced grief and loss of the pregnancy and became "premature parents," suddenly dealing with a vast array of health professionals. Many reported that they felt "transitional" and largely powerless in the health care system. It is significant that feeding was a particularly sensitive and complex issue for the mothers. Similarly, parents of infants with craniofacial anomalies such as clefts of the lip and palate associated with or without congenital syndromes are at increased risk of parental adjustment problems, anxiety, and depression (Kramer, Gruber, Fialka, Sinikovic, & Schliephake, 2008). It is also recognized that parents of children born with any disability may be prone to "cyclical grieving" (Blaska, 1998), increased levels of stress, and problems with adaptation (Hanson & Hanline, 1990).

SLPs' Involvement of Families in Clinical Practice for Pediatric Dysphagia

Dysphagia is regarded as core business for speech-language pathologists in the western world and increasingly so in developing countries. Central to this professional activity is the family. As Morris and Klein (2000 p. 3) stated "the child and family are at the center of every program." Centers of excellence in cerebral palsy around the world, such as the Bobath Centre in London, United Kingdom and the Peto Institute in Budapest, Hungary or specialist residential programs for infants and children with dysphagia, such as at New Visions in Virginia in the United States, have long advocated family-centeredness.

The first epidemiologic research into Australian pediatric dysphagia practice was completed in 2002. The Paediatric Dysphagia National Survey was conducted to ascertain the nature of knowledge, skills, attitudes, and experiences of Australian SLPs including their knowledge and attitude to family-centeredness in relation to their clinical practice (Jakobs, Mathisen, Baines, & Jones, 2003a; Mathisen, 2004). A total of 634 SLP respondents (582 SLPs and 52 SLP students) reported an overall positive attitude toward the role of SLPs with children with dysphagia, but that Australian SLPs do not enter the workforce adequately prepared for the challenges and complexities of pediatric dysphagia practice (Jakobs & Mathisen, 2004).

Respondents reported that their knowledge of dysphagia in children had mostly been through "on the job" learning. Almost half highlighted the need for a specific mentor program in pediatric dysphagia (Jakobs, Mathisen, Baines, & Jones, 2003b). The Paediatric Dysphagia National Survey suggested an overall lack of quality supervision for SLPs already working in the field and that the limited clinical training as students may contribute to feelings of intimidation and incompetence, especially when confronted by a medically complex population and stressed, anxious parents (Jakobs, Mathisen, Baines, & Jones, 2004). Recent attempts to address these shortcomings in new graduates have appeared in the interprofessional literature (Smith & Pilling, 2007) including online learning innovations (Miers, Clarke, Pollard, Rickaby, Thomas, & Turtle, 2007). In Australia, there are calls to formalize specialist recognition in swallowing as in the United States (ASHA Board Recognized Specialist Status in Swallowing and Swallowing Disorders-BRS-S, 2006).

Australian speech-language pathologists reported collaborating more commonly in interdisciplinary teams in rural rather than urban settings (Lobsey, O'Connor, & Perceval, 2005). Speech-language pathologists reported collaborating most commonly with nurses, psychologists, dietitians, physical therapists, occupational therapists, and social workers and less frequently with medical practitioners (GPs and medical specialists). SLPs reported little to no formal preparation in working in these types of clinical settings. One particularly relevant finding was that Australian SLP respondents were overwhelmingly aware of family-centered and family-friendly approaches and its relevance but were unsure of how to apply this knowledge to a caseload of children with dysphagia and their families. The researchers concluded that this finding was related to the paucity of skilled clinical mentors during their clinical education experience.

Families' Views of Involvement in SLP for Pediatric Dysphagia

It is generally accepted by SLPs and their professional partners that the perspective of the parents, siblings, and significant others of infants and children with dysphagia is crucial for successful outcomes, particularly, in regard to families with cultural differences. In this case, a child with dysphagia and his or her supporting family present with a wide range of challenges, such as their attitude toward the child and his or her problems, their relationship to the SLP, and other professionals, the cultural meanings of certain foods and fluids related to their particular cultural background, the foods and fluids used and not used by the family and expectations of recovery or "cure" (Morris & Klein, 2000). Surprisingly, the particular experiences and concerns of families of infants and children with dysphagia have not been thoroughly investigated or reported, except for a recent qualitative study (Stoner, Bailey, Angell, Robbins, & Polewski, 2006). Stoner and her colleagues (2006) interviewed eight parents or guardians of children from 2 to 11 years of age with dysphagia. They reported significant educational concerns and how their child's dysphagia impacted on health status, nutrition, and social-emotional well-being. Stoner et al. (2006) highlighted the heightened potential for family distress and psychosocial dysfunction (also identified by Blaska, 1998; Franklin & Rodger, 2003; Hanson & Hanline, 1990), the unique role of other parents with similar experiences of children with dysphagia as ongoing support networks (Spann, Kohler, & Soenksen, 2003), and the need for professionals to deliver respectful and effective holistic care (reported by Lake & Billingsley, 2000; McWilliam, Lang, Vandiviere, Angell, Collins, & Underdown, 1995, Stoner, Bock, Thompson, Angell, Heyl, & Crowley, 2005). Importantly, the study highlighted the need for adequate preparation in the way health professionals related to families involved in the provision of clinical services including pediatric dysphagia (Jones, 2003). Jones et al. (2003) found that in the context of the provision of Australian rural health care, the need for family-sensitive practitioners from all disciplines was not only desirable but essential. Despite this, little had been done in the way of making this explicit to medical, nursing, and related health care professionals, including speech-language pathology, in their clinical undergraduate or postgraduate education programs.

Nexus Between Research, Clinical Practice, and Families' Views of Pediatric Dysphagia

A holistic, interdisciplinary, family-friendly team is considered best practice in the literature for pediatric dysphagia assessment and management (Morgan & Reilly cited in Cichero & Murdoch, 2006). This includes a detailed medical, nutritional and developmental history, including fine, gross and oral-motor feeding function as well as sensory and communication, environmental, and family factors. As many children with dysphagia are medically complex, no one discipline can be expert in all areas. Regardless of the discipline involved, the quality of the communication with the child's family, set in a context of attachment, security, and trust, is the most important aspect to interprofessionalism within health care (Thompson, 2007).

However, an interdisciplinary focus may be difficult to effect in clinical practice for reasons such as cost, professional territoriality, isolation, ignorance, limited experience, or low expectation of effective teamwork models. Families prefer an environment that is relaxed and naturalistic such as in their homes, preschool, and school settings in addition to the more traditional hospital and outpatient settings (Bell & Alper, 2007).

Few new graduate SLPs have adequate clinical preparation in interdisciplinary teamwork and family-friendly practice. To address this need, the Interdisciplinary Dysphagia Clinic (IDC) was an innovative exercise in applying theory to practice. As a collaborative venture between the University of Newcastle Speech Pathology Program, (the former School of Language and Media), the Faculty of Education and Arts, and the Faculty of Health and Hunter Area Health Service (HAHS), the IDC was established by the author, a speech-language pathologist (Jones, Mathisen, Baines, Dathan-Horder, & Jakobs, 2002; Mathisen, 1999; Mathisen, Dear, King, Muir, Lovell, & Downes, 2005; Mathisen, Lee, King, King, & Dear, 2003). The IDC had three interdependent functions:

- to provide free, family-friendly community service,
- to foster interdisciplinary research opportunities, and
- to provide interdisciplinary clinical education for education and health care students including SLPs

The interdisciplinary approach aimed to ensure safe and optimal nutrition and hydration for maximal growth and development, a valuable parent resource, and a vehicle for advocacy for families (Mathisen, Jakobs, Jones, Baines, & Dathan-Horder, 2002).

This model of service provision, based on similar clinics in Canada, the United States, and United Kingdom was regarded as best practice, enabling families simplified access to a specialized team of medical, education and allied health professionals in a single visit, eliminating the fragmentation of care (Halper, 1993, Wooster Brady, Mitchell, Grizzle, & Barnes, 1998). This model promoted enhanced communication and allowed families living in rural settings equal opportunity to appropriate and timely clinical services for their children. As a result, the model was replicated in various forms in other settings across Australia including private clinics, community health centers, childrens' hospitals, mainstream and specialist educational settings, and tertiary institutions. The IDC largely achieved its research, teaching, and community service goals over 5 years of operation (Mathisen, Dear, King, Muir, Lovell, & Downes, 2005).

Best Practice in Pediatric Dysphagia

Confusion about terminology amongst medical, education, and health professionals may invalidate and bedevil research findings in pediatric dysphagia. Inter-, multi-, and transdisciplinary teams are used interchangeably in the literature despite inherent differences (Scott & Hofmeyer, 2007). Interdisciplinarity generally refers to "activity that goes on in the spaces between disciplines, and particularly the interaction between disciplines which may give rise to new disciplines" (Russell, 2005). Multidisciplinarity brings two or more disciplines together but boundaries are retained (Russell, 2005). Transdisciplinarity refers to activity that transgresses disciplinary boundaries (Nowotny, 2003).

Many health problems are complex. Pediatric dysphagia is frequently a complex health problem that goes underrecognized in the community. As such, best practice requires that an interdisciplinary team manages the condition. Complexity necessarily creates bioethical and legal issues, which may not have been addressed adequately in undergraduate education of SLPs. Complexity also creates the need for a better, more holistic classification system and approach to care (Turnbull, Turnbull, Erwin, & Soodak, 2006). The ICF-CY (WHO, 2007) is a promising direction for dysphagia research and practice in childhood, as it focuses not only on impairment, but also activities, participation, the environment, and well-being of the child and family as a whole.

The demedicalization of health, where the medical profession's long-standing domination in terms of autonomy, social status, and power is being challenged by families armed with increasing access to information and confidence. An emphasis on primary health care and preventative practice as the basis of the health system will result, with a focus on family health and well-being as espoused by the alternative medicine fraternity rather than acute care and hospitals with a focus on disease, the medical model, specialists, and cost blowouts. Expansive social models will continue to grow and reductionist medical models are likely to contract.

Health care in the 21st century is changing rapidly. As sociologists have long known, health care is interdependent on social, demographic, and economic factors, with poverty having the most insidious negative effect on children and their families. In the last decade or so, this reality is being translated into governmental policy in the United States, United Kingdom, and Australia. A broad perspective using an epidemiologic approach to health care provision is outside the knowledge and experience of most health professionals such as SLPs, who focus on the needs of an individual child and family, rather than those of a particular client group. As a result, there is little opportunity for SLPs at present, to accrue evidence about the efficacy and effectiveness of different assessments or treatments for children with dysphagia, even though there is an urgent need to acquire this evidence to justify ethical decision-making and future service provision for children and their families.

Models of Working with Families

There is now widespread promotion of child-centered, family-friendly, and family-centered services, partnership models with parents and increasing client participation, empowerment, and advocacy (Benson, Davies, & Mathisen, 1996; Davis, Day, & Bidmead, 2002; Farrell & Mathisen, 2004; 2005; Gabuthuler, 2005; Mathisen, Sixsmith, & Sixsmith, 1996). The emphasis is on the primacy of the child as part of a family system that is, the neighborhood, community, and cultural system. Similarly, there is a need to focus on SLP services in the context of an entire health system.

In light of wide acceptance of the importance of the first 8 years in a child's life (especially the first 3 years), it is cost effective to provide early intervention to prevent, or at least minimize, later problems and assist in optimal nutrition and brain development. In addition, there is a need to address identified problems of fragmentation of services and an urgent requirement for better collaboration between agencies. Fragmentation of services and treatment approaches is common with children with dysphagia, receiving little or no intervention at one end of the continuum or being overserviced by several different professionals with little or no collaboration at the other end. As a result, parents may have limited knowledge about pediatric dysphagia or remain confused and disempowered with few resources to manage at home or advocate for their child in medical and educational settings.

Management models will continue to impact health care with increasing accountability, quality assurance, and cost-cutting (Deegan, McDonald, & Vajak, 2004). The evidence base for dysphagia in children will be established, providing efficient and effective assessment and interventions that are proven. Outcomes that are functional and meaningful to and defined by the families who use them will be developed (McWilliam, Lang, et al., 1995). SLPs and health and education professionals need to learn to work together for a common purpose, that is, the needs of a common family rather than self-promotion or being seen as "the expert" in pediatric feeding and swallowing. Furthermore, students require inter-professional education, training and clinical experience of pediatric dysphagia to be effective future team members.

Case Study of Family Involvement in Pediatric Dysphagia

The following case study demonstrates a family-centered approach to the complexity of a child with an airway problem and dysphagia, resulting in nutritional compromise and family distress. The significant impact on family functioning and the result of a holistic family-friendly assessment and intervention is demonstrated.

Background

A female toddler of 18 months (Madeleine, not a real name) was referred to the Interdisciplinary Dysphagia Clinic (IDC) by her local SLP, due to increasing concerns about her feeding and continued poor weight gain. She was the youngest of three children who lived at home with both parents. She presented with tracheomalacia (pathologic loss or softening of the tracheal cartilages) (Arvedson & Brosdky, 2002), producing airway collapse to a slitlike opening, resulting in air turbulence or stridor. As a result of the substantial respiratory effort of inspiration, respiratory distress is common, the coordination of breathing, sucking, and swallowing is disrupted, and weight gain is often compromised (Wolf & Glass, 1992).

Madeleine had a long history of recurrent chest infections, aspiration pneumonia and failure to thrive (FTT). On a recent hospital admission, she had been fed nasogastrically for four days (90 mL 3 hourly) and had gained 450 grams. Without enteral feeding, her growth was inadequate (50 grams per week). Despite aggressive antibiotic therapy for chest infections, she ate little at mealtimes, had a poor appetite, and had multiple emergency admissions to hospital with dehydration. Her mother reported long and frustrating mealtime "battles" at home, whereas her father was detached and emotionally unavailable.

The feeding interview with the parents revealed no elimination problems (diarrhea or constipation) but the pediatrician was awaiting test results for celiac disease. Her mother reported that skin blisters would result if certain food types were ingested (e.g., pasta with cheese sauce). However, there was no other suggestion of food allergy. Since birth, a steady decline in weight-for-age had occurred and there was clinical evidence of severe failure to thrive (at birth, Madeleine was at the 90th percentile and was now at the 25th percentile). At 18 months of age, her weight of 10.2 kg was on the 25th percentile and her height of 80 cm was on the 40th percentile. She had been bottle-fed since birth, with long-standing weak sucking and poorly coordinated swallowing, frequent coughing throughout feeds, and fatiguing before the end of a mealtime. She had never cried for demand feeds. She was offered four Pediasure bottle feeds per day, each of 200 mL, to supplement her weight gain. Her mother reported that only 400 mL were typically ingested.

At 10 months of age, the consulting pediatrician requested a modified barium swallow (MBS) study to instrumentally investigate her ongoing dysphagia. Results confirmed a moderate oral-pharyngeal stage dysphagia, characterized by significant difficulty controlling the bolus in the oral cavity, premature spillage over the base of tongue before swallow initiation, and multiple swallows needed to clear residue. There was consistent pooling in the valleculae and piriform sinuses before the swallow but no evidence of penetration or aspiration. At 17 months of age, a second modified barium swallow study was requested but abandoned due to poor cooperation and refusal of all consistencies by the child, despite adequate preparation for the procedure by the SLP and Madeleine's parents.

Family Involvement in Assessment

Mealtime observation at home by the SLP using videotaping for later analysis revealed protracted timing (up to 1 hour per mealtime) and a stressful home environment Crying and force feeding were used by Madeleine's mother due to ongoing anxiety about her decelerating weight. Madeleine was positioned in an appropriate high chair, sitting upright, and preferring to feed herself. She drank thin fluids (typically water or fruit juice) from a trainer cup or used an Avent bottle for formula feeds with a medium flow teat. She finger-fed diced semisolid food textures such as soft chicken, beef, semicooked vegetables, and baked beans and would sometimes nibble on a piece of toast. With assistance from her mother, she could use an open-lipped cup but was unable to regulate the flow rate. She would also walk around the house drinking thin fluids from her trainer cup with a hyperextended neck position.

At clinical assessment, Madeleine's parents provided all previous reports from medical professionals involved including an otolaryngologist, pediatrician, and respiratory physician and gave a thorough case history to the SLP and other IDC team members. After this was completed, Madeleine was taken into an adjoining smaller room with her parents and SLP. Madeleine sat on her mother's knee for reassurance and her father sat beside the SLP on the floor. She was irritable and resistant throughout, when offered various textures of familiar food or drink by her parents or the SLP, with a persistent chesty cough and stuffed-up nose, making nasal breathing difficult. There was evidence of sensory disturbance for example, oral and tactile defensiveness, with no evidence of mouthing or oral-exploratory play on toys.

A standardized oral-motor assessment was completed using the Schedule for Oral-Motor Assessment (SOMA) (Reilly, Skuse, & Wolke, 2000), with moderate oral-motor dysfunction diagnosed. She achieved lip closure and jaw elevation on spoon feeding with better performance on food textures such as roughly mashed banana rather than smooth puree. She had a sustained controlled bite on a biscuit, with evidence of early chewing (vertical jaw excursions). Oral transit times (OTT) were increased to more than 5 seconds for all textures, due to possible inadequate tongue function, which was confirmed by her modified barium swallow results. Of greatest concern was Madeleine's inability to coordinate respiration with swallowing. The increased effort demonstrated and subsequent fatigue were notable due to respiratory compromise. However, she was able to drink thickened fluid (drinking yogurt) from an open cup with less effort and greater coordination.

Refer to Appendix 9A for a Suggested Classification System for a Child with Dysphagia and Appendix 9B for a Sample Interdisciplinary Dysphagia Clinic Report for Madeleine.

In Madeleine's case, dysphagia and subsequent poor weight gain were secondary to the toddler's compromised respiratory functioning (Lefton-Greif & McGrath-Morrow, 2007; Miller & Willging, 2007).

Undiagnosed gastroesophageal reflux disease (GERD) was confirmed using a 24-hour pH study by the consultant gastroenterologist on a subsequent referral as was chronic otitis media (COM) and eustachian tube dysfunction following referral for audiologic assessment. The child was started on a course of antibiotics and LOSEC (antireflux medication) to treat the gastroesophageal reflux disease (GERD) and within two months was showing marked positive behavioral changes.

Family Involvement in Intervention

After counseling was arranged for the parents by the IDC psychologist, maternal anxiety and developing depression regarding feeding were acknowledged and managed effectively. The father was encouraged to take a more active role at mealtimes, which allowed "time out" for Madeleine's mother. She developed a network of support with other mothers of children with dysphagia, which increased her emotional resilience and time with her other two children. Forced feeding was discontinued and the emotional well-being of the family increased.

Despite inconclusive evidence of its effectiveness in the literature (Chang, Lasserson, Gaffney, Connor, & Garske, 2007), the thickening of thin fluids (formula and juice) was recommended with Karicare AR to Level 400-Moderately Thick (Atherton, Bellis-Smith, Cichero, & Suter, 2007) to reduce the likelihood of aspiration pneumonia in future and to support the coordination of breathing with sucking and swallowing (Kirby & Noel, 2007). However, sips of water were permitted to guard against dehydration (Weir, McMahon & Chang, 2005). Prefeeding use of NUK toys, bottle feeding, and cup drinking occurred in an upright supported position only and no extraneous stimuli, such as toys, television, or radio, were allowed at mealtimes. Madeleine was encouraged in all her self-feeding attempts at the beginning of the mealtime which was limited to 20 to 30 minutes only.

Recommendations were given to the parents, for their comments, at the time of assessment and they provided feedback to the IDC team about their feasibility. Families can often be overwhelmed with the number of issues that are addressed at any one time in cases of dysphagia in children. In this instance, it was useful to prioritize the recommendations. As a result, the parents were keen to seek psycho-emotional support for themselves and to return to the pediatrician and GP to begin the referral process for their toddler. SLPs need to be aware that parents, in addition to their involvement with health care professionals are commonly using the Internet to access information and to make contact with each other for emotional support (Leonard, Slack Smith, Phillips, & Richardson, 2003). Madeleine's parents agreed that in 1 month's time, they (and the daycare mother) would work more on individual recommendations regarding the child's feeding and swallowing.

By Interdisciplinary Dysphagia Clinic (IDC) review at 24 months of age, respiratory status and nutritional improvement were noted by the child's growth of new hair, clearance of skin irritation, eruption of additional dentition, and reduced mealtime fatigue. Madeleine's weight of 11.5 kg had increased from the 25th percentile to the 50th percentile. She demonstrated positive affect at mealtimes and was feeding herself pasta of all textures and softened meat strips in a stir fry. Her thickened fluids were successful in preventing any instances of aspiration pneumonia and no dehydration was reported with supervised sips of water. Another follow-up modified barium swallow was requested. Her parents reported improved family functioning and that the daycare mother was reporting similar success. As a result, speech and language development was now more the focus of intervention for her referring SLP. The family decided that a 3-month review by the IDC team was appropriate and they planned their first family holiday with Madeleine and her siblings.

Summary

The widespread use of sophisticated biotechnology in diagnostics and intervention in pediatric swallowing, especially in the rapidly developing area of neonatal and perinatal care, will allow rapid transfer of information resulting in increased cost, training, and specialization. Increasing access to Internet information has the potential to empower families (particularly those in rural and remote settings) to deal more effectively with health and education professionals such as SLPs in pediatric dysphagia. In addition, the development of the first global classification system for children and youth (the ICF-CY) (WHO, 2007) will provide a common coding language, taking into account the impact of environmental (including family) and personal factors on the child, which can be translated across disciplines. These huge advances will fundamentally change the way in which care is delivered with major impact on the child with dysphagia and their family system.

Conclusion

Although the epidemiology of dysphagia in childhood remains ill-defined, it is a common condition, more prevalent in the preschool years and highly variable in expression, from mild and transitory, resolving with time and maturity to complex, lifelong, and life-threatening. Such challenging diversity ideally requires the skills of SLPs working in family-centered practices or family-friendly interdisciplinary team settings. This area of practice may be particularly challenging but is ultimately personally and professionally rewarding. Pediatric dysphagia is an area that is rapidly expanding, given increased medical and surgical interventions, resulting in enhanced survival and low morbidity of preterm and other vulnerable infants and children, in addition to increasing numbers of children diagnosed with lifelong conditions such as autism spectrum disorder (ASD) and cerebral palsy (CP).

Dysphagia in children is unique in that its developing evidence-base straddles many areas of the health and education literature. Families of children with dysphagia can feel isolated, defeated, and lack the confidence to negotiate and advocate for their child. Many are beset with a multitude of other stresses that may preclude effective partnership with professionals. In the last 20 years, SLPs have shown that they have much to give families and vice versa. This is guaranteed to continue in the exciting years ahead.

Acknowledgment. This chapter is dedicated to the children and families of the Interdisciplinary Dysphagia Clinic (IDC) from 2001 to 2006, to the students who learned with us and to the caliber and commitment of the IDC team members. It was a privilege to learn alongside and with Professor Peter Jones, Dr. Peter King, Dr. Olivia Jakobs, Dr. Helen Cornwell, Dr. Mark Lee, Dr. Surinder Baines, Ms. Wendy Dear, Ms. Belinda Downes, Ms. Margaret Muir, Ms. Nadine Farrell, Ms. Katherine Proudfoot, Ms. Gai Lovell, Ms. Domini King, Ms. Diena Grant-Thomson, and Ms. Katrina Dathan-Horder.

References

American Speech and Hearing Association (ASHA). (2006). Board Recognized Specialist Status in Swallowing and Swallowing Disorders-(BRS-S) Retrieved November 10, 2006, from http://www.swallowingdisorders.org/board_recognized_specialists.htm

Arvedson, J., & Brodsky, L. (2002). *Pediatric swallowing and feeding: Assessment and management* (2nd ed.). San Diego, CA: Singular.

Arvedson, J., & Lefton-Greif, M. (2007). Ethical and legal challenges in feeding and swallowing intervention for infants and children. *Seminars in Speech and Language 28*, 232–238.

Atherton, M., Bellis-Smith, N., Cichero, J., & Suter, M. (2007). Texture-modified foods and thickened fluids as used for individuals with dysphagia: Australian standardised labels and definitions. *Nutrition and Dietetics, 64*(Suppl. 2), S53–S76.

Bartlett, S., Kolodner, K., Butz, A., Eggleston, P., Malveaux, F., & Rand C. (2001). Maternal depressive symptoms and emergency use among inner-city children with asthma. *Archives of Pediatric and Adolescent Medicine, 155*, 347–353.

Bell, H., & Alper, B. (2007). Assessment and intervention for dysphagia in infants and children: Beyond the neonatal intensive care unit. *Seminars in Speech and Language, 28*, 213–222.

Benson, J., Davies, K., & Mathisen, B. (1996, May). *Parent-professional partnership: A team approach to therapy.* Paper presented at the Inaugural Conference of the New Zealand Speech-Language Therapists Association and the Australian Association of Speech and Hearing, Auckland, New Zealand.

Blaska, J. K. (1998). *Cyclical grieving: Reoccurring emotions experienced by parents who have children with disabilities.* Department of Child and Family Studies, St. Cloud State University. (ERIC Document Reproduction Service No. ED419349), St. Cloud, MN: Publisher.

Buehler, D., Vandenberg, K., Sweet, N., Sell, E., Parad, R., Ringer, S., et al. (2003). A three-center, randomized, controlled trial of individualized developmental care for very low birth weight preterm infants: Medical, neurodevelopmental, parenting and caregiving effects. *Journal of Developmental and Behavioural Pediatrics, 24*, 399–408.

Burgman, I. (2005). *Reflections on being: Spirituality within children's narratives of identity and disability.* Unpublished Doctoral dissertation, University of Sydney.

Case-Smith, J., Cooper, P., & Scala, V. (1989). Feeding efficiency of premature neonates. *American Journal of Occupational Therapy, 43*, 245–250.

Chang, A., Lasserson, T., Gaffney, J., Connor, F., & Garske, L. (2007). Gastroesophageal reflux treatment for prolonged non-specific cough in children and adults. *Cochrane Database of Systematic Reviews 2006, Issue 4.* Art. *No.CD004823.DOI:10.1002/14651858.CD004823.pub3.*

Davis, H., Day, C., & Bidmead, C. (2002). *Working in partnership with parents: The parent advisor model.* London: The Psychological Corporation.

Deegan, D., McDonald, S., & Vajak, J. (2004). *Parent/caregiver satisfaction with interdisciplinary dysphagia clinic reports: Results of a quality assurance survey.* Unpublished report for the SPTH4010 Advanced Professional Studies Course. Newcastle, Australia: The University of Newcastle.

Dietitians Association of Australia and the Speech Pathology Association of Australia Limited. (2007). The Australian Standardized Terminology and Definitions for Texture Modified Foods and Fluids. *Nutrition and Dietetics, 64*(Suppl. 2), S53–S76.

Drinka, T., & Clark, P. (2000). *Health care teamwork: Interdisciplinary practice and teaching.* Westport CT: Auburn House.

Dunn, W. (2002). *Infant/Toddler Sensory Profile.* San Antonio, TX: The Psychological Corporation.

Farrell, N., & Mathisen, B. (2004, September). *What the people want: Delivery of Australian rural health services-the interdisciplinary approach.* Paper presented at the Australian Student Rural Health Conference, Adelaide.

Farrell, N., & Mathisen, B. (2005, April). *Empowering parents: An interdisciplinary perspective.* Paper presented at 10th National Conference of the Association the Welfare of Child Health. Sydney: AWCH.

Fischer, K. W., & Pare-Blagoev, J. (2000). From individual differences to dynamic pathways of development. *Child Development, 71*(4), 850–853.

Fischer, E., & Silverman, A. (2007). Behavioural conceptualization, assessment and treatment of pediatric feeding disorders. *Seminars in Speech and Language, 28,* 223–231.

Forsyth, B., Leventhal, J., & McCarthy, P. (1985). Mother's perceptions of problems of feeding and crying behaviors: A prospective study. *American Journal of Diseases of Children, 139,* 269–272.

Franklin, L., & Rodger, S. (2003). Parents' perspectives on feeding medically compromised children: Implications for occupational therapy. *Australian Occupational Therapy Journal, 50,* 137–147.

Gabuthuler, S. (2005). Partnership across service delivery models. *ACQuiring Knowledge in Speech Language and Hearing, 7*(2), 53–55.

Galler, J., Harrison, R., Biggs, M., Ramsey, F., & Forde, V. (1999). Maternal moods predict breastfeeding in Barbados. *Journal of Developmental and Behavavioral Pediatrics, 20,* 80–87.

Gisel, E., & Patrick, J. (1988). Identification of children with cerebral palsy unable to maintain a normal nutritional state. *Lancet, 1*(8580), 283–286.

Goldfield, E. (2007). A dynamical systems approach to infant oral feeding and dysphagia: From model system to therapeutic medical device. *Ecological Psychology, 19*(1), 21–48.

Gore, H., & Wood, S. (2006). Assessment and management of feeding and swallowing difficulties. In R. Appleton & T. Baldwin (Eds.), *Management of brain injured children* (2nd ed., pp. 141-150). New York: Oxford University Press.

Halper, A. (1993, June/July). Teams and teamwork: Health care settings. *ASHA Leader*, pp. 34-35, 48.

Hanson, J. L., Jeppson, E., Johnson, B., & Thomas, J. (1997). *Newborn intensive care: Resources for family-centered practice.* Bethesda, MD: Institute for Family-Centered Care.

Hanson, M. J., & Hanline, M. F. (1990). Parenting a child with a disability: A longitudinal study of parental stress and adaptation. *Journal of Early Intervention, 14*, 234-248.

Jakobs, O. (2007). *Paediatric dysphagia and speech pathology in Australia: New innovations in clinical service delivery and tertiary training.* Unpublished doctoral dissertation, The University of Newcastle, Callaghan, Australia.

Jakobs, O., & Mathisen, B. (2004, October). *The competency of Australian speech pathologists in paediatric dysphagia.* Poster presented at the Dysphagia Research Society Meeting, Montreal, Canada.

Jakobs, O., Mathisen, B., Baines, S., & Jones, P. (2003a, May). Paediatric dysphagia and speech pathology in Australia: A summary of research following national survey distribution. *Proceedings of the 2003 Speech Pathology Australia Conference*, Hobart, Tasmania.

Jakobs, O., Mathisen, B., Baines, S., & Jones, P. (2003b, May). *Mentoring undergraduate speech pathology students in paediatric dysphagia: An initiative of the Interdisciplinary Dysphagia Clinic (IDC) team.* Paper presented at the National Conference of Speech Pathology Australia, Hobart, Tasmania.

Jakobs, O., Mathisen, B., Baines, S., & Jones, P. (2004, August–September). Competency in paediatric dysphagia: A professional requirement for speech pathologists in Australia. *Proceedings of the 26th World Congress of the International Association of Logopedics and Phoniatrics*, Brisbane.

Jones, P. (2003, February). *Beyond the clinical placement: Developing rural-based health professional curricula.* Paper presented at the 2003 ANZAME: Association for Health Professional Education, Inaugural NSW State Conference, Newcastle.

Jones, P., Mathisen, B., Baines, S., Dathan-Horder, K., & Jakobs, O. (2002, May). The Interdisciplinary Dysphagia Clinic: *The multi-professional experience-platform for research, clinical practice and learning.* Paper presented at Journey from the Centre: 2002 Speech Pathology Australia Conference, Alice Springs, Northern Territory.

Kenny, D., Koheil, R., Greenberg, J., Reid, D., Milner, M., Moran, R., & Judd, P. (1989). Development of a multidisciplinary feeding profile for children who are dependent feeders. *Dysphagia, 4,* 16-28.

Kirby, M., & Noel, R. (2007). Nutrition and gastrointestinal tract assessment and management of children with dysphagia. *Seminars in Speech and Language, 28,* 180-189.

Kramer, F., Gruber, R., Fialka, F., Sinikovic, B., & Schliephake, H. (2008). Quality of life and family functioning in children with nonsyndromic orofacial clefts at preschool ages. *Journal of Craniofacial Surgery, 19*(3), 580-587.

Lake, J. F., & Billingsley, B. S. (2000). An analysis of factors that contribute to parent-school conflict in special education. *Remedial Special Education, 21,* 240-251.

Lefton-Greif, M., & Arvedson, J. (2007). Pediatric feeding and swallowing disorders: State of health, population trends and application of the International Classification of Functioning, Disability and Health. *Seminars in Speech and Language, 28,* 161-165.

Lefton-Greif, M., & McGrath-Morrow, S. (2007). Deglutition and respiration: Development, coordination and practical implications. *Seminars in Speech and Language 28,* 166-179.

Lefton-Greif, M., & Sheppard, J. J. (2005). Swallowing Dysfunction/Dysphagia in Adults and Children. In W. Hehring (Ed), *Health promotion for persons with intellectual and developmental disabilities: The state of scientific evidence* (pp. 43-59). Washington DC: American Association on Mental Retardation.

Leonard, H., Slack Smith, L., Phillips, T., & Richardson, S. (2003). How is the Internet helping parents of children with rare disorders? *Journal of Paediatrics and Child Health 39*(Suppl.), A1-A16.

Lindberg, L., Bohlin, G., & Hagekull, B. (1991). Early feeding problems in a normal population. *International Journal of Eating Disorders, 10,* 395-405.

Lobsey, N., O'Connor, A., & Perceval, E. (2005). *Interdisciplinary teams in New South Wales Rural Health: Fact or fiction.* Unpublished report. The University of Newcastle.

MacDonald, M. (2007). Mothers of pre-term infants in neonate intensive care. *Early Child Development and Care, 177* (8), 821-838.

Massey, S., Hird, K., & Simmer, K. (2004). Relationship between early feeding and communication development in infants: Birth to 12 months. *Journal of Pediatric Gastroenterology and Nutrition, 39*(2), 227-228.

Mathisen, B. (1999). The paediatric dysphagia clinic. In S. McLeod & L. McAllister (Eds.), *Towards 2000: Proceedings of the 1999 Speech Pathology Australia National Conference* (pp. 223-230). Melbourne: Speech Pathology Australia.

Mathisen, B. (2001). Dysphagia and early language development. *Australian Communication Quarterly, 3*(1), 7-9.

Mathisen, B. (2002). Lara's Story: A clinical profile of gastro-oesophageal reflux disease (GORD). *ACQuiring Knowledge in Speech, Language and Hearing, 4* (2) 95–98.

Mathisen, B. (2003). Re-inventing the delivery of paediatric dysphagia services. *ACQuiring Knowledge in Speech, Language and Hearing, 5,* 79–82.

Mathisen, B. (2004, August–September). How much is enough? A longitudinal study of dysphagia clinical experiences in speech pathology students. *Program and Abstracts of the 26th World Congress of the International Association of Logopedics and Phoniatrics,* Brisbane. Speech Pathology Australia.

Mathisen, B., Dear, W., King, P., Muir, M., Lovell, G., & Downes, B. (2005, November). *The Interdisciplinary Dysphagia Clinic (IDC) 2001–2005: A retrospective.* Paper presented at The Australian Doctors in Developmental Disability National Conference, Newcastle.

Mathisen, B., & Jakobs, O. (2004a, August–September). Epidemiology of children with paediatric dysphagia: The IDC Database. *Program and Abstracts of the 26th World Congress of the International Association of Logopedics and Phoniatrics,* Brisbane. Speech Pathology Australia.

Mathisen, B., & Jakobs, O. M. (2004b, August). *Epidemiology of children with paediatric dysphagia: The Interdisciplinary Dysphagia Clinic database.* Paper presented at the 26th World Congress of the International Association of Logopedics and Phoniatrics, Brisbane, Australia.

Mathisen, B., Jakobs, O., Jones, P., Baines, S., & Dathan-Horder, K. (2002). Client satisfaction with The Interdisciplinary Dysphagia Clinic. In C. Williams & S. Leitão (Eds.), *Journey from the Centre: Proceedings of the 2002 Speech Pathology Australia Conference* (pp. 223–230). Melbourne, Speech Pathology Australia.

Mathisen, B., Lee, M., King, P., King, D., & Dear, W. (2003, November). *The Interdisciplinary Dysphagia Clinic (IDC) research to practice.* Paper presented at the 3rd Annual Primary Health Care Research Conference: Research in Practice-Breaking the Barriers. Corlette. Published online at http://www.newcastle.edu.au/faculty/health

Mathisen, B., & Mathers, M. (2006, April). *Exploring spirituality: Broadening the frontiers of mental health practice.* Poster presented at the Speech Pathology Australia National Conference, Fremantle.

Mathisen, B., Sixsmith, P., & Sixsmith, P. (1996, May). *Partnership with parents—getting it right.* Paper presented at the Inaugural Conference of the New Zealand Speech-Language Therapists Association and the Australian Association of Speech and Hearing, Auckland, New Zealand.

McLeod, S., & Threats, T. (2008). The ICF-CY and children with communication disabilities. *International Journal of Speech-Language Pathology, 10*(1–2), 92–109.

McWilliam, R. A., Lang, L., Vandiviere, P., Angell, R., Collins, L., & Underdown, G. (1995). Satisfaction and struggles: Family perceptions of early intervention services. *Journal of Early Intervention, 19*(1), 43–60.

Miers, M., Clarke, B., Pollard, K., Rickaby, C., Thomas, J., & Turtle, A. (2007). Online interprofessional learning: The student experience. *Journal of Interprofessional Care, 21*(5), 529-542.

Miller, C., & Willging, J. P. (2007). The implications of upper-airway obstruction on successful infant feeding. *Seminars in Speech and Language, 28,* 190-203.

Minkovitz, C., Strobino, D., Scharfstein, D., Hu, W., Miller, T., Mistry, K., et al. (2005). Maternal depressive symptoms and childrens receipt of health care in the first 3 years of life. *Pediatrics, 115*(2), 306-314.

Morgan, A., & Reilly, S. (2006). Clinical signs, aetiologies and characteristics of paediatric dysphagia. In J. Cichero & B. Murdoch (Eds.), *Dysphagia: Foundation, theory and practice* (pp. 391-466). Chichester, UK: Wiley.

Morris, S. E., & Klein, M. (1987). *Pre-feeding skills: A comprehensive resource for mealtime development* (1st ed.). Tucson, AZ: Therapy Skill Builders.

Morris, S. E., & Klein, M. (2000). *Pre-feeding skills: A comprehensive resource for mealtime development* (2nd ed.). Tucson, AZ: Therapy Skill Builders.

Murray, L., & Copper, P. (2003). Intergenerational transmissions of affective and cognitive processes associated with depression: infancy and the pre-school years. In I. M. Goddyer (Ed.), *Unipolar depression: A lifespan perspective* (pp. 17-46). Oxford: Oxford University Press.

Nilsson, E., Lichtenstein, P., Cnattingius, S., Murray, R., & Hultman, C. (2002). Women with schizophrenia: Pregnancy outcome and infant death among their offspring. *Schizophrenia Research, 58,* 221-229.

Nowotny, H. (2003). *The potential of transdisciplinarity. Article 5 in rethinking interdisciplinarity online conference.* Retrieved September 13, 2007, from http://www.interdisciplines.org/interdisciplinarity/papers/5/language/en

Palmer, M., Crawley, K., & Blanco, I. (1993). Neonatal Oral Motor Assessment Scale: A reliability scale. *Journal of Perinatology, 8,* 28-35.

Rahman, A., Iqbal Z., Bunn, J., Lovel, H., & Harrington, R. (2004). Impact of maternal depression on infant nutritional status and illness: a cohort study. *Archives of General Psychiatry, 61,* 946-952.

Reilly, S., & Perry, A. (2001). Is there an evidence base to the management of paediatric dysphagia? *Asia-Pacific Journal of Speech, Language and Hearing, 6*(1), 1-8.

Reilly, S., Skuse, D., Mathisen, B., & Wolke, D. (1995). The objective rating of oral-motor functions during feeding. *Dysphagia, 10,* 177-191.

Reilly, S., Skuse, D., & Poblete, X. (1996). Prevalence of feeding problems and oral motor dysfunction in children with cerebral palsy: A community survey. *Journal of Pediatrics, 129,* 877-882.

Reilly, S., Skuse, D., & Wolke, D. (2000). *Schedule for oral-motor assessment (SOMA).* London: Whurr.

Reilly, S., & Ward, E. (2005). The epidemiology of dysphagia. Describing the problem—Are we too late? *Advances in Speech-Language Pathology, 7*(1), 14-23.

Russell, A. W. (2005). No academic borders? Transdisciplinarity in university teaching and research. *Australian Universities Review, 48*(1), 35–41.

Satter, E. (2000). Foreword. In S. E. Morris & M. Klein (Eds.), *Pre-feeding skills: A comprehensive resource for mealtime development* (2nd ed., pp. v–vii). Tucson, AZ: Therapy Skill Builders.

Scott, C., & Hofmeyer, A. (2007). Acknowledging complexity: Critically analysing context to understand interdisciplinary research. *Journal of Interprofessional Care, 215*, 491–501.

Sheppard, J. J. (2002a). *Dysphagia disorders survey-Pediatric version* (Rev.). Lake Hopatchong NJ (USA ed.): Nutritional Management Associates. Ryde (Australian ed.); Center for Developmental Disability Studies.

Sheppard, J. J. (2002b). *Dysphagia management staging scale (DMSS) (Rev.)*. Lake Hopatchong, NJ (USA ed.): Nutritional Management Associates. Ryde (Australian ed.); Center for Developmental Disability Studies.

Sheppard, J. J., & Fletcher, K. (2007). Evidence-based interventions for breast and bottle feeding in the neonatal intensive care unit. *Seminars in Speech and Language, 28*, 204–212.

Skuse, D., Stevenson, J., Reilly, S., & Mathisen, B. (1995). Schedule for Oral-Motor Assessment (SOMA): Methods of validation. *Dysphagia, 10*, 192–202.

Smith, R., & Pilling, S. (2007). Allied health graduate program—Supporting the transition from student to professional in an interdisciplinary program. *Journal of Interprofessional Care, 21*(3), 265–276.

Spann, S. J., Kohler, F. W., & Soenksen, D. (2003). Examining parents' involvement in and perceptions of special education services: An interview with families in a parent support group. *Focus on Autism and Other Developmental Disabilities, 18*(4), 228–237.

Stoner, J., Bailey, R., Angell, M., Robbins, J., & Polewski, K. (2006). Perspectives of parents/guardians of children with feeding/swallowing problems. *Journal of Developmental and Physical Disabilities, 18*(4), 333–353.

Stoner, J., Bock, S., Thompson, J., Angell, M., Heyl, B., & Crowley, E. (2005). Parental perceptions of interactions between parents of young children with ASD and education professionals. *Focus on Autism and Other Developmental Disabilities, 20*, 39–51.

Strong, J. (2008, February). *Holistic practice without spirituality? Truth and artifice in a child health setting.* Paper presented at the NewMac Postgraduate Symposium, the University of Newcastle, Callaghan.

Sullivan, P., Lambert, B., Rose, M., Ford-Adams, M., Griffiths, P., & Johnson, A. (1998). An epidemiological study of feeding and nutritional problems in children with neurological impairment in Berkshire, Buckinghamshire, Northamptonshire and Oxfordshire [Abstract]. *Journal of Pediatric Gastroenterology and Nutrition, 26*(5), 597.

Thompson, D. (2007). Interprofessionalism in health care: Communication with the patient's identified family. *Journal of Interprofessional Care 21*(5), 561–563.

Threats, T. (2007). Use of the ICF in dysphagia management. *Seminars in Speech and Language, 28*(4), 323-333.

Tuchman, D., & Walter, R. (Eds) (1994). *Disorders of feeding and swallowing in infants and children: Pathophysiology, diagnosis and treatment.* San Diego, CA: Singular.

Turnbull, A., Turnbull, R., Erwin, E., & Soodak. L. (2006). *Families, professionals, and exceptionality: A special partnership* (5th ed.). Columbus, OH: Merrill.

Weir, K., McMahon, S., & Chang, A. (2005). Restriction of oral intake of water for aspiration lung disease in children. *Cochrane Database of Systematic Reviews 2005 Issue 4.* Art. No: CD005303.DOI:10.1002/14651858.CD005303.pubs.

Wolf, L., & Glass, R. (1992). *Feeding and swallowing disorders in infancy: assessment and management.* Tucson, AZ: Therapy Skill Builders.

Wooster, D., Brady, N., Mitchell, A., Grizzle, M., & Barnes, M. (1998). Pediatric feeding: A transdisciplinary team's perspective. *Topics in Language Disorders, 18,* 34-51.

World Health Organization (WHO). (2001). *The International classification of functioning, disability and health (ICF).* Geneva: Author.

World Health Organization (WHO) Workgroup for Development of Version of ICF for Children and Youth). (2007). *International Classification of Functioning, Disability and Health—Version for children and youth: ICF-CY.* Geneva: Author.

Appendix 9A

Using the ICF for a Child with Pediatric Dysphagia

1. **Major Pediatric Dysphagia Diagnostic Categories (Jakobs, 2007)**

   Respiratory

   Behavioral

2. **International Classification of Functioning, Disability and Health (ICF) (WHO, 2001)**

   ICF Classification includes a severity scale

   0 = no impairment (0-4%),

   1 = mild (5-24%),

   2 = moderate (25-49%),

   3 = severe (50-95%),

   4 = complete (96-100%).

Body Structures Codes: Swallowing

s3202 Structure of the palate (high, narrow, vaulting)

s3203 Tongue (difficulty in controlling bolus and premature spillage over base of tongue before swallow initiation)

s330 Structure of the pharynx (loss or softening of tracheal cartilages)

s399 Structures involved in voice and speech, unspecified

also

b440-b449 Respiratory System (tracheomalacia)

and

b810-849 Skin and Related Structures (blisters)

Body Functions Codes: Swallowing

b510 Ingestion functions

b5100 Sucking

b5101 Biting

b5102 Chewing

b5103 Manipulation of food in the mouth

b5104 Salivation

b5105 Swallowing

b51050 Oral swallowing

b51051 Pharyngeal swallowing

b51052 Esophageal swallowing

b51058 Swallowing, other specified

b51059 Swallowing, other unspecified

b5106 Regurgitation and vomiting

B515 Digestive functions

Body Functions Codes: Influences on Eating and Drinking Behaviors

b1301 Motivation

b1302 Appetite

b1670 Receptive language

b250 Taste

b140 Attention

b156 Perceptual functions

b255 Smell

Activities and Participation Codes: Swallowing

d550 Eating

d560 Drinking

Environmental Factors Codes: Swallowing

e1100 Food

e240 Light

e250 Sound

e310 Immediate family

e410 Individual attitudes of immediate family members

e450 Individual attitudes of health professionals

e580 Health services, systems and policies

Personal Factors Codes: Swallowing

Age

Gender

Race

Personality traits

Coping style

Family upbringing

Appendix 9B

Sample Interdisciplinary Dysphagia Clinic Report

Speech Pathologist:
Pediatrician:
Special Needs Dentist:
Occupational Therapist:
Dietician:
Psychologist:

INTERDISCIPLINARY DYSPHAGIA CLINIC REPORT

Name: Madeleine   **Date:** September 20, 2008
Address:
Phone: **DOB:**   **Age:** 18 months
Height: 80 cm (40th percentile)   **Weight:** 10.2 kg (25th percentile)

Past Medical History: Tracheomalacia, aspiration pneumonia, recurrent chest infections, Failure to thrive (FTT)

Issues/Concerns Addressed at Today's Visit:

Medical/Development   □ Adequate   □ Improving   ■ Other
Sees Pediatrician and ENT since birth for medical care and community SLP. Has been referred to allergist for metabolic testing for celiac disease.

Dental   □ Adequate   □ Improving   ■ Other
Has beginning caries in primary dentition. Evidence of possible gastroesophageal reflux disease (GERD).

Growth/Weight   □ Adequate   □ Improving   ■ Other
Growth has decelerated since birth. Weight has decreased to cross three percentiles (FTT).

Diet/Nutrition   □ Adequate   □ Improving   ■ Other
Madeleine has been nasogastrically-tube fed and has a history of dehydration. She is on four Pediasure bottle feeds per day, each

275

of 200 ml, to supplement her weight gain but only 400 ml is ingested. She is using a trainer cup to drink thin fluids and an Avent bottle with a medium flow teat.

A fussy eater who prefers to feed herself and appears to be orally and tactile defensive. She has never mouthed toys and appears to have missed out on normal oral exploratory play. Her diet is limited but includes textural preferences such as dry toast, finger-fed semisoft chicken, and cooked vegetable pieces.

Swallowing/Oral Motor   □ Adequate   □ Improving   ■ Other

The Schedule for Oral Motor Assessment (SOMA) (Reilly et. al., 2000) was completed, incorporating the Australian standardized definitions and terminology for texture-modified foods and fluids (Dietitians Association of Australia and The Speech Pathology Association of Australia Limited, 2007).

Moderate-severe oral-motor dysfunction was diagnosed with the following results:

Foods

Texture C (Smooth Pureed) (apple puree): Within normal limits for self-fed purees.

Texture B (Minced and Moist) (cottage cheese): Refused.

Texture A (Soft) (cooked carrot piece): Could bite and use early chewing (vertical jaw movement/munching) with oral stasis and delayed swallow.

Unmodified-Regular Food (Farex biscuit): Could bite and use early chewing (vertical jaw movement/munching) with delayed swallow.

Fluids

Level 400-Moderately Thick (Trainer cup with slow flow thickened fluid): Stridor reduced, coordination improved with controlled bolus and no coughing.

Unmodified-Regular Fluid (Trainer cup with water): Stridor, coughing, and uncoordination evident if allowed to self-feed.

Unmodified-Regular Fluid (Open lipped cup with water): Small sips were swallowed effectively but needed supervision and encouragement from parents for optimal flow rate and minimal stridor.

Modified Barium Swallow (MBS) results

10 months: Moderate-severe oral-pharyngeal stage dysphagia confirmed.

17 months: Abandoned due to noncooperation.

Positioning/Equipment   ☐ Adequate   ☐ Improving   ■ Other

Infant/Toddler Sensory Profile (Dunn, 2002) completed. Evidence of sensory avoidance.

She sits upright in a high chair for mealtimes with the TV and/or radio on. Also roams around during the day with a trainer cup of thin fluid to self feed.

She is right hand dominant. Requires assistance with open-lipped cup to control flow rate. Enjoyed pretend play to feed a toy.

Behavior/Self-Feeding   ☐ Adequate   ☐ Improving   ■ Other

Wary and difficult to engage with SLP. Happy to be fed by parent, especially mother. Irritable at mealtimes with aversive behavior (e.g., crying and avoidance/refusals) if fed by SLP or father. Strongly motivated to hold a spoon, biscuit and trainer cup to self-feed.

Communication   ☐ Adequate   ☐ Improving   ■ Other

Speech, receptive and expressive language development appear significantly delayed or disordered and require thorough assessment by local SLP. No words heard but gestures used (negation and pointing). High likelihood of chronic otitis media and/or eustachian tube dysfunction associated with GERD.

Education   ☐ Adequate   ☐ Improving   ■ Other

Attends day care 1 day per week when mother works part-time. Day-care mother has major problems feeding her, usually takes bottles of Pediasure only.

IDC Recommendations

☐ Medical

Suggest referral to pediatric gastroenterologist regarding possible gastroesophageal reflux disease (GERD).

Full audiologic assessment is recommended.

Collaboration with local GP, paediatrician, and SLP regarding metabolic and celiac disease testing and developmental assessment including speech and language.

Investigate psychological and social support networks for parents.

Follow up Modified Barium Swallow study requested.

☐ **Dental**

Regular dental checks are required.

☐ **Growth/Weight/Nutrition**

Ongoing local dietetic support to be organized.

Suggestions regarding using foods that are calorie-dense to improve weight gain. Appears to be orally-defensive and hypersensitive to textures in the mouth. Consider using techniques to increase tolerance for a wider variety of textures in her mouth at the table, by creating a playground at the table using toys to be fed by Madeleine. No fights or coercion to be used at mealtimes.

If no progress after review, may need to consider percutaneous endoscopic gastrostomy (PEG) feeding with oral supplementation.

☐ **Swallowing/Oral Motor**

Mealtimes to be 20 to 30 minutes only with self-feeding at beginning and help from mealtime partner (parent or day-care mother) at the end where necessary.

Suggest using NUK and oral exploratory toys for example, Chewy Tubes and Tubing to increase intraoral tolerance for new food textures. Encourage fingers in mouth and different foods for self-feeding. Madeleine enjoyed deep vibration around her face.

☐ **Positioning/Equipment**

Follow-up occupational therapy is recommended to assist with some of the sensory issues and review of overall developmental status including visual-motor skills recommended.

☐ **Education**

It would be useful for Madeleine's parents, the daycare mother, and the IDC team to meet together to ensure consistency with feeding goals across environments (home and daycare).

For IDC Review in 1 month.

Recommendations shared with and approved by the parents.

Chapter 10

Working with Families of Children with Hearing Loss

Alice Eriks-Brophy

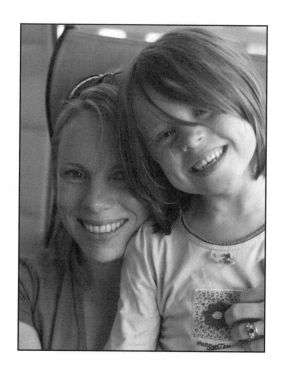

Introduction to Childhood Hearing Loss, Communication Options, and Family Involvement: The Realities of Diagnosis

Permanent bilateral hearing loss is present in 1 to 6 of 1,000 newborns. Hearing impairment present at birth or occurring in early childhood frequently is described as representing a significant barrier to the natural acquisition, development, and use of spoken language. Indeed, historical references to individuals with significant hearing loss referred to them as being "deaf and dumb," implying a basic inability to develop speech. Regrettably, such negative and dated perspectives on the potential of individuals with hearing loss to develop communication continue to exist in the general public. Fortunately, advances in the field of childhood hearing loss that include the early diagnosis of hearing loss through neonatal hearing screening programs, the early enrolment of families into communication intervention programs to establish a mode of communication, and the early fitting of hearing aids or a cochlear implant for families desiring such technologies have the potential to moderate these potential negative effects and consequences of childhood hearing loss.

The major effects of a hearing loss on speech and language development in children vary widely and depend on a multitude of factors including the degree and configuration of the loss, the amount and type of residual hearing, the age at which hearing loss occurred, the age of identification of the hearing loss, the age at enrolment in intervention, the age at amplification, emotional and cognitive factors associated with the child, the presence of additional handicaps, and environmental facilitators and barriers.

Available communication intervention options for children with hearing loss traditionally have been divided into oral versus gestural approaches. These approaches can be further divided into subcategories depending on the degree to which they encourage or discourage the use of oral versus signed language. The goals of these early intervention programs range from integration with hearing peers to education fostering a Deaf culture identity (Schwartz, 1996). The numerous philosophies surrounding the language education of children with hearing loss has led to the field being perceived as fraught with controversy and animosity between proponents of the differing approaches. Families of deaf and hard-of-hearing children and indeed the children themselves have often been caught in the middle of political and highly charged emotional debates between professionals. Fortunately, professional communication regarding the advantages and disadvantages of the various communication options available along with increased professional sensitivity toward the perspectives of other stakeholders in the intervention process have increased in recent years.

At the present time, fundamental decisions regarding the choice of the most appropriate communication option for a child and the associated intervention paradigms and technologic supports are being left more and more in the hands of parents, who are provided with assistance and information in arriving at an informed choice. However, this more family-focused approach is not without its inherent difficulties.

As between 91 and 93% of all children with hearing loss are born to hearing parents (Northern & Downs, 2002), parents rarely have any familiarity with hearing loss prior to the diagnosis of their child. The identification of hearing loss in a child can lead to significant disruption in family roles and increased family stress. The diagnosis often comes as a shock to parents and often is accompanied by a period of grieving for the loss of the hoped-for child (Gregory, 1995; Luterman, 1987; Marschark, 1997; Marschark & Clark, 1998; Moeller, 2007; Pollack, Goldberg, & Caleffe-Schenke, 1997). Although such reactions are a normal part of adapting to the hearing loss, families who experience prolonged difficulty in accepting the diagnosis of hearing loss and whose emotions and feelings of guilt become overwhelming have less energy and motivation to participate in early intervention (Luterman, 1987). This situation has direct negative consequences for the child's progress across multiple domains of development, including the acquisition of language. As part of most early intervention programs, parents therefore are provided with counseling and support in order to arrive at an acceptance of their child's diagnosis and to enable them to take an active part in the management of their child's hearing loss. Through parent guidance sessions, therapists counsel parents through the stages of grieving and engage families in discussions surrounding their stress levels, coping styles, and support systems (Cole, 1992; Estabrooks, 1994; Meadow-Orlans et al., 2003; Schuyler & Rushmer, 1987). Addressing parental issues and concerns and achieving a balance between parents' needs and those of the child with hearing loss are seen as essential components in facilitating parental involvement in early intervention programs for children with hearing loss (Pipp-Siegel & Biringen, 2000).

At the time of diagnosis parents often are asked to integrate a great deal of information and make a number of important fundamental decisions while at the same time coming to terms with their child's diagnosis. Families may be presented with information regarding hearing loss in general, the variety of communication options to promote language development in their child, and the forms of technology available to make sound available for language development and environmental awareness. Many families experience significant stress at this time, and their ability to be involved in the decision-making process may be negatively affected. In addition, parents may need to access a wide variety of services and schedule numerous appointments with a variety of professionals in order to respond to their child's need. These services generally are not available at the same site. Necessary services include appointments in audiology to determine the exact degree and configuration of the child's hearing loss, to develop the child's audiogram, and to discuss potential candidacy for a cochlear implant if the child is eligible. The child generally will be fitted with hearing aids soon after diagnosis, necessitating visits to the hearing aid acoustician for hearing aid fitting and earmold impressions required for the use of hearing aids. These ear molds may need to be changed often as the infant grows very quickly. Communication intervention may be provided by a variety of professionals including teachers of the deaf and hard of hearing, certified Auditory-Verbal therapists, and speech-language pathologists (SLPs). Service delivery may be organized through home visits or through family visits to a clinic or service agency. School boards may be involved in service provision as well. Parent groups, play groups, and family support services are available in a variety of settings and across a variety of communication options. Generally, however, service agencies promote a single communication option, making access to information on alternative choices complicated for parents and transitions between service agencies difficult.

Historical Overview of Parental Involvement in Early Intervention Programs for Children with Hearing Loss

Family Involvement in Gestural Approaches to Language Development

Historically, the majority of children with profound hearing losses were described as being unable to benefit from amplification and oral intervention approaches, and typically were enrolled in programs that emphasized gestural approaches to communication. In North America, such approaches include the use of American Sign Language (ASL), the language of the culturally Deaf community, along with artificial sign systems structured to more closely resemble oral English, including Seeing Essential English (SEE1) and Signing Exact English (SEE2). Many of these children were enrolled in residential schools for the Deaf, where a variety of gestural approaches were used to support learning. As children spent a large portion of their time away from home, the parents of these children often did not learn to use sign language beyond a rudimentary level. In many cases, this led to a breakdown in communication between the Deaf child and the family, precluding any sort of effective parental involvement. Many personal accounts of Deaf adults who experienced this situation in their upbringing reflect a mixture of conflicting emotions surrounding their family's inability to communicate with them directly.

Family Involvement in Aural Approaches to Language Development

Traditionally, children with profound hearing losses of 95 dB or greater were described as being unable to develop spontaneous oral communication and unable to access their own vocalizations or the majority of environmental sounds. However, advances in hearing aid technology and changes in candidacy requirements for cochlear implantation have resulted in greatly increased access to oral communication and spoken language through the use of such technology. Children identified through neonatal hearing screening programs are often fitted with hearing aids by 3 months of age, and children with severe to profound hearing losses who meet the selection criteria are currently receiving cochlear implants as young as 12 months of age.

At the present time, results from neonatal hearing screening programs indicate that parents of children with hearing loss, the majority of whom are themselves hearing, are choosing aural/oral intervention approaches for their children. As an example, the Ontario Neonatal Hearing Screening program known as the Infant Hearing Program (IHP), offers families a choice between three communication options: American Sign Language (ASL), Auditory-Verbal therapy (AVT), a strictly oral intervention approach, and a combined oral-gestural program referred to as a dual approach. The Ontario IHP offers communication intervention to children with moderate to profound hearing loss from time of diagnosis until the age of school entry and to children with lesser degrees of hearing loss if they are not meeting their communication milestones. Statistics obtained from the IHP for 2006/2007 indicate that, of 335 children with permanent hearing impairment (bilateral, unilateral, any degree) diagnosed in Ontario, 6 families chose dual programs, 15 chose ASL, and 240 chose AVT (S. Weber, personal communication, September 2007). Although these statistics are likely to vary somewhat in other regions of North America, they do provide some evidence that the vast majority of parents are currently choosing communication options that place some emphasis on oral language development.

Many children with hearing loss can develop age-appropriate speech, language, and literacy skills and be fully integrated into regular classrooms if they are identified early, fitted with appropriate hearing technology, and provided with early language intervention (Dettman, Pinder, Briggs, Dowell, & Leigh, 2007; Stacey, Fortnum, Barton, & Summerfield, 2006; Uchanski & Geers, 2003; Yoshinaga-Itano, 2000). Other factors proposed to impact directly on the ability of children who are deaf or hard of hearing to acquire effective oral communication skills include degree of hearing loss, age of diagnosis, any delay in fitting the child with appropriate hearing technology, and the presence of any additional handicapping conditions. Furthermore, certain recognized authorities in the field of hearing loss such as Moeller (2000), Calderon (2000), Calderon and Greenberg (1997), Meadow-Orlans, Mertens, and Sass-Lehrer (2003), and Yoshinaga-Itano (2000) have emphasized the role of family or parental involvement (PI) as an important mediating factor in achieving positive language outcomes for children with hearing loss. Some of these researchers have argued that parental involvement may supercede degree of hearing loss as a key component of early intervention programs for children with hearing loss, and may potentially be a critical variable in predicting the outcomes of early intervention for these children.

Parental involvement in early intervention and school-based education for children with hearing loss is being highly encouraged and, in some contexts, is an expected part of intervention. In fact, in some programs, families may be dismissed from intervention programs due to a perceived lack of parental involvement. Nevertheless, empirical evidence to support the critical role of parental involvement in achieving high outcomes in speech and language development for children with hearing loss is currently lacking. Because parental involvement encompasses such a wide variety of behaviors, activities, and goals, it remains difficult to substantiate claims that parental involvement is central to intervention outcomes and successful development of children's communication. Furthermore, there is as yet no consensus in the field with respect to an operational definition of parental involvement, those domains and behaviors that might most effectively indicate positive parental involvement, and the means by which parental involvement might be objectively measured in early intervention programs for children with hearing loss.

Researchers in the domain of communication disorders in particular generally agree that early intervention programs that directly involve parents result in improved speech and language outcomes for the child. For example, McLean and Woods Cripe (1997) conducted a systematic review of 56 studies examining the efficacy of center-based versus home-based early intervention approaches for children with speech and language disabilities, with the implication that home-based approaches contained a higher parental involvement component. They concluded that the specific child and family variables associated with the proposed effectiveness of the home-based programs were not adequately described in the studies they reviewed. Thus, although parental involvement in early intervention is proposed by many researchers as being a critical variable in predicting outcome, there is currently little empirical evidence to support this notion, particularly in the field of childhood communication disorders. The meta-analysis conducted by White, Taylor, and Moss of the evidence supporting the importance of parental involvement from 172 intervention studies in early intervention (1992, p. 91) concluded that, "[t]here is no convincing evidence that the ways in which parents have been involved in early intervention result in more effective outcomes." White, Taylor, and Moss (1992) conclude that, although the evidence provided by the research they reviewed was not sufficient to conclude that parental involvement was a crucial component of effective early intervention programs, this did not mean that parental involvement is *not* an important mediating factor in achieving positive outcomes. The authors called for experimental research that is methodologically sound and that allows evidence-based conclusions to be drawn with respect to the potential benefits of parental involvement in terms of cost, benefits for family members, and potentially improved outcomes from early intervention programs that include strong parental involvement components versus those that do not.

The current state of evidence in support of the role of parental involvement in achieving speech and language outcomes for preschool children with hearing loss and other communication difficulties is no more compelling than that reviewed above. This situation is due, in part, to a lack of consistent operationalization of the construct of parental involvement. Although some studies have focused on attitudinal components of parent involvement, defining parental involvement in terms of parental expectations for the child's progress in the development of communication skills, other studies have defined parental involvement primarily in behavioral terms, including carryover of intervention activities into the home environment, or attendance and behavior during intervention sessions. Such differences in definition and measurement of parent involvement make it difficult to assess the impact of parental involvement across different studies assessing outcomes of early intervention programs for children with communication disorders, including those designed for children with hearing loss.

In addition to a lack of evidence in support of the crucial role of parental involvement in early intervention, as yet no objective measure to evaluate parental involvement in early intervention for children in general and children with hearing loss in particular currently exists. As stated by White et al., "[c]urrent measurement techniques assess only general dimensions of family functioning and are not well established in terms of their psychometric properties" (1992, p. 119). In lieu of objective measures, clinicians working with children with hearing loss and other communication difficulties typically have relied on such variables as rate of parental attendance to intervention sessions, parental "enthusiasm" in participating in intervention, upkeep of the child's amplification devices, regularity of completion of homework, variables associated with parenting style and family interaction patterns, and parental facility in the communication mode of the child as indicators of parental involvement (Meadow-Orlans, Mertens, & Sass-Lehrer, 2003). In addition to being highly subjective, such measures might be influenced by a number of factors not directly associated with or indicative of parental involvement per se. These factors might include family constellation, family illness, geographic location and distance from the intervention center, socioeconomic status, cultural background, and other ecologic factors. The role of these factors in defining and evaluating parental involvement has not as yet been determined.

A systematic review of the evidence supporting the role of parental involvement in early intervention programs for children with hearing loss is currently being conducted by the author. The review is examining the following questions: Is parental involvement a mediating factor in achieving positive speech and language outcomes for preschool children identified with hearing loss? Can parental involvement be measured objectively? What specific parental behaviors are associated with improved speech and language outcomes in these children? To date, over 65,000 searches based on an elaborate concept map containing key words relevant to the review questions have been conducted in the electronic databases of CINAHL, ERIC, and PsycInfo. Evidence collected through the systematic review process to date suggests that there currently is insufficient empirical evidence to support claims regarding the mediating effects of parental involvement in achieving improved speech and language outcomes for preschool children with hearing loss. However, as stated by White, Taylor, and Moss (1992), this does not mean that parental involvement does not have a mediating effect, but rather that the current research does not allow any cause-effect relationships to be drawn with respect to the role of parental involvement due to methodological weaknesses and the lack of studies containing sufficient quantitative data to permit statistical analyses to be carried out.

Current State of the Assessment of Parental Involvement in Aural/Oral Approaches to Language Development

Two articles specifically addressing the role of parental involvement in early intervention for children with hearing loss constitute the state of the evidence in favor of parental involvement as a determining factor in outcomes of childhood aural rehabilitation. The first and most commonly cited is a study by Moeller (2000) who investigated the relationship between age at enrollment in intervention and language outcomes for a group of 112 deaf and hard-of-hearing children. As part of this study, Moeller developed a rating scale evaluating family involvement in the early intervention program that was completed by the clinician involved with the family. Parental perceptions of their own involvement were not examined. The scale consists of five possible ratings of family participation and an associated list of variables proposed to characterize the level and quality of involvement in the early intervention program, ranging from a rating of 1, equivalent to "limited and far below average participation" to a rating of 5 indicating "ideal participation." Numerous factors are associated with each rating, and include parental acceptance of the child's hearing loss, parental stress level, active engagement in intervention sessions, regularity of session attendance, parental advocacy efforts, effectiveness of parental communication strategies as a language model for the child, familiarity with and fluency in the child's mode of communication, and additional supports available to parents through extended family and other agencies. Each of these variables is rated as part of a global profile and cannot be separated from the whole. In the study, ratings were provided retrospectively for each family by two independent clinicians who had been directly involved with the family. Interrater reliability using Cohen's kappa was reported as being high for the oral and total communication programs in which the children were enrolled. Multiple regression and correlational analyses indicated that parental involvement was an important contributor to language outcomes for children with hearing loss, as family involvement contributed the most unique variance in the regression analysis and was highly correlated with age of enrolment in the early intervention program, accounting for vocabulary and verbal reasoning skill levels. On the basis of these findings, Moeller concluded that active involvement of families in the child's early intervention program enhances communication skill development for young children with hearing loss. She points out, however, that more refined tools that include greater specification and verification of the constructs used in measuring parental involvement in her rating scale are needed in order to draw definitive conclusions regarding the specific role of parental involvement in enhancing communication development for children with hearing loss.

DesJardin (2003) reported on the development of scale to assess parental self-efficacy and involvement in early intervention programs for young children with hearing loss. Self-efficacy or self-confidence is argued to be an important component of family-centered early intervention, as it focuses on competencies and parenting practices that are proposed to have a positive impact on child outcomes (Bandura, 1982; Epstein, 1995; Hoover-Dempsey & Sandler, 1995, 1997). DesJardin points out that, although these components have been proposed as essential components in theoretical models of parental involvement developed in the educational literature, they have not been incorporated into the construct of parental involvement associated with early intervention for children with hearing loss. In her *Scale of Parental Involvement and Self-Efficacy (SPISE)*, DesJardin uses 10 items to assess parental self-efficacy, and 11 items to assess parental involvement. Both parental self-efficacy and parental involvement are broken down into two domains: self-efficacy/parental involvement and amplification use; and self-efficacy/parental involvement and speech and language development. Five to six items per domain are rated by parents on a 1 to 7 Likert scale, resulting in a total mean score. Each item can be examined to gain insights into parental perceptions of their role in the early intervention program, their confidence in working with their child to develop speech and language skills, and the use of amplification technology. No details are provided with respect to the development of the scale, the construct validity of the items within each scale, or the demographic characteristics of the children and families with whom the scale was pilot tested. DesJardin concludes that the SPISE provides clinicians with information on parents' beliefs and competencies in providing intervention to their young children with hearing loss. However, the predictive validity of the SPISE to distinguish between involved/efficacious and uninvolved/inefficacious families and the impact of these variables on child outcomes remains undetermined. Furthermore, there is little overlap in the variables associated with parental involvement proposed by Moeller (2000) and those contained in Desjardin's (2003) parental involvement subscales of the SPISE. This highlights the fact that those factors that might be most highly associated with parental involvement in early intervention programs for children with hearing loss have not as yet been established with any degree of consistency or reliability.

Definitions and Parameters of Parental Involvement in Early Intervention Programs for Children with Hearing Loss

No concise definition of parental involvement currently exists in the literature on early intervention programs for children with hearing loss. Those authors who define the construct of parental involvement do so in terms that are ambiguous and open to subjective interpretation. Parental involvement tends also to be defined in terms of type(s) of involvement. For example, DesJardin (2003, p. 397) defines parental involvement as the "extent to which parents are involved in the specific parenting responsibilities or tasks that professionals recommend to develop their child's auditory and speech-language skills." Simser (2001, p. 49) defines parental involvement as "parental participation in intervention sessions and follow-up at home." The construct is undefined in the studies reported by Moeller (2000) and Calderon (2000). Furthermore, theoretical models that may serve to underpin the concept of parental involvement in early intervention as opposed to school contexts have not as yet been elaborated in any detail. Existing school-based theoretical frameworks examining the construct of parental involvement, the factors influencing parental involvement, and the means of promoting parental involvement such as those developed by Epstein (1995), Hoover-Dempsey and Sandler (1995, 1997), and Bronfenbrenner (1979) have not yet been adequately applied to parental involvement in early intervention programs for children with hearing loss. Questions such as the amount and type of parental involvement necessary to ensure positive communication outcomes, and the domains of parental involvement that might be predictive of such outcomes remain unanswered.

Variables Affecting Parental Involvement in Intervention for Children with Hearing Loss

A number of variables have been proposed to affect family involvement in communication intervention for children with hearing loss, although none of these have been addressed in the early intervention program literature on outcomes for children with hearing loss. These include such variables as parental education levels, parental progression through the stages of the grieving process typically associated with a diagnosis of hearing loss, parents' ability to access and integrate new knowledge, parents' ability to manage technology such as hearing aids, cochlear implants, and FM systems; and parents' flexibility in their time schedules permitting them to attend intervention sessions where they will learn to communicate with their child using gesture alone, a combination of gesture and spoken language, or spoken language alone, depending on their preference. Additional factors that might affect parental involvement include such variables as parental knowledge of hearing loss and amplification (as indicated by Desjardin, 2003), aspects of parental stress, parental acceptance of their child's diagnosis, individual child and family characteristics, aspects of the parent-child relationship, elements of the clinician-family relationship, and ecologic factors including access to the early intervention program site, geographic location of residence, and transportation issues. A limited amount of primarily anecdotal evidence indicates that cultural differences in perceptions of parental involvement and the counseling practices inherent to many early intervention programs may impact participation and involvement for parents representing minority culture backgrounds.

Cultural Differences in Perceptions of Parental Involvement

There is now considerable evidence pointing to important cultural differences in parental reaction to childhood disability in general, and to deafness in particular, that have a clear impact on the evaluation of parental involvement in early intervention programs. These reactions include a strong social stigma associated with hearing loss, the search for a cure through traditional healers and folk rituals, remedies and/or religion; and beliefs related to the etiology of the child's hearing loss (Callaway, 2000; Goldbart & Mukherjee, 1999a, 1999b; Grant, 1993; Huff & Kline, 1999; Lynch & Hanson, 1992; Odom, Hanson, Blackman, & Kaul, 2003). For some families, participation in intervention efforts for the child with a disability such as hearing loss may be perceived as useless, and parents may be reluctant to engage in discussions surrounding their child's diagnosis. Such cultural differences in the concepts, beliefs, and reactions to hearing loss would be expected to have a strong impact on parents' perceptions of the goodness of fit of the early intervention program to their and their child's needs, the effectiveness of counseling and intervention, as well as their willingness and ability to participate in such activities. In the face of these beliefs, misjudgements of minority culture parents and of their participation in their child's early intervention program may arise that may contribute to deficit interpretations of parental involvement for minority culture families involved in early intervention programs for their children with hearing loss.

A study examining attitudes, perceptions, and values of education among immigrant Hmong parents of children with hearing loss indicated that, although these parents valued education and wanted to be involved in their children's programs, they were unsure of how to become involved, had limited knowledge of the practices and procedures inherent to their child's programs, and felt the language and customs of the educational and intervention context in which they found themselves to be "entirely alien" (Wathum-Ocama & Rose, 2002). Eriks-Brophy and Crago (1993) report a similar reaction from an Inuk mother of a child with profound hearing loss enrolled in an early intervention program emphasizing the development of spoken language. This mother described the strategies demonstrated during the session as "not feeling right" within the context of the communicative patterns valued by her culture, and was unable to follow through with these suggestions despite a strong desire that her child learn to speak.

A recent nationwide survey in the United States of parents of children with hearing loss in early intervention programs corroborate these findings with respect to multicultural and second language families. Meadow-Orlans et al. (2003) indicate that parents of children with hearing loss from minority culture backgrounds reported lower levels of satisfaction with services provided to their children as compared to majority culture parents. These minority culture parents expressed perceptions of encountering both cultural and linguistic barriers to participation in intervention and access to service. They also experienced and maintained higher stress levels associated with their child's diagnosis and participation in intervention than did majority culture parents. A study of families enrolled in an early intervention approach focused on the development of spoken language conducted by Easterbrooks, O'Rourke, and Wendell (2000) indicated that children of parents reporting satisfactory outcomes from their early intervention program were primarily white, had fewer additional disabilities than the general population of deaf students, tended to come from families with small numbers of children where mothers were well-educated and did not work outside the home, and had annual income levels well in excess of the U.S. national average (Easterbrooks et al., 2000). Thus, the need for an instrument to assess parental involvement in a culturally sensitive manner is becoming an issue of urgent concern.

The ultimate goal of any early communication intervention program for children with hearing loss is to meet the needs of both the child and the family. The current context of early communication intervention for children with hearing loss includes increasing diversity in the North American population, a high incidence of hearing loss in children from minority culture backgrounds, and an increasing popularity in the selection of aural/oral intervention approaches for families of children with hearing loss identified through current screening efforts. The examination of parental perceptions of their involvement in such intervention programs as well as the speech and language outcomes of preschool children from majority and minority culture backgrounds enrolled in these approached therefore is of considerable importance.

Clinical Practice: SLPs' Involvement of Families in Childhood Hearing Loss

In an attempt to begin to address the numerous unresolved issues associated with defining and assessing parental involvement in early intervention programs for children with hearing loss, a study is being undertaken by the author to examine practicing clinicians' definitions of parental involvement and to identify factors that might have an influence on parental involvement (Eriks-Brophy, 2008). The study is being carried out in two phases, the first consisting of a review and verification of variables proposed to influence the construct of parental involvement in early intervention programs for preschool children with hearing loss, and the second consisting of a more formal verification of these variables using focus group interviews with clinicians and parents of children with hearing loss. To date, three focus groups have been conducted with professionals providing early intervention to families of children with hearing loss in the greater Toronto area, a large, multicultural urban center in Ontario, Canada. The objectives of the focus groups were to discuss definitions of parental involvement, to identify factors that might have an influence on parental involvement and to rate the importance of the 60 variables potentially influencing parental involvement that had been derived from the first phase of the study. Twenty-seven professionals providing oral/aural rehabilitation services to families in the greater Toronto area have participated in the three focus groups. One-third of the participants worked exclusively in early intervention programs. Two-thirds worked in school settings at the time of the focus groups, but had prior experience working with families in early intervention programs. The professionals provide a variety of communication options to the families with whom they were involved, ranging from auditory-verbal therapy to combined gestural and oral approaches to language development. Years of experience of the participants varied from 2 years to over 20 years of involvement with families of children with hearing loss. All but three of the participants represented majority culture backgrounds and spoke English as their first language. Two of the participants themselves had prelingual hearing loss and had participated in early intervention programs as children.

Results obtained from the focus groups conducted to date indicated that parental involvement contained several key components that included:

- involvement in audiologic management,
- working collaboratively with the professional,
- engaging in effective and meaningful communication with the professional,
- active and ongoing participation in their child's program and in intervention sessions,
- working with their child at home to support the early intervention program,
- knowledge of the early intervention program and the goals set out for their child, and
- maintaining a balance between "work" and "play" in home activities.

Factors identified as having an influence on parental involvement included:

- parent's motivation,
- parental acceptance of the hearing loss,
- cultural and second language issues,
- socioeconomic status,
- parental education levels,
- family structure and the presence of other siblings in the family,
- the presence of a supportive network for the family,
- the child's temperament and attitude,
- familiarity with the health care and educational systems,
- time commitments outside the early intervention program, and
- parental confidence in working with their child.

All participants agreed that parental involvement was essential to child outcomes, but used only informal measures to assess parental involvement. These measures included: homework completion, session attendance, parents' questions during sessions, and active participation in sessions. Perceived benefits of parental involvement included:

- generalization of speech and language skills,
- increased progress in therapy,
- increased motivation, and
- the empowerment of the parent and the child.

Implications for the lack of parental involvement included:

- lack of progress,
- decreased generalization of skills learned in therapy,
- decreased effectiveness of therapy, and
- poor rapport between parents and professionals.

Obstacles to parental involvement identified by the participants included:

- differing perceptions of parental involvement between parents and clinicians,
- difficulties associated with access to service,
- issues affecting family functioning including lack of time and lack of resources in the home,
- lack of parental education,
- individual differences in parental progression through the stages of the grieving process,
- multicultural and second language contexts, and
- "hard to reach" families.

With respect to multicultural and ESL families in particular, the participating professionals reported that these families often felt overwhelmed with the information and expectations associated with early intervention programs and school-based programs. Many of the participants felt that the language demands of the intervention program had the potential to exceed the parents' second language abilities, causing them to experience significant additional stress. Some of the participants expressed the opinion that minority culture parents had differing expectations regarding the eventual benefits of the program and, in some cases, a lack of confidence with respect to program and parental involvement demands. All of these obstacles were perceived as having a potentially negative impact on outcomes for children from multicultural and second language backgrounds. The participants indicated that additional knowledge about working effectively with multicultural families and understanding their perceptions and experiences of involvement would benefit their practice.

Clearly, additional information is needed to understand parental involvement and, through such understanding, enhance family-centered early intervention services. The research questions and associated methodology currently are being used in focus groups with families of children with hearing loss enrolled in early intervention programs containing a significant parental involvement component in order to determine potential areas of match/mismatch and differences in perceptions of parental involvement between parents and clinicians. It is likely that there will be important differences in parental versus clinician perceptions of parental involvement. It is hoped that the research will provide insights into the core variables that might be included in the development of an objective tool to measure parental involvement in early intervention programs for children with hearing loss.

Case Study of Family Involvement in Childhood Hearing Loss

The case example presented below is fictional but incorporates the realities of parents who receive a diagnosis of hearing loss for their child through current neonatal hearing screening efforts. Such programs exist in most large North American birthing hospitals and in other countries around the world including Australia and the United Kingdom, although the process described in the case is representative of that currently in place in Ontario, Canada. The case example is presented from the perspective of hearing parents, as these represent 93% of the families into which children with hearing loss are born.

Background—Demographic Details About Child and Family

Marie and Ron were anxiously awaiting the birth of their first child. The pregnancy had been uneventful and Marie had been able to continue working in her position as a legal assistant until 2 weeks prior to her due date. Ron had arranged to take the first week after the birth off from his position as a computer analyst. When baby Laura arrived, perfectly on time, Ron and Marie were ecstatic. Their baby girl was perfect in every way, just as they had hoped and expected she would be. Neither of them gave it much thought when they were asked to provide consent for the administration of a routine hearing screening when Laura was 27 hours old, on the morning of the day Marie and Laura were to leave the hospital. The screening was carried out at Marie's bedside by a hospital screener who described the screening process and equipment that would be used. The initial screen was carried out using distortion product otoacoustic emission (DPOAE) equipment, where a small probe was inserted into Laura's ears, one at a time, and some soft sounds were played. The process was so noninvasive and so quick that Laura never woke up. The screener reported that Laura had a "refer" result on the DPOAE screen and that second test would be carried out using automated auditory brainstem response (ABR) equipment, also at the bedside. Small electrodes were attached to Laura's forehead and behind each ear to record the brain's response to soft sounds played into Laura's ears. Again, Laura slept peacefully throughout the screening. When the screener told them that Laura had again received a "refer" result, Marie and Ron were surprised but not overly alarmed. They felt that hearing loss was something that happened to old people, and so could not be an issue with their newborn baby. The screener informed them that the results did not necessarily mean that Laura had a hearing loss, but that they would need to bring Laura in for a second level of hearing screening in 2 weeks' time at a screening site in their community. The time interval would allow any debris that might still be left in Laura's ears after the birth to clear. The screener provided them with a pamphlet titled, "Your Baby Needs a Hearing Assessment," as well as the address of the closest local screening clinic to attend. Marie and Ron left the hospital with only vague feelings of concern about Laura's hearing, but were firm in their intention to take Laura to the community screening, just to be sure.

Family Involvement in the Assessment

Two weeks later, Laura was again screened using the ABR equipment and again received a "refer" result in both ears. Marie and Ron were told that Laura would now need to be seen for a more complete audiologic assessment at a large pediatric hospital in the city. They were provided with an appointment date for 5 days later. It was a long and stressful wait for the day of the audiologic appointment to arrive. The audiologist informed Ron and Marie what tests would be performed. She showed them the equipment that would be used and how noninvasive the testing was. When the audiologist conducted the assessment, she verified that Laura had not been upset in any way, and had slept throughout the testing. When she then informed them that the tests showed that Laura had a severe hearing loss in both ears, both Marie and Ron were in shock. No member of their families had ever had any hearing problems, other than Ron's elderly grandfather who had worn a hearing aid in later life. The audiologist arranged for Marie and Ron to meet with a family support worker associated with the screening program, who would be able to provide them with more information. The audiologist then asked if they had any questions. Both parents asked if the test results could be incorrect. After all, Laura was only 7 days old. How could she cooperate on a hearing test? Was there not some mistake? What did a severe hearing loss mean? Would Laura ever be able to hear anything? Would she be able to talk? The audiologist carefully and respectfully responded to all of their questions, but Marie and Ron were not reassured. They left the hospital thinking only one thing, "Our baby is deaf!"

The diagnosis of hearing loss set in motion a long series of meetings and appointments, beginning with the family support worker, Jody, who came to their home and calmly answered all of their questions about hearing loss, the types of communication options available, and the various services and resources in their local community. In the meantime, Ron had spent a great deal of time searching the Internet about deafness, and was confused and frustrated by the contradictory information that was available and the differences in communication options that were represented. Jody explained this information to them in an unbiased way and, over a number of meetings, provided them with the information they were looking for in order to arrive at some important decisions. Both Marie and Ron wanted Laura to have the chance to hear and, they hoped, to talk, just like other children. They wanted Laura to get hearing aids or maybe a cochlear implant so she would be able to be integrated into a regular school. Appointments for additional audiologic assessments were arranged, and Marie and Ron were directed to a local center where oral communication intervention was provided. Before Laura was even fitted with her hearing aids, they became involved in weekly therapy sessions where they began to learn more about hearing loss, the development of auditory skills in babies, how to take care of the hearing aids, and how to provide Laura with the best possible language and listening environment. The therapist, Stephanie, told them that they would be Laura's first and most important teachers, and that she would help them to develop the skills to provide Laura with the best possible language models. At the center they met several other parents whose children had hearing loss, and were reassured by their positive attitudes and their children's progress in oral language development. The day Laura got her hearing aids was a difficult one for both Marie and Ron. Laura was now 5 months old. The aids looked so big on Laura's little head, and really accentuated the fact that she had a hearing loss. Marie was tempted to take them off when they left the audiologist's office; she felt people would stare at her baby and would know there was something wrong. Ron convinced her to leave them on, as that was the only way Laura would ever be able to hear.

Family Involvement in Intervention

Laura and Marie started to attend weekly hour-long sessions at the local early intervention center, where Stephanie involved Marie in activities to develop Laura's listening skills, to make the link between sounds and words, and to show Marie how to use everyday events and activities as auditory and language-learning experiences. Marie decided to take a temporary leave of absence from her job in order to be able to attend the sessions. Ron arranged with his employer to attend every third session and was actively involved in the home activities Marie was learning at the center. Within 4 weeks of wearing her hearing aids, Laura began to show indications that she was hearing and responding to sound. She smiled when she heard her mother's voice, blinked and startled to sounds in the environment, and began to vocalize in response to her parents' playful input. Marie and Ron learned that these were positive indicators that Laura's hearing aids were providing her with good acoustic input. Stephanie encouraged Marie and Ron to keep track of Laura's language and listening development using a checklist, and provided them with activities and language that would promote these skills. Each therapy session was used to demonstrate auditory and communication skills, with Marie and Ron actively involved in interacting in the session and practicing the activities. Stephanie encouraged them to create exciting learning environments where listening, speech, language, thinking, and communication could be integrated following natural developmental patterns.

Marie and Laura also attended regular audiologic appointments, with the goal to obtain a complete and accurate audiogram of Laura's residual hearing ability across all the frequencies, thus ensuring optimal amplification. Laura also required many appointments with the hearing aid acoustician for new earmolds and with the audiologist for hearing aid adjustments. Jody, the family support worker, remained in regular contact with Marie and Ron to follow Laura's progress and to ensure they also were doing fine. Although both Ron and Marie had periods of sadness about Laura's hearing loss and often wondered why this had happened to their daughter, they generally felt optimistic about Laura's progress and her potential to develop speech and language. They felt comfortable enough with Stephanie to discuss these issues and received additional support by enrolling in a support group for parents with hearing loss held at the intervention center. Stephanie recommended that Laura might benefit from contact with other children, so Marie and Laura went to a local playgroup for infants and toddlers in the neighborhood. Marie was thrilled when she began to notice that at 18 months Laura seemed to be verbalizing and approximating words, communicating in much the same way as the other children in the playgroup. At 24 months, Stephanie decided to administer the Preschool Language Scale-4th Edition, a standardized test of expressive and receptive language. This was the first time Marie was asked to sit on the other side of the two-way mirror and observe her child and the SLP without taking part in the interaction. The results showed that Laura was functioning at close to age-equivalent levels in her receptive language and was delayed by 6 months in her expressive language when compared to her peers with typical hearing. Because Laura had received her hearing aids at 5 months, her hearing age was equivalent to 19 months, making her performance close to what would be expected for the amount of time she had been wearing her hearing aids. Ron, Marie, and Stephanie were thrilled. Laura continued to receive weekly language and auditory stimulation through her therapy sessions until age 3. At that time, her language skills were within normal limits for her chronologic age, and her intervention sessions were reduced to a frequency of once every 3 to 4 months, allowing Stephanie to monitor her progress.

Family Involvement in Discharge Planning

When Laura reached age 4, a formal assessment conducted at the intervention center indicated that her language abilities were within 6 months of the range expected for her age, her articulation skills were generally at age level with a few residual speech production errors that were developmentally appropriate, and she was beginning to exhibit some preliteracy abilities and interests. A case conference was held with Stephanie, Ron, Marie, and an itinerant teacher from the local school board, where discharge plans were discussed. As Laura would soon begin attending junior kindergarten the itinerant teacher was introduced to the family and a transition plan for Laura's school entry was arranged. The itinerant teacher would work with Laura in the school setting as needed and would provide support to the receiving classroom teacher. Stephanie recommended that Laura obtain an FM system to be used in school. The itinerant teacher investigated possible classroom placements in the local school, met with the classroom teacher to inform her about Laura's needs as a student with hearing loss, and provided the teacher with specific strategies to facilitate Laura's learning in the regular classroom, including how to use the FM system. Although they were aware that the need for regular audiologic follow up and changes in ear molds would continue to exist, Laura and Ron were especially pleased that their daughter was able to communicate at a level permitting her to attend her local school with her friends from the neighborhood. On discharge from the early intervention center, Ron and Marie were asked to provide feedback regarding the services they had received and their overall satisfaction with Laura's intervention program. Although both parents agreed that it had been a long and challenging road, their and their therapist's intensive and extensive involvement in Laura's language and auditory skill development had led to the best possible outcome. As Marie stated in her discharge interview:

> When you're doing lessons at home every day, and trying to get to meetings, and trying to get more information on how to do the job better, and going for tests, and going for medical appointments, and having

left a full time job that I really loved and making *this* my full time job, and really wanting to do everything I could do for her. . . . It was a very interesting time, a very interesting time. I sometimes think now, "Did we have to really? Did we have to do so much?" But you know what? You wouldn't change it!

Summary and Conclusions

Understanding those parental behaviors that have a positive mediating effect on speech and language outcomes for children with hearing loss would enhance therapy, would potentially increase speech and language development, and would provide specific suggestions for parents to help them work more effectively with own children in increasing speech and language abilities. The predictive value of parental involvement on speech and language outcomes for children with hearing loss is an important question for clinicians, researchers and parents, and has the potential to influence government policy on funding for provision for early intervention speech-language pathology services using a family-based model. Although researchers in the domain of communication disorders generally agree that early intervention programs that directly involve parents result in improved speech and language outcomes for the child, unfortunately, the research evidence in favor of parental involvement generated to date suggests that there is currently little empirical support for claims regarding the facilitative effects of parental involvement in achieving improved speech and language outcomes for preschool children with hearing loss. In spite of this, given the importance attributed to parental involvement in early intervention for children with hearing loss, a number of important issues remain. First, objective, measurable indicators of parental involvement are required. These indicators must be culturally sensitive in order to prevent bias in clinical evaluations of parental involvement that may contribute to misjudgements and erroneous reasons for dismissal from an early intervention program where parental involvement is a central component. The selected indicators of parental involvement must be relevant to the field of early intervention for children with hearing loss and should not be based exclusively on factors derived from the educational literature. This implies that an appropriate theoretical context for the description of the role of parental involvement in early intervention must be developed. Additional empirical evidence is required to demonstrate that children with hearing loss benefit from parental involvement in their early intervention programs in a measurable way. To accomplish this, instruments assessing parental involvement will need to be developed that will permit the examination of specific domains of parental involvement in conjunction with specific domains of outcome. Furthermore, a tool examining parental involvement should provide clinicians with specific information related to which domains associated with parental involvement might need to be improved versus those that constitute strengths for individual families and should assist families in improving their parental involvement if this is a real issue.

With respect to multicultural issues in parental involvement in particular, several questions need to be addressed. First, what do families from other cultures understand by the concept of parental involvement? Furthermore, is there a potential for bias or misrepresentation of parental involvement when current clinical definitions and their associated behaviors are applied to families from other cultures? Can we assume that families from other cultures will be comfortable in following our definitions and expectations of parental involvement? Finally, the question of potential differences in outcome of intervention attributable to cultural bias in parental involvement requires careful examination. An ongoing research study currently is examining the role of cultural background in parental perceptions of their involvement in early intervention programs for children with hearing loss (Eriks Brophy & Corter, in progress). Results of the study have the potential to increase our awareness and understanding of the various forms of parental involvement that might be demonstrated in early intervention programs and to enhance cultural sensitivity in service delivery for preschool children with hearing loss and their families.

The best evidence in favor of the importance of parental involvement in early intervention must be measurable and unbiased if parental involvement truly is to become accepted as a predictive factor of outcome. The development of an objective, culturally sensitive measure of parental involvement in early intervention programs for preschool children with hearing loss is required to accomplish this. Research reported here represents a preliminary step in the development of such a tool. It is hoped that such a tool would contribute to the generation of clear evidence in support of the important role of parental involvement as an important mediating factor in achieving positive language outcomes for children with hearing loss.

References

Bandura, A. (1982). Self-efficacy in human agency. *American Psychologist,* *37,* 122-147.

Bronfenbrenner, U. (1979). *The ecology of human development.* Cambridge, MA: Harvard University Press.

Calderon, R. (2000). Parental involvement in deaf children's education programs as a predictor of language, early reading, and social-emotional development. *Journal of Deaf Studies and Deaf Education, 5,* 140-155.

Calderon, R., & Greenberg, M. (1997). The effectiveness of early intervention for deaf children and children with hearing loss. In M. Guralnick (Ed.), *The effectiveness of early intervention* (pp. 455-482). Baltimore: Paul H. Brookes.

Callaway, A. (2000). *Deaf children in China.* Washington, DC: Gallaudet University Press.

Cole, E. (1992). *Listening and talking: A guide to promoting spoken language in young hearing-impaired children.* Washington, DC: Alexander Graham Bell Association for the Deaf.

DesJardin, J. (2003). Assessing parental perceptions of self efficacy and involvement in families of young children with hearing loss. *Volta Review, 103*(4), 391-409.

Dettman, S., Pinder, D., Briggs, R., Dowell, R., & Leigh, J. (2007). Communication development in children who receive the cochlear implant younger than 12 months: Risks versus benefits. *Ear and Hearing, 28*(2,Suppl.), 11S-18S.

Easterbrooks, A., O'Rourke, C., & Wendell, T. (2000). Child and family factors associated with Deaf children's success in auditory-verbal therapy. *Pediatric Otology, 21*(3), 341-344.

Epstein, J. (1995). School/family/community partnerships: Caring for the children we share. *Phi Delta Kappan, 76*(9), 705-707.

Eriks-Brophy, A. (2008). *Parental involvement in communication outcomes for children with hearing loss.* Manuscript in preparation.

Eriks-Brophy, A., & Crago, M. (1993). Feeling right: Approaches to a family's culture. *Volta Review, 95*(5), 123-130.

Estabrooks, W. (1994). *Auditory-Verbal therapy: For parents and professionals.* Washington, DC: A.G. Bell.

Goldbart, J., & Mukherjee, S. (1999a). The appropriateness of Western models of parental involvement in Calcutta, India. Part 1: Parent's views on teaching and child development. *Child: Care, Health and Development, 25*(3), 335-347.

Goldbart, J., & Mukherjee, S. (1999b). The appropriateness of Western models of parental involvement in Calcutta, India. Part 2: Implications of family roles and responsibilities *Child: Care, Health and Development, 25*(3), 348-358.

Grant, J. (1993). Hearing-impaired children from Mexican American homes. *Volta Review, 95*(5), 131–135.

Gregory, S. (1995). *Deaf children and their families.* Cambridge, UK: Cambridge University Press.

Hoover-Dempsey, K.., & Sandler, H. (1995). Parental involvement in children's education: Why does it make a difference? *Teachers College Record, 97,* 310–331.

Hoover-Dempsey, K., & Sandler, H.. (1997). Why do parents become involved in their children's education? *Review of Educational Research, 67,* 3–42.

Huff, R., & Kline, M. (1999). *Promoting health in multicultural populations.* Thousand Oaks, CA: Sage.

Luterman, D. (1987). *Deafness in the family.* Boston: Little Brown.

Lynch, E., & Hanson, M. (1992). *Developing cross-cultural competence.* Baltimore: Paul H. Brookes.

Marschark, M. (1997). *Raising and educating a deaf child.* New York: Oxford University Press.

Marschark, M., & Clark, M. D. (Eds.). (1998). *Psychological perspectives on deafness* (Vol. 2). Mahwah, NJ: Lawrence Erlbaum Associates.

McLean, L., & Woods Cripe, J. (1997). The effectiveness of early intervention for children with communication disorders. In M. Guralnick (Ed.), *The effectiveness of early intervention* (pp. 349–428). Baltimore: Paul H. Brookes.

Meadow-Orlans, K., Mertens, D., & Sass-Lehrer, M. (2003). *Parents and their deaf children.* Washington, DC: Gallaudet University Press.

Moeller, M. (2000). Early intervention and language development in children who are deaf and hard of hearing. *Pediatrics, 106*(3), E43.

Moeller, M. (2007). Current state of knowledge: Psychosocial development in children with hearing impairment. *Ear and Hearing, 28*(6), 729–739.

Northern, J., & Downs, M. (2002). *Hearing in children.* Baltimore: Lippincott, Williams and Wilkins.

Odom, S., Hanson, M., Blackman, J., & Kaul, S. (2003). *Early intervention practices around the world.* Baltimore: Paul H. Brookes.

Personal communication, Stacey Weber, Senior Program Consultant, Early Years Programs Strategic Policy and Planning Division, Ministry of Children and Youth Services, September 10, 2007.

Pipp-Siegel, S., & Biringen, Z. (2000). Assessing the quality of relationships between parents and children: The emotional availability scales. *Volta Review Monograph, 100*(5), 237–249.

Pollack, D., Goldberg, D., & Caleffe-Schenck, N. (1997). *Educational audiology for the limited-hearing infant and preschooler.* Springfield, IL: Charles C. Thomas.

Schuyler, V., & Rushmer, N. (1987). *Parent-Infant habilitation: A comprehensive approach to working with hearing-impaired infants and toddlers and their families.* Portland, OR: Infant Hearing Resource.

Schwartz, S. (1996). *Choices in deafness: A parents' guide to communication options*. Bethesda, MD: Woodbine House.

Simser, J. (2001, Fall). Parents: The essential partner in the habilitation of children with hearing impairment. *The Listener*, pp. 47-53.

Stacey, P., Fortnum, H., Barton, G., & Summerfield , A. (2006). Hearing-impaired children in the United Kingdom, I: Auditory performance, communication skills, educational achievements, quality of life, and cochlear implantation. *Ear and Hearing, 27*(2), 161-186.

Uchanski, R. M., & Geers, A. E. (2003). Acoustic characteristics of the speech of young cochlear implant users: A comparison with normal-hearing agemates. *Ear and Hearing, 24*(1Suppl.), 90S-105S.

Wathum-Ocama, J., & Rose, S. (2002). Hmong immigrants' views on the education of their deaf and hard of hearing children. *American Annals of the Deaf, 147*(3), 44-55.

White, K., Taylor, M., & Moss, V. (1992). Does research support claims about the benefits of involving parents in early intervention programs? *Review of Educational Research, 62*, 91-125.

Yoshinaga-Itano, C. (2000). Successful outcomes for deaf and hard of hearing children. *Seminars in Hearing, 21*, 309-325.

Chapter 11

Working with Families to Facilitate Emergent Literacy Skills in Young Children with Language Impairment

A. Lynn Williams and Martha J. Coutinho

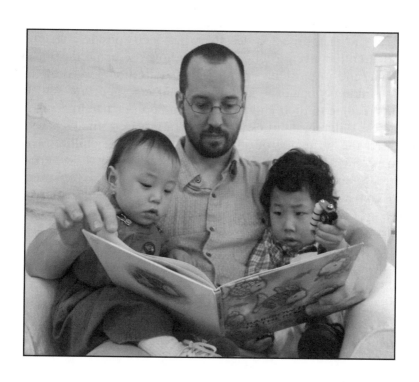

Research: Historical Overview of Family Involvement in Emergent Literacy

Historical Overview

Emergent literacy skills are an important part of children's early language development and are influenced long before children start formal instruction (Adams, 1990; Snow, Burns, & Griffin, 1998). They encompass a range of skills, including sensitivity to the phonological structure that underlies oral and written language, knowledge of the function and form of print, and recognition of words as discrete elements of written and spoken language. Specifically, emergent literacy includes the components of phonological awareness, alphabet knowledge, print awareness, and oral language. Although most children acquire these skills through interactions with their environment and with adults, some children—particularly those at risk—do not acquire these foundational skills. Reading books is the single best source for children to gain most of their knowledge about oral and written language, but reading alone is insufficient for children experiencing difficulties. For these children more explicit intervention is required.

For the past three decades, there has been considerable interest in and attention given to understanding how the home literacy environment, and in particular parent-child shared book-reading, influences children's language acquisition and emergent literacy skills. Parents reading to their children is a common practice in many families across different cultures. A number of research studies have documented the influence of storybook exposure on children's early language and literacy skills (cf., Kaderavek & Sulzby, 1998; Roberts, Jurgens, & Burchinal, 2005; Senechal & LeFevre, 2002); however, the exact contributions of parent-child storybook reading to later language and literacy skills still is not certain. Furthermore, less is known about the benefits of shared book-reading for children with language impairment (LI).

Table 11–1 summarizes studies of parents reading to children with LI. The importance of studying shared book-reading of parents with children with language impairment is demonstrated in the observed differences between parents of children with language impairment and parents of typically developing (TD) children that have been reported.

Table 11–1. Studies of Parents (Without Training [white boxes] and With Training [shaded boxes]) Reading to Children with Language Impairment (LI)

Study	Participants	Study Aim(s)	Key Finding(s)
Pellegrini, McGillicuddy-DeLisi, Sigel, & Brody (1986)	60 parents—4-year-old children with LI; 60 parents—4-year-old children who were typically developing (TD)	Descriptive study of maternal reading behaviors	Differences observed between parents of children with LI and mothers of TD children. Parents of LI children gave more nonverbal support and used simpler questions than parents of TD children.
Evans & Schmidt (1991)	1 mother—3-year-old preschooler with LI and 1 mother—2-year-old preschooler who was TD	Descriptive study of maternal-child reading interactions	Differences in maternal reading behaviors observed between mothers. The mother of child with LI controlled more of the interaction than mother of TD child.
Schneider & Hecht (1995)	28 mothers—4-year-old children with LI	Descriptive study of maternal reading behaviors	Differences in children's attention to storybook reading influenced maternal interactions. With children who produced few on-task utterances, mothers made fewer requests for their children to participate. For children who were actively engaged, mothers made more requests for them to participate, but fewer requests for extended verbal contributions.
Kaderavek & Sulzby (1998)	1 mother and 3-year-old preschooler with LI	Descriptive study of maternal reading behaviors	Maternal reading style was characterized as being directive with questioning. The child did not initiate and was resistive to shared book reading.

continues

Table 11–1. *continued*

Study	Participants	Study Aim(s)	Key Finding(s)
Ezell & Justice (1998)	12 mothers— 4-year-old preschool children with LI	Descriptive study of maternal reading behaviors and print awareness	Maternal questions focused on pictures rather than print. There was a negative correlation between rate of maternal questioning and children's expressive vocabulary.
Rabidoux & MacDonald (2000)	20 mothers— 2-year-old children with LI	Descriptive study of material reading behaviors	Mothers used a teaching role during reading activities while their children were more passive, but attentive.
Crowe (2000)	5 mothers— 3-year-old preschoolers with LI	Descriptive study of maternal reading behaviors and child participation	Although there was considerable variation across mothers in rate of behaviors, maternal reading behaviors were characterized primarily by pointing, reading, and asking closed-ended questions. Children's participation was characterized by labeling and pointing to pictures.
Justice & Kaderavek (2003)	11 mother-child dyads; children were 4 years old with LI	Descriptive study of parent-child storybook interactions that focused on maternal control features (topic initiation and contingency response)	Individual differences were observed across dyads, but generally mothers and children had balanced topic control, reciprocity, and contingency.
Hockenberger, Goldstein, & Haas (1999)	7 mother-child dyads (3 Head Start children with mild-moderate developmental disabilities and 4 Head Start children at-risk)	Descriptive study of maternal commenting during joint book reading.	All mothers increased use of specific comments and 4 children showed improved emerging literacy skills on a standardized measure.

Table 11–1. *continued*

Study	Participants	Study Aim(s)	Key Finding(s)
Crain-Thoreson & Dale (1999)	32 4-year-old children with language delays; 10 parents; 7 staff members	Experimental study with children assigned to one of 3 groups: (1) Parent; (2) Staff/practice; or (3) Staff/control to examine linguistic performance as a result of Dialogic Reading program	Children in all 3 groups produced longer utterances and more different words and participated more in shared book reading. The magnitude of change was positively correlated with the magnitude of change in adult behavior.
Crowe, Norris, & Hoffman (2000)	3 mothers—3-year-old children with LI	Descriptive study that examined effects of Complete Reading Cycle (CRC) training on parent and child communicative participation during story reading.	Notable changes in mothers' reading behaviors with concomitant changes in children's communicative behaviors (increased verbal turns, MLU, and semantic complexity)
Skibbe, Behnke, & Justice (2004)	5 mothers—4-year-old children with LI	Descriptive study of parent-implemented PA intervention that examined maternal scaffolding.	Children whose mothers used more directive and responsive scaffolds performed better on more PA tasks than children whose mothers used fewer scaffolds.
Crowe, Norris, & Hoffman (2004)	6 caregiver-child dyads; 3-year-old children with LI	Descriptive study of interactive reading routine training program on communicative participation and lexical diversity of utterances during shared reading.	Children significantly increased the frequency of communicative turns, total number of words, and number of different words produced during shared reading.

continues

Table 11–1. *continued*

Study	Participants	Study Aim(s)	Key Finding(s)
Justice & Skibbe (2005)	2 groups of mothers— 4-year-old children with SLI (experimental and control groups)	Experimental study of the effects of shared reading activities that incorporated explicit print concepts	Both groups made gains in their print concept performance, but the print-focused children (experimental group) gained an average of 13 standard score points compared to the control group that gained an average of 7 standard score points. This demonstrated the importance of explicit and systematic targeting of skills for slowly progressing learners.
Justice, Kaderavek, Bowles, & Grimm (2005)	22 prekindergarten children with LI— parents assigned to experimental or comparison groups	Experimental study of a 10-week parent-implemented PA intervention program directed at rhyme and alliteration tasks.	Experimental group made significant gains in rhyme awareness, but not alliteration. The magnitude of PA change was influenced by the children's age and speech and language impairment.

Shaded boxes represent studies of trained parents.
LI = language impairment, TD = typically developing.

Specifically, parents of children with language impairment provided more nonverbal support and used simpler questions (Pellegrini, McGillicuddy-DeLisi, Sigel, & Brody, 1986) and controlled more of the interaction (Evans & Schmidt, 1991) than parents of TD children.

As shown in Table 11–1, most of the earlier studies were descriptive studies that characterized the reading interactions of parents and children with LI, whereas the later studies reported the effects of parent training on parent-child interactions during shared reading activities. Taken together, the descriptive studies of parents reading to their children without training document that, although shared book-reading involves a shared context with balanced topic control, reciprocity between parent and child, and topic contingency (Justice & Kaderavek, 2003), most of the interaction is directive with closed-ended questions, pointing, and reading by the parents; the children engage in more passive participation characterized by labeling and pointing (Crowe, 2000; Ezell & Justice, 1998; Kaderavek & Sulzby, 1998; Rabidoux & MacDonald, 2000).

With training, however, parents learned to actively engage their children through specific questioning strategies (Crowe, Norris, & Hoffman, 2000, 2004; Whitehurst, Fischel, Lonigan, Valdez-Menchaca, Arnold, & Smith, 1991), scaffolding (Skibbe, Behnke, & Justice, 2004), and specific commenting (Hockenberger, Goldstein, & Haas, 1999). The descriptive and experimental studies demonstrate the potential of parent-child shared storybook reading as an important context for developing early language and literacy skills and facilitating intervention goals. Collectively, these studies report that changes in parental reading behaviors resulted in increases in child linguistic behaviors. Specifically, children increased the frequency of communicative turns, total number of words, and semantic complexity during shared storybook reading as a result of parent training (Crain-Thoreson & Dale, 1999; Crowe, Norris, & Hoffman, 2000, 2004). In addition, children achieved gains in phonological awareness skills (Justice, Kaderavek, Bowles, & Grimm, 2005; Skibbe, Behnke, & Justice, 2004) and print awareness (Justice & Skibbe, 2005) following parent training.

Therapist-Centered Approaches

The clinician-directed interventions generally are focused on the phonological awareness component of emergent literacy. These interventions typically utilize behaviorist-oriented approaches that involve shaping, repetition, and a hierarchical mastery of discrete skills.

There have been a few studies on phonological awareness interventions with children who have phonological or language impairments and included goals that addressed rhymes, beginning and final sounds, and segmentation and blending activities. These therapist-centered approaches utilized either one-on-one interventions (Gillon, 2000) or classroom-based interventions (van Kleeck, Gillam, & McFadden, 1998) with little or no parental involvement.

The results from this growing body of work indicate that phonological awareness skills can be facilitated in clinical and classroom settings using explicit intervention activities that are carefully structured and implemented by well-trained clinicians and teachers. However, the opportunities for children to interact with staff-administered interventions is limited compared to parent-administered interventions. In fact, Fey, Cleave, Ravida, Long, Dejmal, and Easton (1994) contend that increased parental access to effective intervention should be considered to promote generalization of treatment effects as an alternative to clinician-directed interventions. Using parents as intervention agents is endorsed by policymakers as a viable and cost-effective alternative to clinician-directed activities that incorporate one-on-one or classroom-based interventions.

Family-Centered Approaches

Parent-implemented interventions are consistent with the trend toward more naturalistic approaches in phonological awareness intervention (Justice & Ezell, 2002; Justice & Pence, 2004; Skibbe, Behnke, & Justice, 2004) and emergent literacy in general (Crain-Thoreson & Dale, 1999; Dale, Crain-Thoreson, Notari-Syverson, & Cole, 1996). It is not surprising, then, that studies on parent training have gained considerable attention as an important and powerful context for facilitating intervention goals. Several studies have reported that parent training resulted in changes in maternal reading behaviors that had a concomitant increase in the children's communicative behaviors (Crain et al., 1999; Crowe et al., 2000, 2004), phonological awareness skills (Skibbe et al., 2004; Justice et al., 2005) print awareness (Justice & Skibbe, 2005), and emerging literacy skills in general (Hockenberger et al., 1999).

An example of a parent-implemented intervention approach that has been used with children with language impairment is the Complete Reading Cycle (CRC) described by Crowe et al. (2000, 2004). The CRC is a responsive interactive reading approach that teaches parents to establish a joint focus, elicit a response, provide a response, and give feedback. In the studies examining CRC, parents were encouraged to comment and question, and they could assume the role of initiator or responder during shared storybook reading. In both studies using parent-child dyads, Crowe and colleagues reported the children with language impairment showed increased communicative behaviors in terms of frequency of communicative turns, MLU, and semantic complexity.

Skibbe et al. (2004) reported on a parent-implemented phonological awareness intervention program that involved maternal scaffolding to explicitly facilitate rhyme, onset distinction, and segmentation skills with their 4-year-old children with language impairment. Five mother-child dyads participated in the 12-week book-reading intervention. The mothers read one new book four times each week for the 12 weeks. Nine structured teaching tasks that included questions that specifically addressed each of the three targeted phonological awareness skills (3 questions per skill area) were designed for each book. The intervention paradigm incorporated the following four features: (1) explicit phonological awareness instruction occurred within the context of the books; (2) phonological awareness intervention encompassed a range of skills in each book-reading session (rhyme, onset distinction, and segmentation); (3) the intervention stimuli for the phonological awareness tasks were derived directly from the storybooks; and (4) the intervention utilized maternal scaffolding to support the children's learning. The results of the intervention indicated that the mothers used a range of scaffolds, but tended to use phonological cues that provided models of phonological concepts, and praise that provided affirmation of their children's performance. The authors noted that children whose mothers used more directive and responsive scaffolds performed better on more phonological awareness tasks than children whose mothers used fewer scaffolds.

In a similar parent intervention paradigm, Justice and Skibbe (2005) reported the results of a print-focused intervention that involved parents reading one new book a week for 12 weeks. In this intervention, parents systematically and explicitly targeted print concepts that involved three specific targets (differentiate print from pictures, point to the title of the book, and print directionality). They compared the results of the experimental group of parents reading to their 4-year-old children with language impairment and a control group of parents who read to their children with the same frequency, but who did not systematically or explicitly address print targets in their storybook readings. The researchers reported that, whereas both groups demonstrated improved performance in print concepts, the print-focused children achieved an average of 13 standard score points compared to the average of 7 points gained by the control children. These findings demonstrated the importance of explicit and systematic targeting of skills, rather than simply shared book reading, in order for children with language impairment to learn print concepts.

Evidence Base of Effectiveness of Family Involvement

Evidence-based approaches are those that have empirically demonstrated efficacy or effectiveness. One framework for evaluating the level of empirical support for the effectiveness of family-based emergent literacy interventions is the research continuum described initially by Fey (2002) and repeated in McCauley and Fey (2006). According to Fey, programmatic research on a particular intervention approach progresses along a continuum of research that includes at the lowest level *exploratory studies*, which then proceeds to *efficacy studies*, and finally leads to *effectiveness studies*. Related to emergent literacy, exploratory studies represent first tier investigations that involve systematic observation of children to identify factors that appear to contribute the most to literacy acquisition in specific areas. The next stage in the research continuum involves efficacy studies, which utilize experiments in which an independent variable, such as an intervention approach, is manipulated within a highly controlled laboratory or clinical environment. The emphasis of efficacy studies is internal validity with a small, homogeneous group of participants, random assignment, and carefully trained interventionists. Following the outcome of several efficacy studies with internal validity that support positive effects for the intervention, the final tier in research involves effectiveness studies. At this level of research, there is a shift from focusing on internal validity to documenting external validity, or the generalization of effects to a broader population within a typical setting. In sum, intervention approaches that have empirically demonstrated efficacy or effectiveness are classified as evidence-based.

Using this framework, Justice and Pullen (2003) described the available empirical research on adult-child shared storybook reading research as having probable efficacy for influencing young children's emergent literacy development. In particular, two types of adult-child storybook reading interventions were classified as being efficacious approaches: dialogic reading and print referencing.

Dialogic reading is an intervention approach first described by Whitehurst and colleagues as a method for adults to actively engage with children using specific questioning strategies to facilitate oral language skills (cf., Whitehurst, Arnold, Epstein, Angell, Smith, & Fischel, 1994; Whitehurst, Epstein, Angell, Payne, Crone, & Fischel, 1994; Whitehurst, Zevenbergen, Crone, Schultz, Velting, & Fischel, 1999). These studies largely have been conducted with at-risk children, as well as some children with developmental delays, and have been limited to the impact of this approach on children's oral language skills, in particular, vocabulary and mean length of utterance. Additional research is needed to evaluate the clinical viability of this approach across a range of emergent literacy domains with children who have language impairment and to examine its benefits relative to other methods of shared book-reading.

The second efficacious adult-child storybook approach is print referencing. Similar to the dialogic approach, adults use a shared storybook context, but with an emphasis to improve children's knowledge of print concepts. As described in the studies that were previously discussed, adults use verbal and nonverbal strategies in book-reading activities to facilitate the child's print awareness. Verbal strategies include explicit questions about print, whereas nonverbal behaviors include tracking print while reading. As with dialogic reading, a number of studies have shown that print referencing is a promising intervention with probable efficacy for facilitating emergent literacy skills in at-risk preschool children. As in the dialogic reading approach, additional studies are needed to determine its efficacy for children with special needs.

To summarize, adult-child storybook approaches (dialogic reading and print referencing) have evidence that support their probable efficacy, but more studies need to be done with parents and children with language impairment across a range of emergent literacy domains. At this point, the available evidence base for parent-implemented interventions with preschool-aged language impairment children provides support to classify these as *promising interventions.*

Clinical Practice: SLPs' Involvement of Families in Emergent Literacy Interventions

As the discussion of the studies in the previous sections indicates, there is a movement toward utilizing parent-implemented storybook interventions. These studies further indicate that parents provide an ideal context for intervention. They have much more time with the children than a clinician would and they interact with them in many different settings. Furthermore, the use of storybook reading has been shown to be a powerful intervention context for children with language impairment for several reasons (Hockenberger et al., 1999; Justice & Kaderavek, 2003; Justice & Pullen, 2003). First, shared storybook reading has a highly routinized and contextualized nature that is predictable and provides children with repeated opportunities for practice. Second, storybook reading establishes joint attention between the child and parent and provides a controlled context in which to interact. Third, the book illustrations support the saliency of the adult language used during reading and connect to the majority of child utterances that occur during book reading, which are directly related to the illustrations. Fourth, shared storybook reading has social valence as it provides an interesting and motivating activity for preschool children. Fifth, storybooks can be used to explicitly address a range of emergent literacy behaviors, including phonological awareness and print concepts. Finally, books and shared storybook reading provide a practical context for intervention as an inexpensive, available, and easily portable activity that is highly adaptable across different themes and topics to capture differences in children's interests.

There are cautions, however, in parent-implemented interventions. Crowe et al. (2004) stressed that the speech-language pathologists' training of parents must be sensitive to parent and child behaviors during shared reading in order to determine the reciprocal effects of the actions of one upon the other and identify the appropriate level of intervention. In other words, a rigid training program may not fit all parents and children interactional patterns. Hockenberger et al. (1999) reported that only four of the seven mothers in their study participated throughout the intervention project in completing weekly tapes, meeting with the research assistant on a regular basis, and being responsible for the book reading sessions with their children. Therefore, the researchers recommended a more family-centered approach that included having the mothers participate in the planning stages of the intervention program and develop their role in the intervention in order to increase their sense of collaboration and responsibility.

Families' Views of Involvement in SLP for Facilitating Emergent Literacy Skills

Families' perceptions of their delivery of intervention generally have not been reported. One exception is the study by Justice et al. (2005) in which parents were the intervention agents in a phonological awareness intervention program that lasted 10 weeks. In this intervention, the parents in the experimental group read one new book four times a week for the 10-week period and implemented two phonological awareness tasks at the end of each storybook reading. The tasks addressed rhyme awareness and beginning sound awareness using a "search and find" activity in which the children were asked to find another word in the book that shared the specific phonological characteristics with the target word (either rhyming or same beginning sound). Parents in the comparison group also used "search and find" tasks that focused on vocabulary by asking the child to find a particular object in the book. A five-item questionnaire was given to the parents in both groups to determine their perceptions about the effectiveness of their intervention with their children. The questions examined the parents' enjoyment of the reading sessions, how useful they perceived the sessions to be to their children's language skills, and finally how much their children enjoyed the sessions. Parents completed a 5-point Likert-type scale anonymously at the end of the intervention program. For the experimental and comparison groups, parents indicated that they enjoyed the reading sessions (5.0 and 4.5, respectively) and also that the children enjoyed the reading sessions (4.7 and 4.6, respectively). However, the parents in both groups rated the helpfulness of the sessions to their children's language development slightly lower (3.4 and 3.8, respectively).

Other reports of families' perceptions of involvement in intervention are largely provided in terms of fidelity of implementation of the intervention. Hockenberger et al. (1999) reported that only four of the seven mothers participated as requested throughout the project in returning weekly tapes, meeting with the research assistant, and implementing the book-reading sessions. Even with this subset of mothers who completed the project, some missed appointments without prior cancellation or forgot to turn in their weekly audiotapes. Hockenberger et al. suggested that a more family-centered approach that involved the parents in the planning stages of the project likely would facilitate greater parental involvement and commitment to the program.

Importantly, the Hockenberger et al. report on treatment fidelity points out the need to understand the social and cultural values and beliefs related to literacy and adult-child interactions in working with families. Although emergent literacy has been described as a "sociocultural process" due to the strong influences of the social and cultural contexts on children's emergent literacy development (Justice & Pullen, 2003), relatively few studies have examined cultural differences in home literacy experiences and parent-child shared book-reading practices. The few studies that have been conducted have examined home literacy practices in African American families (Anderson-Yockel & Haynes, 1994; Roberts, Jurgens, & Burchinal, 2005), Puerto Rican families (Hammer, Miccio, & Wagstaff, 2003), Dutch families (Bus, Leseman, & Keultjes, 2000), and Chinese families (Johnston & Wong, 2002). These studies indicate differences in the frequency and nature of shared book-reading between parents and children from western, Caucasian families. For instance, Hammer et al. (2003) reported that the home literacy environment of bilingual Puerto Rican families had on average fewer than 10 adult or children's books in the homes and the mothers engaged in adult literacy activities about once a month. Anderson-Yockel and Haynes (1994) reported that African American mothers used significantly fewer questions during shared book-reading than did Caucasian mothers. Johnston and Wong (2002) reported important differences between mothers from western cultures and Chinese mothers with regard to interactions with storybooks that reflect differences in childrearing beliefs. Their survey results indicated that Chinese mothers seldom read to their preschool children, and they were more likely to use picture books and flash cards to teach their child new words. Finally, differences in home literacy experiences have also been reported relative to socioeconomic status. A number of studies have described a lower storybook reading frequency for low-income families compared to middle-income families (cf., Anderson & Stokes, 1984).

This research, as well as that of others (e.g., Sonnenschein & Munsterman 2002), indicates that both parent-child literacy interactions and the perceptions of the parent and children of literacy events are strongly influenced by social and cultural factors. These beliefs can influence many of the factors related to how children and adults participate in and perceive the storybook reading activities, such as the frequency of shared reading, as well as the interaction between adults and children. It is therefore important for speech-language pathologists to consider families' beliefs and practices in utilizing parent-implemented storybook interventions. Based on the social systems perspective (Bronfenbrenner, 1979), such differences in interactions and beliefs could be expected to impact early intervention outcomes that utilize parent-child shared book-reading as an intervention context.

Nexus Between Research, Clinical Practice, and Families' Views of Emergent Literacy Interventions

From the review of parent-implemented storybook interventions, it is clear that shared parent-child book-reading can be a powerful and successful context to facilitate early language and literacy skills for children with language impairment. Based on the compilation of findings across the studies, the following implications are summarized for "best practices":

1. Train parents until they achieve a high level of fidelity in implementation of the intervention activities (Justice et al., 2005) to utilize specific behaviors in their shared reading sessions, such as asking open-ended questions (Crowe, Norris, & Hoffman, 2004; Elias, Hay, Homel, & Freiberg, 2006), making specific comments during joint reading (Hockenberger et al., 1999), giving children time to respond during interactive storybook reading (Crain-Thoreson & Dale, 1999), and implementing directive and responsive scaffolding to facilitate children's acquisition of specific emergent literacy skills (Skibbe et al., 2004);

2. Develop specific goals and associated training activities that structure the intervention activities to be implemented by the parents (Justice et al., 2005; Justice & Skibbe, 2005);

3. Implement frequent and repeated book readings several times per week that utilize predictable routines and permits more active child communicative participation (Justice & Kaderavek, 2003);

4. Adapt the intervention strategies to fit the existing reciprocal interactions for particular parent-child dyads to maximize effective parent-child interactions that promote reciprocity and balance in book-reading interactions, and reduce problem interaction behaviors, such as frequent topic shifts (Justice & Kaderavek, 2003); and

5. Recognize the impact of social and cultural influences and utilize a family-centered approach that involves parents in the planning of activities from the beginning (Hockenberger et al., 1999; Johnston & Wong, 2002; Justice & Kaderavek, 2003).

Kaderavek and Justice (2002) summarize "best practices" and "potential pitfalls" in using adult-child shared storybook reading as an intervention context. These are summarized in Table 11–2.

Table 11–2. Summary of "Best Practices" and "Potential Pitfalls" in Using Shared Storybook Reading as an Intervention Context

Factors	Potential Pitfalls	Best Practices
Interest and Engagement in Books	• As some children with LI may actually dislike interacting with books, it is important to assess children's orientation and motivation toward book-reading.	• Determine child's interest in books by asking them to describe their feelings about book reading; ask parents to describe their child's behaviors during book-reading activities; examine child's engagement during book-reading and play activities. • Use a different intervention context (e.g., play-based interactions) and address low orientation to books as a parallel goal.
Parent Reading Behaviors	• One intervention strategy will not "fit" all parent-child dyads and may actually reduce the parents' sensitivity to their children's needs during the shared reading activity.	• Adapt the intervention strategies to fit the existing reciprocal interactions for particular parent-child dyads in order to maximize effective parent-child. Interactions that promote reciprocity and balance in book-reading interactions, and reduce problem interaction behaviors, such as frequent topic shifts.
Promoting Generalization	• Books provide one context for learning new concepts and rules. Consequently, a child may view the book-reading activities as the context in which particular concepts are practiced and not generalize them to other contexts.	• Create different contexts that utilize new concepts that were present in the storybooks through naturalistic play activities. • Reverse reader-listener roles so that the child gradually assumes the parent role of some of the book-reading exchanges.
Social and Cultural Influences	• Differences in home literacy experiences and cultural values exist from western, middle-class Caucasian cultures that can result in a mismatch in shared book-reading expectations and interactions.	• Structure shared book-reading interactions to incorporate familiar books or book genres and incorporate interactive styles that are familiar to the children based on observations of parent-child storybook interactions.

Table 11–2. *continued*

Factors	Potential Pitfalls	Best Practices
Social and Cultural Influences *continued*		• Incorporate practices that are harmonious with the family's culture. Specifically, Johnston and Wong (2002) suggested alternative intervention strategies: a. Use family photo albums or create scrapbooks of family adventures to tell and retell personal narratives, b. Use rich cultural heritage of religious or historical oral storytelling to encourage retelling and inferencing.

Source: Adapted from Kaderavek and Justice (2002).

In summarizing this section of the chapter on "best practices," it is important to note that many of the interventions described have incorporated treatment packages with multiple components, such as asking open-ended questions, and having parents repeat, expand, and recast the child's utterances. Others, most notably Hockenberger et al. (1999), involved a single-component intervention strategy, such as commenting. Therefore, as Hockenberger and colleagues suggest, it may not be necessary to train parents to use a larger set of strategies to obtain desired outcomes.

Case Study of a Parent-Implemented Shared Storybook Intervention

The following case study is based on an enhanced dialogic reading approach (EDR) that was used with low-income families and their 4-year-old children, as described by Williams (2006). Although the children in this study were typical language learners, the approach could be employed with children who have language impairment. EDR is based on the dialogic reading approach described by Whitehurst and his colleagues (Whitehurst, Arnold, et al., 1994; Whitehurst, Epstein, et al., 1994; Whitehurst et al., 1999), but differed in the focus and intensity of the parent training and intervention activities. Different from the dialogic reading approach, EDR focused on strategies to improve oral language skills *and* phonological sensitivity (rhyming, sound awareness, sound manipulation, print awareness, and alphabet knowledge). EDR also involved longer training sessions with the families: 90 minute sessions for 5 weeks compared to two 30-minute instructional sessions that typically are completed in the dialogic reading approach.

Parents were recruited to participate in the 5-week shared reading program through a low-income (Title 1) preschool in northeastern Tennessee in the United States. Eight families participated in the program, which included six mothers, one father, and one mother and father dyad. Ethnicity of the parents was African American (2) and Caucasian (6). The families were primarily employed in nonmanagement and blue-collar jobs in which at least one parent had completed high school. None of the parents had a college degree. The parents completed a Home Screening Questionnaire (Frankenberg & Coons, 1986) that included questions regarding discipline practices and home environment. Scores on the questionnaire were reported as "non-suspect" or "suspect" based on the parent's answers. "Suspect" indicated that the child was considered "at risk" for language and learning problems based on his/her home environmental characteristics. Two of the eight children received a rating of "suspect."

The first of the weekly training sessions provided instruction to the parents on the dialogic reading strategies of using interactive question strategies (CROWD and PEER). CROWD is an acronym that represents the five question types parents were taught to use during shared book-reading sessions (Completion, Recall, Open-ended, Wh-, and Distance questions). PEER represents the interaction strategies of Prompt, Evaluate, Expand, and Repeat. The later training sessions focused on instructional activities used to facilitate specific aspects of phonological sensitivity through shared book-reading.

The major difference between the dialogic reading approach and EDR was the modification of the CROWD questions to train phonological sensitivity rather than solely focus on oral language skills. For example, a completion question in the dialogic reading approach with the book, *The Hungry Thing*, might be "The Hungry Thing pointed to a sign that said _____ [feed me]." In comparison, a completion question in the EDR approach that focuses on rhyming might be "Shmancakes' sounds like 'fancakes' sounds like _____ [pancakes]." CROWD questions were used to address different levels of phonological sensitivity, such as rhyme identification, rhyme generation, sound awareness, and sound substitution. In EDR, CROWD questions were also designed to address print knowledge, including tracking and print awareness. An example of a CROWD question for print knowledge would be "Where would you start reading on this page?" or "Point to a word on this page."

The weekly meetings included a variety of activities in training the parents, which involved a brief presentation of the information, followed by demonstrations, role play, and a question and answer period. The specificity, focus, and redundancy of the training provided support to the parents in learning the concepts and strategies to facilitate their children's phonological sensitivity through book-reading. Specific activities were given to the parents each week, along with sample questions to ask with each book that included all five CROWD question types. Specific questions and page numbers were given to support parents' implementation of the EDR program. The format of the 90-minute weekly sessions is outlined below.

- Parents report on previous week's book and home activities (what worked and what did not work well); trainers and parents reviewed any questions about the week's activities (15 minutes)
- Overview of the topic for current week (5 minutes)
- Present information for topic current week (15 minutes)
- Show videotape demonstration of a parent and child reading the selected book for the week using CROWD questions (5 minutes)
- Break time with snacks (10 minutes)
- Distribute new book and handout with the sample CROWD questions (10 minutes)
- Role-play with parents or parents with each other to practice the new book with the sample questions (15 minutes)
- Question and answer (10 minutes).

Books and toys that focused on a particular aspect of phonological sensitivity were provided each week to the families. The books were selected on the basis of the specific aspect of phonological sensitivity that was being targeted for the week and toys were selected to correspond with the books and provide an expansion of the book-reading activities. Table 11–3 summarizes the books, toys, and emergent literacy targets that were addressed each week.

Parents were asked to complete and return a weekly reading log that included the frequency and type of CROWD questions asked, the number of times the book was read, and whether the toys were used with the book. The log also asked parents to indicate what activities worked well or not, and if they had any questions or suggestions regarding the week's activity.

The children, four boys and four girls, were tested just prior to beginning the EDR program and again at the end of the 5-week program. Tests that evaluated a range of phonological awareness skills were administered to each child. These included the *Phonological Awareness Literacy Screening-Pre-Kindergarten* (PALS-PreK; Invernizzi, Sullivan, & Meier, 2001) and the *Preschool Comprehensive Test of Phonological and Print Processing* (Pre-CTOPPP; Lonigan, Torgesen, & Rashotte, 2002). Speech and language measures were also completed using the

Table 11–3. Weekly Books, Toys, and Emergent Literacy Skills Targeted in the Enhanced Dialogic Reading Program

Week	Book	Toys	Emergent Literacy Skill
Week 1	*Cock-A-Doodle-Moo* by Bernard Most	Plastic farm animals	Sound substitution and rhyming
Week 2	*The Hungry Thing* by Jan Slepian and Ann Seidler	Plastic food	Rhyming and sound substitution
Week 3	*The Cow That Went Oink* by Bernard Most	Plastic farm animals	Sound awareness and sound manipulation (addition, deletion)
Week 4	*The Disappearing Alphabet* by Richard Wilbur	Plastic or magnetic alphabet letters	Print awareness and rhyming
Week 5	*Henny Penny* by Paul Galdone	Plastic farm animals	Rhyming

Source: From Williams and Coutinho (2003).

Goldman-Fristoe Test of Articulation-2 (Goldman & Fristoe, 2000) and transcription of a 20-minute language sample that was analyzed using the *Systematic Analysis of Language Transcripts* (SALT; Miller & Chapman, 2000). Williams and Coutinho (2003) reported the results of the parent-implemented storybook program, which indicated that the short, focused training was effective in increasing the children's emergent literacy skills. These results indicate that even though there was a short time period between test administrations, significant changes in emergent literacy skills occurred following a focused, short-term parent training program. Furthermore, the areas that demonstrated significant changes were those that were specifically targeted in the parent-implemented program (i.e., emergent literacy skills involving phonological sensitivity). A summary of the children's pre- and post-training performance on the test measures is presented in Table 11–4.

Table 11–4. Children's Test Performance Pre- and Post-Enhanced Dialogic Reading Training on Emergent Literacy, Speech, and Language Measures

Test Measure	Pre-Training Mean (standard deviation)	Post-Training Mean (standard deviation)
Phonological Awareness Literacy Screening-Pre-Kindergarten (PALS-PreK)	84.5 (9.6)	91.8 (5.45)**
Preschool Comprehensive Test of Phonological and Print Processing (Pre-PCTOPPP)	69.0 (10.2)	80.0 (7.85)*
Goldman-Fristoe Test of Articulation-2 (GFTA-2)	66.5 (25.2)	69.1 (25.9)
Mean Length of Utterance (MLU)	4.26 (.55)	4.88 (.85)
Total Number of Words (TNW)	522 (116)	498 (126)
Number of Different Words (NDW)	175 (22.9)	168 (20.6)

*significant at $p = .02$.
**significant at $p = .01$.
Pre-CTOPPP and PALS-PreK (mean raw scores with Pre-CTOPPP ceiling at 130 and PALS-PreK ceiling at 131); MLU, TNW, and NDW (mean values based on *Systematic Analysis of Language Transcripts* [SALT] analyses).
Source: From Williams and Coutinho (2003)

In addition to the child testing, parents were videotaped reading to their children before the EDR training and again after completing the 5-week program. Parent and child engagement variables of initiations and responses were examined in these videotaped shared book-readings. Table 11–5 summarizes these data and indicates that parents significantly increased their initiations (questioning) and responses during shared storybook reading. The children had a significant increase in their responses, which was directly related to the parents' increase in initiations using the CROWD questioning strategies.

Together, these findings show that the parent training program demonstrated a first order effect in parents being able to effectively change their interactive book-reading strategies. This change resulted in a second-order effect with their children demonstrating an increase in their emergent literacy skills. Follow-up studies with these families revealed that the parents reported that they continued to use the dialogic reading strategies with their children 6 months after the EDR training (Adams, Davis, Norby, Rothrock, Williams, & Coutinho, 2004); and even 18 months after completing the training when their children were enrolled in first grade (Chalk, Eggers, King, Rouse, Williams, & Coutinho, 2005).

The specificity and structured support provided in the weekly training sessions and the materials given to the parents promoted a sense of understanding and accomplishment for the parents and fostered compliance with implementing the home program. All parents completed the program and high attendance was maintained through-

Table 11–5. Frequency of Parent-Child Interaction Behaviors During Pre- and Post-Training Videotaped Shared Storybook Reading Sessions

Interaction Behavior	Pretraining	Post-Training
Parent Initiations	10.87	36.5
Child Initiations	4.12	8.5
Parent Responses	6.12	19.75
Child Responses	5.62	22.25

out the 5-week program. Even with serious health and family issues that arose during the training period, parents returned from hospital admissions and family deaths to complete the program. The importance of this type of structure and parental support in implementing the home literacy program cannot be overstated and is considered key in developing an intervention program that can be successfully delivered by parents.

Summary and Conclusions

This chapter focused on the rich intervention context of parent-child shared storybook reading to facilitate emergent literacy skills in children with language impairment. The advantages, best practices, and cautions of parent-implemented intervention were described, along with the research evidence that supports this as a promising intervention approach with probable efficacy. A case study that utilized an EDR program was described for low-income families that provided sufficient structure and support and resulted in significant changes in parental behavior which led to significant increases in their children's emergent literacy skills.

In conclusion, Johnston (2008) eloquently states that children's language and literacy development depend on a number of factors; none of which on their own is sufficient to guarantee competency in these skills. That is, shared book-reading alone does not provide a *sufficient* context for children to acquire these skills. Similarly, shared book-reading may not even be *necessary* for children to develop emergent literacy skills, a fact borne out in cross-cultural studies. Yet, as presented in this chapter, parent-implemented storybook reading provides a powerful intervention context when developed and structured in ways that honor the families' culture, values, and beliefs.

Acknowledgments. We would like to acknowledge the library assistance of Amanda Arnold and Olisa Horton as we worked on this chapter. We are also greatly appreciative of the parents and children at Fairmont Elementary School for their participation in the enhanced dialogic reading program.

References

Adams, M. J. (1990). *Beginning to read: Thinking and learning about print.* Cambridge, MA: MIT Press.

Adams, M., Davis, T., Norby, J., Rothrock, W., Williams, A. L., & Coutinho, M. (2004, November). *A shared storybook parent reading program for low-income preschoolers.* Presentation to the American Speech-Language-Hearing Association Annual Convention, Philadelphia.

Anderson, A. B., & Stokes, S. (1984). Social and institutional influences on the development and practice of literacy. In H. Goelman, A. Oberg, & F. Smith (Eds.), *Awakening to literacy* (pp. 158–184). Portsmouth, NH: Heinemann.

Anderson-Yockel, J., & Haynes, W. O. (1994). Joint book-reading strategies in working-class African American and white mother-toddler dyads. *Journal of Speech and Hearing Research, 37*, 583–593.

Brofenbrenner, U. (1979). *The ecology of human development: Experiment by nature and design.* Cambridge, MA: Harvard University Press.

Bus, A. G., Leseman, P. P. M., & Keultzjes, P. (2000). Joint book reading across cultures: A comparison of Surinamese-Dutch and Dutch parent-child dyads. *Journal of Literacy Research, 32*, 53–76.

Chalk, K., Eggers, T., King, N., Rouse, J., Williams, A. L., & Coutinho, M. (2005, November). *Enhanced dialogic reading intervention: A follow-up study.* Presentation to the American Speech-Language-Hearing Association Annual Convention, San Diego, CA.

Crain-Thoreson, C., & Dale, P. S. (1999). Enhancing linguistic performance: Parents and teachers as book reading partners for children with language delays. *Topics in Early Childhood Special Education, 19*(1), 28–39.

Crowe, L. K. (2000). Reading behaviors of mothers and their children with language impairment during repeated storybook reading. *Journal of Communication Disorders, 33*, 503–524.

Crowe, L. K., Norris, J. A., & Hoffman, P. R. (2000). Facilitating storybook interactions between mothers and their preschoolers with language impairment. *Communication Disorders Quarterly, 21*, 131–146.

Crowe, L. K., Norris, J. A., & Hoffman, P. R. (2004). Training caregivers to facilitate communicative participation of preschool children with language impairment during storybook reading. *Journal of Communication Disorders, 37*, 177–196.

Dale, P. S., Crain-Thoreson, C., Notari-Syverson, A., & Cole, K. (1996). Parent-child bookreading as an intervention for young children with language delays. *Topics in Early Childhood Special Education, 16*, 213–235.

Elias, G., Hay, I., Homel, R., & Freiberg, K. (2006). Enhancing parent-child book reading in a disadvantaged community. *Australian Journal of Early Childhood, 31*(1), 20–25.

Evans, M. A., & Schmidt, F. (1991). Repeated maternal book reading with two children: Language-normal and language-impaired. *First Language, 11,* 269-287.

Ezell, H. K., & Justice, L. M. (1998). A pilot investigation of parents' questions about print and pictures to preschoolers with language delay. *Child Language Teaching and Therapy, 16,* 273-278.

Fey, M. E. (2002, March). *Intervention research in child language disorders: Some problems and solutions.* Presentation to the 32nd Annual Mid-South Conference on Communciative Disorders, Memphis, TN.

Fey, M. E., Cleave, P. L., Ravida, A. I., Long, S. H., Dejmal, A. E., & Easton, D. L. (1994). Effects of grammar facilitation on the phonological performance of children with speech and language impairments. *Journal of Speech and Hearing Research, 37,* 594- 607.

Frankenberg, W. K., & Coons, C. E. (1986). Home Screening Questionnaire: Its validity in assessing home environment. *Journal of Pediatrics, 108,* 624-626.

Galdone, P. (1968). *Henny Penny.* New York: Clarion Books.

Gillon, G. T. (2000). The efficacy of phonological awareness intervention for children with spoken language impairment. *Language, Speech, and Hearing Services in Schools, 31,* 126-141.

Goldman, R., & Fristoe, M. (2000). *Goldman-Fristoe Test of Articulation-2.* Circle Pines, MN: American Guidance Service.

Hammer, C. S., Miccio, A. W., & Wagstaff, D. A. (2003). Home literacy experiences and their relationship to bilingual preschoolers' developing English literacy abilities: An initial investigation. *Language, Speech, and Hearing Services in Schools, 34,* 20-30.

Hockenberger, E., Goldstein, H., & Haas, L. S. (1999). Effects of commenting during joint book reading by mothers with low SES. *Topics in Early Childhood Special Education, 19*(1), 15-27.

Invernizzi, M., Sullivan, A., & Meier, J. (2001). *Phonological Awareness Literacy Screening- Prekindergarten.* Virginia State Department of Education. Charlottesville, VA: Curry School of Education.

Johnston, J. R. (2008). *Reading to kids: Course material and exam questions.* Retrieved February 14, 2008, from http://www.speechpathology .com/ceus/preview_text_course.asp?class_id=2760

Johnston, J. R., & Wong, A. (2002). Cultural differences in beliefs and practices concerning talk to children. *Journal of Speech, Language, and Hearing Research, 45,* 916-926.

Justice, L. M., & Ezell, H. K. (2002). Use of storybook reading to increase print awareness in at-risk children. *American Journal of Speech-Language Pathology, 11,* 17-29.

Justice, L. M., & Kaderavek, J. N. (2003). Topic control during shared storybook reading: Mothers and their children with language impairments. *Topics in Early Childhood Special Education, 23*(3), 137-150.

Justice, L. M., Kaderavek, J., Bowles, R., & Gimm, K. (2005). Language impairment, parent- child shared reading, and phonological awareness: A feasibility study. *Topics in Early Childhood Special Education, 25*(3), 143–156.

Justice, L. M., & Pence, K. L. (2004). Addressing the language and literacy needs of vulnerable children: Innovative strategies in the context of evidence-based practice. *Communication Disorders Quarterly, 25*(4), 173–178.

Justice, L. M., & Pullen, P. C. (2003). Promising interventions for promoting emergent literacy skills: Three evidence-based approaches. *Topics in Early Childhood Special Education, 23*(3), 99–113.

Justice, L. M., & Skibbe, L. (2005, November). *Explicit literacy instruction during book reading: Impact on preschoolers with SLI.* Presentation to the American Speech-Language-Hearing Association Annual Convention, San Diego, CA.

Kaderavek, J., & Justice, L. M. (2002). Shared storybook reading as an intervention context: Promises and potential pitfalls. *American Journal of Speech-Language Pathology, 11*, 395–406.

Kaderavek, J. N., & Sulzby, E. (1998). Parent-child joint book reading: An observational protocol for young children. *American Journal of Speech-Language Pathology, 7*, 33–47.

Lonigan, C., Wagner, J., & Rashotte, C. (2002). *The Preschool Comprehensive Test of Phonological and Print Processing.* Tallahassee, FL: Florida State University.

McCauley, R. J., & Fey, M. E. (2006). *Treatment of language disorders in children.* Baltimore: Paul H. Brookes.

Miller, J. F., & Chapman, R. S. (2000). *Systematic Analysis of Language Transcripts* [computer software]. Language Analysis Laboratory, Waisman Center, University of Wisconsin-Madison.

Most, B. (1996). *Cock-a-doodle-moo.* Orlando, FL: Harcourt Brace.

Most, B. (1990). *The cow that went oink.* Orlando, FL: Harcourt Brace.

Pellegrini, A. D., McGillicuddy-DeLisi, A. V., Sigel, I. E., & Brody, G. H. (1986). The effects of children's communicative status and task on parents' teaching style. *Contemporary Educational Psychology, 11*, 240–252.

Rabidoux., P. C., & MacDonald, J. D. (2000). An interactive taxonomy of mothers and children during storybook interactions. *American Journal of Speech-Language Pathology, 9*, 331–344.

Roberts, J., Jurgens, J., & Burchinal, M. (2005). The role of home literacy practices in preschool children's language and emergent literacy skills. *Journal of Speech, Language, and Hearing Research, 48*, 345–359.

Schneider, P., & Hecht, B. (1995). Interaction between children with developmental delays and their mothers during a book-sharing activity. *International Journal of Disability, Development and Education, 42*(1), 41–56.

Senechal, M., & LeFevre, J. (2002). Parental involvement in the development of children's reading skill: A five-year longitudinal study. *Child Development, 73*(2), 445–460.

Skibbe, L., Behnke, M., & Justice, L. M. (2004). Parental scaffolding of children's phonological awareness skills: Interactions between mothers and their preschoolers with language difficulties. *Communication Disorders Quarterly, 25*(4), 189–203.

Slepian, J., & Seidler, A. (1967). *The hungry thing.* New York: Scholastic.

Slepian, J., & Seidler, A. (1993). *The hungry thing goes to a restaurant.* New York: Scholastic.

Slepian, J., & Seidler, A. (1993). *The hungry thing returns.* New York: Scholastic.

Snow, C., Burns, M. S., & Griffin, P. (1998). *Preventing reading difficulties in young children.* Washington, DC: National Academy Press.

Sonneschein, S., & Munsterman, K. (2002). The influence of home-based reading interactions on 5-year-olds' reading motivations and early literacy development. *Early Childhood Research Quarterly, 17*, 318–337.

van Kleeck, A., Gillam, R. B., & McFadden, T. U. (1998). A study of classroom-based phonological awareness training for preschoolers with speech and/or language disorders. *American Journal of Speech-Language Pathology, 7*, 65–76.

Whitehurst, G. J., Arnold, D. S., Epstein, J. N., Angell, A. L., Smith, M., & Fischel, J. (1994). A picture book reading intervention in day care and home for children from low-income families. *Developmental Psychology, 30*, 679–689.

Whitehurst, G. J., Epstein, J. N., Angell, A. L., Payne, A. C., Crone, D. A., & Fischel, J. E. (1994). Outcomes of an emergent literacy intervention in Head Start. *Journal of Educational Psychology, 86*, 542–555.

Whitehurst, G. J., Fischel, J. E., Lonigan, C. J., Valdez-Menchaca, M. C., Arnold, D. S., & Smith, M. (1991). Treatment of early expressive language delay: If, when, and how. *Topics in Language Disorders, 11*, 55–68.

Whitehurst, G. J., Zevenbergen, A. A., Crone, D. A., Schultz, M. D., Velting, O. N., & Fischel, J. E. (1999). Outcomes of an emergent literacy intervention from Head Start through second grade. *Journal of Educational Psychology, 91*, 261–272.

Wilbur, R. (1997). *The disappearing alphabet.* Orlando, FL: Harcourt.

Williams, A. L. (2006). Integrating phonological sensitivity training and oral language within an Enhanced Dialogic Reading Approach. In L. M. Justice (Ed.), *Clinical approaches to emergent literacy intervention* (pp. 261–294). San Diego, CA: Plural.

Williams, A. L., & Coutinho, M. (2003, November). *Contexts for facilitating emergent literacy skills.* Presentation to the American Speech-Language-Hearing Association Annual Convention, Chicago.

Index